HEALTH RADAR'S
ENCYCLOPEDIA OF
Natural Healing

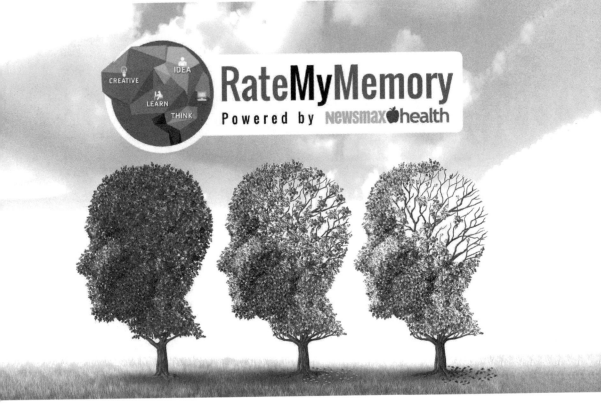

Is it Normal Forgetfulness?
Or Something More Serious?

You forget things — names of people, where you parked your car, the place you put an important document, and so much more. Some experts tell you to dismiss these episodes.

"Not so fast", says Dr. Gary Small, director of the UCLA Longevity Center, medical researcher, professor of psychiatry, and a *New York Times* best-selling author.

Dr. Small says that most age-related memory issues are normal but sometimes can be a warning sign of future cognitive decline.

Now Dr. Small has created the online RateMyMemory Test — allowing you to easily assess your memory strength in just a matter of minutes.

It's time to begin your journey of making sure your brain stays healthy and young!

Test Your Memory Today:

MemoryRate.com/Healing

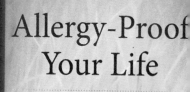
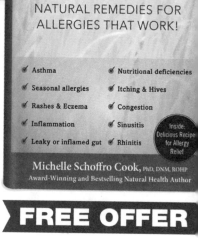
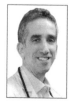

HEALTH RADAR'S ENCYCLOPEDIA OF
Natural Healing

Health Breakthroughs to Prevent and Treat
Today's Most Common Conditions

NICK TATE

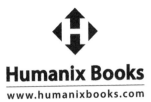

Humanix Books
www.humanixbooks.com

Humanix Books

Health Radar's Encyclopedia of Natural Healing
Copyright © 2017 by Humanix Books
All rights reserved

Humanix Books, P.O. Box 20989, West Palm Beach, FL 33416, USA
www.humanixbooks.com | info@humanixbooks.com

Library of Congress Control Number: 2017935104

Cover Design: Design by Tom Lau
Interior Design: Scribe Inc.

Humanix Books is a division of Humanix Publishing, LLC. Its trademark, consisting of the word "Humanix," is registered in the Patent and Trademark Office and in other countries.

Disclaimer: The information presented in this book is meant to be used for general resource purposes only; it is not intended as specific medical advice for any individual and should not substitute medical advice from a health care professional. If you have (or think you may have) a medical problem, speak to your doctor or health care practitioner immediately about your risk and possible treatments. Do not engage in any therapy or treatment without consulting a medical professional.

ISBN: 978-1-63006-082-4 (Trade Paper)
ISBN: 978-1-63006-083-1 (E-book)

Printed in the United States of America
10 9 8 7 6 5 4 3 2 1

CONTENTS

Part II: Disease Directory

INTRODUCTION

For one hundred years, the primary focus of conventional medicine has been to *treat* diseases—such as cancer, cardiovascular disease, diabetes, and dementia—using drugs, surgery, and radiation. In fact, the US *health care* system is a bit of misnomer; it's really more of *disease* care model.

By contrast, alternative medicine practitioners have sought to *prevent* diseases from developing in the first place—emphasizing what we might call *well* care, which boosts the body's inherent immune defenses with natural therapies, herbs, healthy practices, and other treatments.

Today, we stand on the brink of a new era in modern medicine that brings together both approaches—conventional and alternative—that aim to prevent, manage, and treat diseases by harnessing our natural healing systems and immune defenses.

Great strides have been made in the fields of genetics, immunotherapy, and stem cell treatments in recent years that have allowed millions of Americans to take advantage of this cutting-edge medical science. At the same time, scientific researchers are increasingly confirming the benefits of centuries-old alternative healing practices that have been shown to boost wellness and longevity.

This book showcases the best of both worlds, providing a comprehensive compendium of the latest scientifically proven advances in the emerging field of natural medicine. Taken from the pages of Newsmax's well-regarded *Health Radar* newsletter and the company's other health publications, this anthology spotlights the most effective and promising conventional and alternative therapies to treat, manage, and even prevent the fifty top causes of death, disease, and disability in the United States and around the world.

In its pages, you will learn the following:

- How breakthroughs in immunotherapy are saving the lives of many cancer patients and providing a more effective and less harmful alternative to the three leading treatment options—surgery, radiation, and chemotherapy—that have been the primary methods of combatting cancer for decades
- The promising ways stem cell research is leading to new treatments for heart disease, the nation's number-one killer; diabetes; cancer; Alzheimer's disease; and other maladies, offering hope to the millions of Americans who are grappling with such disorders
- How to take advantage of new genetic tests that can identify your individual health profile and potential predisposition to hundreds of diseases and conditions—information that can help you prevent, manage, and treat them effectively
- The ways modern-day scientific researchers are confirming what traditional and alternative medicine practitioners have known for centuries about the disease-fighting capability of herbs, botanical medicines, and natural healing methods
- The most effective medical foods, health-boosting diets, and nutritional approaches that have been found to increase longevity, cuiled from researchers who have traveled the world to identify the key nutrients that contribute to a long and healthy life
- Why exercise is better than drugs for a host of maladies and the best workout strategies for treating, managing, and preventing diabetes, cardiovascular disease, Alzheimer's, certain forms of cancer, and other obesity-related disorders that cost the nation $150 billion in health care expenditures every year
- The common traits of cancer patients who have experienced what scientists call "radical remission"—unexplained recoveries not tied to chemo, surgery, radiation, or other treatments—based on the latest research
- Proven methods for maintaining your mental edge as you age, including promising new approaches to preventing or slowing the progression of Alzheimer's and other forms of dementia that afflict more than five million Americans
- What works—and what doesn't—when it comes to alternative medicine, based on analyses of thousands of expert studies
- Effective treatments and remedies for hundreds of common afflictions, diseases, and disorders
- How hidden toxins and chemical contaminants put your health—and your life—at risk and what you can do to avoid them
- Critical health and wellness screenings and tests you should undergo based on your age and medical history, as well as procedures you should avoid that might do more harm than good

- Commonsense strategies for maximizing your health care dollar in a post-Obamacare world, including ways to make sensible decisions to boost your health and wellness with off-the-grid health care approaches

In short, this book has been designed to be an owner's manual for your body and mind, offering a best-of-both-worlds analysis of alternative and conventional approaches to treating hundreds of health conditions. It offers a practical consumer's guide—chock full of simple tips and clear-eyed advice—to the most powerful natural, nontoxic approaches to living a long, healthy, and happy life.

PART I

New Frontiers of Medicine

1

IMMUNOTHERAPY

Better than Chemo, Radiation, Surgery, and Other Conventional Cancer Treatments

At ninety-one, former president Jimmy Carter became the most well-known beneficiary of a new type of immunotherapy that all but cured him of an advanced form of cancer that doctors had initially predicted would kill him in a matter of months. The approach, which boosts the body's natural defenses to fight disease, is more effective than conventional radiation, surgery, and chemo. Many specialists believe it represents the greatest medical advance in decades.

Immunotherapy: Harnessing the Body's Natural Defenses to Fight Disease
For nearly a century, the idea of enlisting the natural power of the body's immune system to combat cancer and other illnesses has been the dream of conventional doctors and alternative medicine practitioners alike. Now that dream is becoming a reality with the advent of immune-boosting drugs like Keytruda, the medication used to eradicate former president Jimmy Carter's cancer in 2016.

The US Food and Drug Administration (FDA) green-lighted Keytruda (also known as pembrolizumab) in late 2015 for patients with a genetically linked form of lung cancer. But other studies have found it to also be effective against melanoma, lymphoma, and leukemia, as well as breast, bladder, and colorectal cancers.

As a result, Keytruda has become the therapeutic poster child for a new generation of treatments designed to work with the body's immune defenses to combat cancer.

And while Carter might be the most famous beneficiary of this new line of treatments, he is just one of many cancer survivors who are benefitting. Oncologists say that Keytruda—and similar drugs—offers the tantalizing prospect of extending the lives of tens of thousands of patients with late-stage cancer, with research showing that it is safer and more effective than chemo.

The FDA's approval of Keytruda was a historic milestone in medicine. It marked the first time an immunotherapy drug has been designated a first-line treatment for patients with advanced cancer and a high concentration of a specific protein called PD-L1 in their tumors.

But experts say that this is just the beginning of a new era in medicine that will fundamentally change how cancer—and other health conditions—will be treated in the years ahead.

Targeting More Cancer Types
According to the American Association for Cancer Research (AACR), more Americans are benefiting from immunotherapy than ever before. The organization's 2016 Cancer Progress Report noted that a growing number of different types of cancer are being treated with immunotherapy.

The AACR reported that immunotherapy drugs accounted for four of the thirteen new cancer treatments approved since 2015—including Keytruda. The drug is one in a new class of immunotherapy drugs called "checkpoint inhibitors" that have been approved for melanoma, lung cancer, bladder cancer, head and neck cancer, Hodgkin lymphoma, and kidney cancer.

"The promise of immunotherapy for cancer therapy has never been greater, and the opportunity to make significant progress in this critical area is real," says AACR president Dr. Nancy Davidson.

Such treatments not only help cancer patients live longer but also improve their quality of life. Today, a record 15.5 million cancer survivors are now living in the United States, an increase of 1 million people since 2014.

Still, cancer remains the second leading cause of death in the United States, pointing to the need for more research into immunotherapy and other treatments, says Dr. Margaret Foti, chief executive officer of the AACR. "Research has made tremendous advances against cancer," Foti notes. "However, we need to accelerate the pace of progress because it is unacceptable that one American will die of cancer every minute of every day this year."

Davidson adds, "And in fact, if the necessary funding is provided, we will accelerate the pace of progress and, in turn, markedly reduce morbidity [illness] and mortality from cancer."

Immunotherapy: At a Glance

Drug companies, federal health agencies, universities, and US researchers are investing billions of dollars into immunotherapy treatments. Hundreds of clinical trials are under way to attempt to identify the most promising lines of therapy to replace or complement conventional chemo, radiation, and surgery.

Here's a closer look at some of the key questions and answers about the promise and challenges in the field based on the latest information from the National Cancer Institute (NCI).

What Is Immunotherapy?

Immunotherapy is any type of treatment that enlists the immune system to fight diseases. Some forms of immunotherapy—such as allergy shots—have been around for decades. But the latest and most exciting developments in the field have been in the area of cancer treatment.

Unlike chemotherapy, radiation, and surgery (treatments that kill tumors by poisoning, burning, or cutting them out), immunotherapy works by an entirely different method—by strengthening the cells of the immune system to help them attack the cancer. In doing so, it has fewer negative side effects and does not damage healthy tissues.

Are Drugs the Only Type of Immunotherapy?

Actually, no. But drugs are the most widely used form of cancer immunotherapy—specifically, the new class of medications called "checkpoint inhibitors." Four such drugs have been approved by the FDA, including Keytruda (pembrolizumab), the medication used to treat former president Jimmy Carter, manufactured by Merck; Yervoy (ipilimumab) and Opdivo (nivolumab), made by Bristol-Myers Squibb; and Tecentriq (atezolizumab), by Genentech.

Such drugs are delivered intravenously and put the brakes on a process that cancer cells use to evade the immune system, allowing killer T-cells to attack the tumor. They target "checkpoint proteins" (such as PD-1 and CTLA-4) that cancer cells sometimes enlist to avoid being attacked by the immune system.

But drugs aren't the only form of immunotherapy. Others include the following:

VACCINES. Unlike typical vaccines—used to prevent the flu, pneumonia, and childhood diseases—cancer vaccines are used to treat or eradicate the disease after it has developed by arming the immune system to attack tumors. But like traditional vaccines, cancer shots are often made from actual tumor cells that are "killed" and then used to create a vaccine that can target other tumors when reinjected.

The FDA has approved a vaccine called Provenge to treat prostate cancer. A second, called Bacillus Calmette-Guérin (BCG), is made from a weakened form of the bacteria that causes tuberculosis and is used to treat bladder cancer by causing an immune response against cancer cells. BCG is also being studied in other types of cancer.

Other vaccines enlist "dendritic cells"—special cells that help the immune system recognize cancer cells—and reengineered viruses, bacteria, or yeast cells that have been altered so they no longer cause disease but still provoke a strong natural defense against tumors.

In addition, Duke University researchers are developing a promising experimental vaccine that uses a weakened polio virus to provoke a strong immune system response to target brain cancer.

ADOPTIVE CELL TRANSFER. This form of immunotherapy is highly specialized and involves reengineering a cancer patient's own T-cells—a type of white blood cell that is part of the immune system—to more aggressively fight his or her cancer. Researchers take T-cells from a cancer patient and isolate those that are most active against tumors or modify their genes to make them better able to find and destroy cancer cells. They then grow large batches of these hyperaggressive T-cells in the lab and reintroduce them intravenously to the patient.

MONOCLONAL ANTIBODIES. These drugs are designed to bind to specific targets in the body—such as tumor cells—and can cause an immune response that destroys cancer. Some tag cancer cells so it is easier for the immune system to find and destroy them. Others are engineered to attach to cancer cells and immune system T-cells alike, so they can be used individually in a one-two combination to direct T-cells to tumors. One drug that harnesses this approach is called Blincyto, and the FDA has approved it to treat leukemia.

CYTOKINES. These proteins, which are made by the body's cells, play a key role in normal immune functions and the ability to respond to cancer. The two main types of cytokines used to treat cancer are called interferons and interleukins.

OTHERS. Some other forms of immunotherapy are being studied to try to boost specific parts of the immune system, including T-cells and so-called tumor-infiltrating lymphocytes.

How Successful Is Immunotherapy?

Despite the strides made over the past decade to research and develop new forms of immunotherapy, there has been a widely varying degree of success. Studies show that up to four in ten patients are helped by checkpoint inhibitors, but greater survival rates have been seen in those with melanoma and those who have used two drugs in combination.

Cell therapy has led to remissions in 25 to 90 percent of patients with lymphoma or leukemia, with some remissions lasting for years.

Does Insurance Cover Immunotherapy?

Because the therapy is so new and experimental, in some cases, insurers have not covered the full costs for treatment, which is expensive. Keytruda, for instance, carries an annual price tag of about $150,000. And even in cases where an oncologist prescribes it and insurance covers it, copayments are often very high.

One option is for patients to enroll in clinical trials, in which case, the drugs and other forms of therapy are provided free of charge.

For information on ongoing clinical trials and immunotherapy, visit the following websites:

- The National Institutes of Health (NIH) clinical trials website: http:// clinicaltrials.gov
- The NCI immunotherapy website: https://www.cancer.gov/about-cancer/ treatment/types/immunotherapy

You can also visit the websites of the makers of these immunotherapy drugs: Keytruda (pembrolizumab) was developed by Merck (Merck.com), Tecentriq (atezolizumab) was developed by Genentech (Gene.com), and both Yervoy (ipilimumab) and Opdivo (nivolumab) are made by Bristol-Myers Squibb (BMS.com).

Other Recent Advances in Immunotherapy

CANCER GENE MAP. Scientists at the Sanford Burnham Prebys Medical Discovery Institute (SBP) recently identified 122 new genetic regions that affect the immune response to cancer. The findings, published in *Cancer Immunology Research*, could inform the development of future immunotherapies.

"By analyzing a large public genomic database, we found 122 potential immune response drivers—genetic regions in which mutations correlate with the presence or absence of immune cells infiltrating the tumors," said lead author Eduard Porta-Pardo, PhD, a postdoctoral fellow at SBP. "While several of these correspond to proteins with known roles in immune response, many others offer new directions for cancer immunology research, which could point to new targets for immunotherapy."

UNIVERSAL VACCINE. German scientists have discovered how to rewire immune cells to fight any type of disease—raising the prospect of developing a universal cancer vaccine. The new potential therapy involves injecting tiny particles of genetic code into the body that link up with immune system cells and teach them to recognize specific cancers.

Although scientists have shown previously that is it is possible to engineer immune cells outside the body so they can spot specific types of cancer, this is the first time it has happened inside cells, and the genetic code could be programmed for any form of the disease. Custom-made vaccines would be designed—based on the genetic profile of a particular patient's cancer cells—to fight the disease and keep it from recurring.

Tests in mice showed that the vaccine triggered a strong immune response, while trials in three skin cancer patients demonstrated that the treatment could be tolerated. The study was carried out by researchers from Johannes Gutenberg University, Biopharmaceutical New Technologies, Heidelberg University Hospital, and the Cluster for Individualized Immune Intervention.

NATURAL KILLER CELLS. An experimental therapy that revs up the immune system's cancer-fighting ability might help treat some leukemia patients facing a grim prognosis. The treatment involves infusions of "natural killer" (NK) cells taken from a healthy donor and chemically "trained" to go after tumor cells.

Researchers at Washington University in St. Louis found that of nine patients with acute myeloid leukemia (AML) who received the therapy, four went into complete remission for as long as six months.

IMMUNOTHERAPY DRUGS. Oregon Health and Science researchers who treated ten men with advanced prostate cancer using Keytruda have reported promising results in some of those patients—suggesting that it might be an effective alternative to conventional treatments in at least some cases.

Three of the first ten participants enrolled in the ongoing clinical trial experienced rapid reductions in prostate-specific antigen (PSA), an early measure of treatment effect. Imaging scans also showed that tumors shrank in two of these three men, including metastatic liver tumors in one patient. Two of the three participants who responded to the treatment gained relief from cancer pain and were able to stop taking opiate pain medication. Although the drug did not work for all the men, those who experienced positive results clearly benefited, researchers said.

OTHER NEW MEDICATIONS. The new immunotherapy drug called nivolumab might be more effective than conventional chemotherapy for people with advanced head and neck cancers. An international phase III trial found that more than twice as many cancer patients taking nivolumab were alive after one year compared with patients receiving chemotherapy.

Patients receiving the immunotherapy drug also had fewer side effects than those undergoing conventional chemo, according to the findings presented at the European Society for Medical Oncology 2016 Congress in Copenhagen and published in the *New England Journal of Medicine* by scientists from the Institute for Cancer Research in London.

Can the Polio Virus Cure Cancer?

An experimental immunotherapy program at Duke University is using a surprising new weapon in the war on cancer—infusions of the polio virus that have successfully been used to treat patients with inoperable brain tumors.

While the doctors and researchers spearheading the effort are reluctant to use the words "cancer cure" to describe the work, the early success of the innovative effort is at least the next best thing. If ongoing clinical trials of the technique continue to prove promising, it could become a new way to treat cancer—alongside surgery, radiation, and chemotherapy.

"The idea of targeting cancer with viruses has been around for at least a hundred years," notes Dr. Matthias Gromeier, one of the lead investigators heading up the new anticancer research at the Preston Robert Tisch Brain Tumor Center at Duke, whose work gained wide attention from a spot on *60 Minutes*. "However, valid strategies of using 'oncolytic' (cancer-fighting) viruses emerged only recently. This is mostly due to technological advances in genetic engineering of viruses."

The Duke project involves injecting a genetically engineered poliovirus—known as PVS-RIPO—into deadly brain tumors. Early testing involving primates and human patients has found that PVS-RIPO homes in on cancer cells and destroys them without harming healthy tissues.

Gromeier explains that the Duke team essentially disarmed the virus through genetic manipulation, so it cannot cause polio, while maintaining its ability to infect, target, and kill certain cells—specifically, brain tumor cells.

"To work against cancers in patients, oncolytic viruses must target cancer cells for infection, and they must kill them. At the same time, they must be safe," says Gromeier, a professor of neurosurgery, molecular genetics, and microbiology at Duke, who has been working on the polio virus project for twenty-five years.

"Accomplishing this is very difficult scientifically, and only very few viruses are suitable as cancer-fighting agents in the clinic. We achieved this feat by genetic engineering to remove poliovirus's inherent disease-causing ability."

Gromeier explains that the resulting PVS-RIPO virus "naturally infects [and] kills cancer cells, but not normal cells, because its ability to grow (and kill) depends on biochemical abnormalities only present in cancer cells."

He adds that tests in patients have proven that PVS-RIPO has "no ability to cause poliomyelitis, and no ability to change back to wild-type poliovirus that can cause poliomyelitis."

The treatment targets a form of brain cancer called glioblastoma, which is what killed Senator Ted Kennedy in 2009. It is a particularly virulent cancer, killing about twelve thousand Americans every year—60 percent of whom die within two years of diagnosis, according to the American Brain Tumor Association.

PVS-RIPO works by not only infecting and killing brain tumor cells directly but also recruiting the patient's own immune response against the cancer, Gromeier explains.

Once brain tumors are infected with PVS-RIPO, a patient's immune system recognizes and targets the virus and kills the cancer cells. Just how PVS-RIPO harnesses the power of the body's own defenses to attack tumors that were infused with the virus is a major research goal of Gromeier's laboratory.

The research is still in early stages—undergoing what's known as a "phase I" clinical trial of the technique in cancer patients with glioblastoma. Since 2012, at least five patients have been treated, according to Duke.

One of the first patients in the trial died six months following PVS-RIPO infusion due to tumor regrowth. But none of the others have had any toxic side effects, indicating that PVS-RIPO is safe. What's more, four are still alive, and at least two are cancer-free three years after receiving the infusion of polio virus, the researchers said.

Now they are conducting additional FDA-approved phase II and phase III studies with larger groups of cancer patients, including adults and children. If they prove as promising as the first two cases, the approach could lead to wider use of cancer-fighting viral agents in brain cancer. Gromeier believes that the approach might be promising for combatting other forms of cancer as well.

"Because PVS-RIPO naturally targets and destroys cancer cells from most common cancer types (pancreas, prostate, lung, colon, and many others), it can be directed against these cancers as well," Gromeier says. "To establish this in the clinic, we plan future clinical trials in patients with cancers other than brain tumors."

If those follow-up studies prove successful, the FDA could give the approach a so-called breakthrough status to fast-track its development.

Duke isn't the first or only research institution investigating the use of viruses to kill cancer. More than one hundred years ago, physicians first reported unexpected cancer remissions in patients who came down with the flu, and by the 1950s, scientific research into the idea began in earnest.

New genetic engineering techniques developed in just the last two decades have allowed scientists to modify viruses to target cancer. Nearly a dozen biotech companies and research institutions are experimenting with these genetically engineered viruses.

Biotech giant Amgen has been working on a herpes virus–based treatment (called T-VEC) for melanoma. And several smaller companies—including Oncolytics Biotech DNATrix and Oncos Therapeutics—are reportedly conducting their own research.

Ten Functional Foods That Destroy Cancer Cells

The new breed of immunotherapy drugs isn't the only way to boost your immune system's ability to fight cancer. Certain foods contain powerful compounds that can fight many dreaded diseases. Some might prevent and even control the growth of cancer cells in the body.

"The main mechanism behind these foods is their anti-inflammatory properties," notes Dr. Dimitri Alden, a renowned New York City–based cancer surgeon. "Inflammation causes cancer cells to grow and spread, so by eating these foods, you can prevent this process."

Here are ten of the most recognized functional foods that destroy cancer cells:

1. **Grapes and red wine.** Resveratrol, the powerful ingredient found in grapes and wine, is an extremely powerful antioxidant. It also inhibits cyclooxygenase-2 (COX-2) production, which is related to cancers and other types of inflammation. COX-2 inhibitors such as resveratrol have been shown to decrease the incidence of cancer along with precancerous growths.

2. **Sea vegetables.** These delicious treats from the sea include nori, arame, kombu, and wakame. They contain a variety of antioxidant and anti-inflammatory compounds that prevent and reverse the damage done by foods and other factors that cause inflammation and oxidative stress—two known contributing factors to many types of cancers.

3. **Turmeric.** The miracle ingredient in this spice is curcumin, which is found in most Indian dishes. Curcumin is an extremely powerful antioxidant and anti-inflammatory that reduces the metastases of tumors and

might destroy or prevent their growth in the first place. Alden says that the spice inhibits the formation of new blood vessels in cancer cells—a crucial step in delaying development.

4. **Green tea.** Green tea owes its cancer-destroying abilities to a group of plant flavonoids known as catechins. One of these catechins, epigallocatechin gallate (EGCG), is the most powerful anti-inflammatory and also disrupts the development of cancer cells.

5. **Cruciferous vegetables.** We all know that veggies are healthy, but cruciferous vegetables like broccoli, arugula, cabbage, cauliflower, and kale contain chemicals called glucosinolates that create compounds that fight cancer. According to the Linus Pauling Institute, they work by eliminating carcinogens before they can damage DNA.

6. **Garlic.** According to researcher Dr. Carmia Borek, PhD, many populations have used garlic as a remedy for cancer for thousands of years. The NCI says that garlic might reduce the risk of stomach, colon, esophageal, and breast cancer. The Iowa Women's Study revealed that women who consumed the most garlic had a 50 percent lower risk of colon cancer. Borek recommends taking aged garlic extract (AGE) for the most consistent cancer-fighting benefits.

7. **Hemp oil.** Hemp oil speeds up the healing process throughout the body and also raises melatonin levels. Melatonin has been shown to reduce or even completely stop the growth of certain types of cancers, so the extra production of it thanks to hemp oil is a great asset in your body's fight against cancer. Hemp oil can be consumed through gelcaps or even directly out of the bottle.

8. **Mushrooms.** These tasty fungi have antiviral and anticancer effects that have been proven through numerous in-vitro and animal research studies. Mushrooms have been used for more than five thousand years in ancient and traditional medicines due to their powerful effects on a number of diseases and conditions, including cancer.

9. **Ginger.** Certain compounds found in ginger make it a powerful anti-inflammatory and antioxidant that reduces oxidative stress that your body has to fight daily. Studies have shown that ginger can reduce cancerous tumors by as much as 56 percent and have also shown it to be a more effective remedy than traditional medical treatments like chemotherapy with certain types of cancers.

10. **Tomatoes.** These red fruits and the products made from them contain lycopene, a compound known for its ability to destroy cancer cells.

Scientific studies show that lycopene helps prevent prostate, lung, and stomach cancers. This powerful antioxidant offers a double whammy, as it also reduces your risk of heart disease by lowering "bad" low-density lipoprotein (LDL) cholesterol and blood pressure.

2

GENETICS

Using the Body's Own DNA to Diagnose, Treat, and Even Prevent Chronic Diseases

Half of Americans carry one or more gene defects that hike their risk of a heart attack or stroke—the leading causes of death in the United States. That increased cardiovascular risk is roughly as much as heavy smoking. Millions more Americans are genetically predisposed to cancer, diabetes, and other major killers. Yet most don't know that tests are available to unmask these hidden genetic mutations. But gene testing is revolutionizing the US health care system and placing the diagnosis, management, and treatment of hundreds of ailments in the hands of patients themselves.

Is It in Your Genes? New DNA Tests Offer Up a Goldmine for Health
The science of genetics has revolutionized US health care in ways that are transforming how doctors diagnose, manage, and treat health conditions that were once death sentences for millions of Americans.

Just a generation ago, only a few tests were available to screen newborns for genetically inherited diseases like Down syndrome or cystic fibrosis. Today, tests are available for more than thirty-five thousand diseases related to more than ten thousand conditions, according to the National Institutes of Health (NIH) Genetic Testing Registry (GTR).

But this rapidly expanding field of amazing medical science leaves many puzzling over how much we want to know about our genetic heritage and how best to use that information to improve our health, longevity, and quality of life.

Here's a primer on this new frontier in medicine and the pros and cons of genetic testing.

What Can Our Genes Tell Us?

Genomics allows us to find out all sorts of information about ourselves, our ancestors, and our children. Genetic tests offer insights into trivial conditions—baldness, for instance—as well as serious diseases, such as cystic fibrosis, breast cancer, or heart disease.

While a positive genetic test for baldness might not have serious implications for your health, some screenings allow us to understand our risk for serious diseases. In response, we can make lifestyle modifications to combat the disease or be more conscientious about diagnostic medicine.

If you know that you're genetically predisposed to develop breast cancer, for example, you might be sure to undergo regular mammograms to detect the first signs of a tumor. You might also keep your weight down, eat a healthy diet, get regular exercise, and limit your alcohol—all of which can reduce your odds of developing breast cancer, regardless of your genetic risks.

Depending on your personal situation, you might want to seek genetic counseling as well as test results. If, for instance, you need to know your status as a carrier for cystic fibrosis before you have a baby, medical centers with genetic counselors can interpret complicated test data for you. If you are merely curious about certain traits and your ancestry, your best option might be an organization like 23andMe, which is approved by the US Food and Drug Administration (FDA) to provide genetic tests and information without genetic counseling.

Keep in mind that the results of genetic testing can either put your mind at ease or give you something new to worry about. On the plus side, a test might give you important information about how to prevent or treat a particular condition. But it might also put you in a position where you have to make hard decisions about your future, your desire to have children, and your family's health.

If your motivation for testing is more than curiosity, consider using a medical center, says Robin Schwartz, assistant professor of genetics and genome sciences at University of Connecticut Health Center. The advantage of genetic counseling is that you can develop a plan, cope with difficult decisions, and figure out where your support is.

"People also have expectations that when we do a test, we'll know everything, but we don't," she explains. "There are people who want info and those who don't. They may be afraid of how they'll cope with information. Not everyone is made the same, and some people can adjust to trauma or bad news more easily."

Rapid Advances in Recent Years

The science of genetic testing has evolved dramatically over the past four decades, as has counseling. That's particularly true in the case of genetic disorders like cystic fibrosis.

"What we would have said in 1978 is very different from what we say now," Schwartz explains. "Genetic testing has helped a great deal in understanding different diseases and how this information can be used in clinical practice.

"Not everyone has the same mutation, and we can look at specific mutations and how they can be treated. This can make a very serious disease not as serious. We can also tap into the expertise of colleagues across the country."

The same is true for other health conditions, such as breast cancer and diabetes. Certain forms of these diseases respond better to particular treatments, depending on a patient's genetic makeup. "Testing is not just to see if you have the gene for breast cancer," Schwartz says. "Everyone has these genes. It is to determine what one's risk is based on family history."

In addition, most people with diabetes and heart disease have a family history of these conditions, but genes aren't the only factor to consider when deciding how best to treat and manage them. "Families have similar exercise and eating habits, and you may have modifiable factors," Schwartz notes. "There is common 'garden variety' testing for cardiovascular risk, such as triglycerides, cholesterol, and family lifestyle, but there are also genetic findings that have to do with the heart. Now we have a lot more genetic testing, and we can decide if something is a significant risk or not.

"There may be rhythm problems, cholesterol metabolism issues, problems with the heart muscle, the way pulmonary arteries work—and some of these are not as rare as we thought. Genetic testing can really help people. We can intervene to reduce risk, and medical intervention can save lives."

Gene Testing for Children and Adults

The most common genetic test is the one doctors routinely use to screen newborns for forty different conditions or metabolic disorders.

"Early intervention can significantly alter the course of these diseases," Schwartz explains. "When a baby is born with specific symptoms, it can be extremely helpful in treatment and mitigating other family members' risks.

"As we gain more knowledge, we work in nearly all areas of health care. It is not just in terms of testing, but evaluating familial testing and risk. We overlap research with public health, testing, analysis of a family history, determining inheritance pattern and coordinating testing based on guidelines. The roles of genetic counselors are expanding. It takes more expertise to interpret genetic test results, and we often consult with patients and their doctors. It helps them to make decisions."

23andMe, the giant genetics counseling business that helps people trace their ancestry, also provides genetic tests that might lead the average person to a fuller understanding of conditions that impact their daily living.

Dr. Emily Drabant Conley, PhD, vice president of business development for 23andMe, notes that the company offers consumers genetic tests without requiring genetic counseling. "They are not required to talk to a genetic counselor, and ours is the only FDA-cleared test on the market where consumers can access results without medical assistance," she says. "We had to demonstrate that people can understand genetic results on their own. Our tests are accessible to everyone, and we don't provide a diagnosis."

23andMe offers three areas of testing: carrier status, wellness, and traits. Customers can be tested for carrier status for thirty-five different diseases, like sickle cell anemia, Tay-Sachs disease, and cystic fibrosis, before deciding whether to have children. Wellness tests include information about things like lactose intolerance, how you respond to caffeine, and the connection between saturated fat and your body weight.

The third area of testing is for traits, like baldness or sneezing in sunlight. In addition, the company also provides ancestry breakdowns and gives people the opportunity to connect with living relatives. "It's a neat way to flesh out the family tree," Conley says.

Although 23andMe has been offering consumer genetic tests for almost a decade, it took a while before the FDA allowed the company to give reports on medical conditions. In part, that is because of concerns about the complexities and uncertainties in the interaction among genes, lifestyle, and other factors in the development of health conditions.

There's a common saying among genetic specialists about many health conditions that are hereditary: genes load the gun, but lifestyle pulls the trigger. "There are some complicated genetic conditions, and these might include genetics but also environment and lifestyle," Conley says. "There are some physician-ordered tests for complex things, but genetics are more a part of the everyday discourse. We try to provide people with as much information as possible, but what they do with the results is up to the individual.

"Some of those reports today are not related to the entire spectrum of what you might have. All answers to tests can be different depending on family history."

Q&A: Genetic Testing at a Glance

Q: Where can I get more information on genetic tests that are available?

A: Where you go for genetic-testing information depends, in part, on the kind of questions you have. If you are looking for specific traits, a commercial testing center like 23andMe can help. If you are trying to determine carrier status before having a baby, you might want to seek out an accredited center or a genetic counselor recommended by your doctor or health care facility.

- To find a genetic counselor, consult the National Society of Genetic Counselors (http://www.nsgc.org; 312-321-6834).
- For general information and a list of accredited programs, contact the Accreditation Council for Genetic Testing (http://www.gceducation.org; 913-222-8668).

Q: What does genetic testing cost and will insurance cover it?

A: As genetics has gained prominence in many medical fields, insurance companies have moved to cover many tests that are medically warranted. For instance, if your doctor believes that you are a candidate for early intervention in the case of a particular disease, like colon or breast cancer, your insurer is likely to pay for genetic testing. But an insurance company might not cover a test if it isn't clear that it will be of value to the patient.

Also worth noting,

- The US Centers for Disease Control and Prevention (CDC) has developed policies and guidelines for when genetic tests are warranted (http://www.cdc.gov/genomics/gtesting/).
- Positive genetic testing results are not the same as having a preexisting condition. It's also worth noting that people with preexisting conditions cannot be denied insurance coverage under existing federal law.
- Costs of tests can range from $100 to more than $2,000.
- For more information about genetic test coverage and reimbursement, see https://www.genome.gov/19016729/coverage-and-reimburasment-of-genetic-tests/.

Q: Who has access to genetic testing results?

A: The NIH keeps databases with genetic test information, but the details can't be linked to specific patients. Federal laws, like the Common Rule and the Health Insurance Portability and Accountability Act (HIPAA) keep consumers' information safe and private.

To check on specific aspects of privacy and testing, consult https://www .genome.gov/27561246/privacy-in-genomics/.

Q: Who regulates genetic testing?

A: The FDA has the authority to regulate genetic tests, but with the rapid increase in different kinds of tests, the agency has only been able to regulate a small number of these.

The Centers for Medicare and Medicaid Services (CMS) also has some authority to regulate clinical testing, and the Federal Trade Commission (FTC) monitors advertising claims for accuracy.

Q: What kinds of tests are available?

A: A wide number of tests are available to consumers. Among them,

Prenatal testing. Such tests were among the first developed and are commonly used during pregnancy to identify fetuses that might have genetic disorders and problems.

Newborn screening. Babies are tested a few days after birth to determine if they might be predisposed to have certain diseases.

Carrier testing. This lets you know that you carry certain genetic mutations, defects, or variations that could be passed on to your children and make them more likely to develop a particular condition. Carriers often don't have any symptoms.

Diagnostic screening. Such testing can determine if you have a genetic condition that might be making you ill now or in the future. Having this information might change the way you treat or manage the disease.

Predictive testing. This can give you information about your risk of developing a disease and might be combined with lifestyle modifications to counteract it.

Pharmacogenomic testing. If you and your doctor want to know how certain medicines might be processed by your body, this test can provide valuable guidance, including details on the likelihood that the drug will help or hurt you.

Preimplantation screening. This type of testing is used to find genetic changes in embryos that were created using techniques like in-vitro fertilization. Embryos that have no genetic mutations are implanted in a uterus to begin a pregnancy.

Forensic testing. DNA testing is also used by criminal investigators for legal purposes and to settle paternity suits.

Q: How is genetic testing done?
A: Samples of blood, hair, saliva, skin, or other tissue are used for genetic analysis. Newborns are tested with a small blood sample taken from the baby's heel. Amniotic fluid that surrounds the fetus during pregnancy can be used for testing before birth. For more information, visit the National Society of Genetic Counselors website: http://aboutgeneticcounselors.com/Genetic-Testing/How-Does-the-Testing-Process-Work.

Q: Which genetic tests are most common?
A: BRCA1 and 2, a test for breast and ovarian cancer, is often done to determine if a woman has a higher likelihood of developing these cancers. Of all cases diagnosed each year, 5 to 10 percent are due to these and other gene mutations.

Other common tests include hereditary nonpolyposis colorectal cancer (HNPCC) testing to screen for colorectal cancer, multiple assessments for genes that might contribute to cancer or diabetes, and those performed to determine if a patient will benefit from a certain chemotherapy drug or course of treatment.

Tests for genetic diseases can pinpoint the following:

- autism
- Crohn's disease
- cystic fibrosis
- Down syndrome
- hemophilia
- Huntington's disease
- neurofibromatosis
- Parkinson's disease
- prostate cancer

- sickle cell disease
- skin cancer
- achondroplasia
- familial hypercholesterolemia
- fragile X syndrome
- spinal muscular atrophy

Ethical, Legal, and Social Implications of Genetic Testing

When the Human Genome Project (HGP) was started, it was clear that there would be ethical issues to consider. A portion of the HGP budget was allocated for research on ethics, legalities, and social implications.

As clinical research has expanded, the Ethical, Legal and Social Implications (ELSI) Research Program has continued to review questions on these issues related to the use of DNA in the courtroom, the use of stored genetic samples, and the privacy of individuals involved.

Based on the ELSI's work, here are some key issues to consider if you're contemplating genetic screening.

Insurance Coverage and Reimbursement of Genetic Tests

- BRCA1 and 2 testing for breast cancer and HNPCC testing for colorectal cancer can help doctors make an effective plan for screening and preventive measures—but not all insurance policies will cover the costs. If you're considering such tests, it's a good idea to make sure your insurance policy will pay for them.
- Some tests can help physicians decide whether to treat patients with specific chemotherapy drugs—to keep them from suffering needlessly from toxic drugs that might have no effect. But an insurance company might not cover such testing if it isn't clear that it will be of value to the patient. To help clarify the situation, the CDC is developing policies and guidelines for when tests are warranted.
- The Affordable Care Act (ACA; Obamacare) passed in 2010 bars insurance companies from rejecting coverage for individuals with preexisting conditions. As a result, a genetic test that might identify someone with a predisposition for a particular health condition cannot be used to deny, rescind, or limit insurance coverage.
- Coverage for preventive care and screening is required under ACA, and determining high-risk people and subsequent care has been a big step forward in genetic testing.

- Some people purchase life insurance based on family history, and once insurance is purchased, you can't be dropped on the basis of genetic testing.
- Private testing, like 23andMe, now costs $199, so people have the opportunity to do initial testing before deciding to pursue more complex testing at a medical facility.

Privacy in genomics is considered in the following situations, among many others:

- Balancing the importance of privacy and the value of sharing data broadly is critical.
- The NIH has a number of databases that allow researchers to share information that is not linked to individuals.
- Some populations might be discriminated against if they are linked by genetics to specific conditions.
- When physicians collect specimens in medical settings—like blood spots from newborns—family members have been known to protest, even though such information might be useful to other families.
- Federal laws like HIPAA help keep consumer information safe.

Regulation of Genetic Tests
- The FDA has the authority to regulate genetic tests, but with the tremendous increase in different kinds of tests, they have only been able to regulate a small number of these.
- If you elect to use 23andMe, the FDA oversees tests like carrier status, but not all tests require FDA approval or genetic counseling.
- The CMS and the FDA regulate clinical testing, while the FTC monitors advertising claims.

Resources from NIH on Genetic Testing

An excellent resource for information on genetic testing can be found at the NIH GTR (http://www.ncbi.nih.gov/gtr/).

- The GTR provides information on more than 35,000 diseases relating to 10,480 health conditions offered by a total of 475 labs.
- Information is available on any particular test's purpose, methodology, and validity, as well as evidence of the test's usefulness.

Resources defining the clinical relevance of genetic variants can be found here:

- Clinical Genome Resource (ClinGen) Program (https://www .clinicalgenome.org/)
- Clinical Variation (ClinVar) Archive (https://www.ncbi.nlm.nih.gov/ clinvar/)
- Electronic Medical Records and Genomics (eMERGE) Network (https:// emerge.mc.vanderbilt.edu/)
- National Human Genome Research Institute (https://www.genome.gov/)

Genetic Testing: Fast Facts

- In the 1950s and 1960s, deoxyribonucleic acid (DNA) was discovered as the basis of human cells, and scientists came to learn that genes were the basis for DNA.
- No two human beings share the same genes or DNA, and this discovery led to the research that continues in genetics today.
- The HGP, completed in 2003, estimated that each human has between twenty thousand and twenty-five thousand genes.
- Diseases are not caused by genes but by mutations (sometimes called variants or defects) that make a gene function improperly. The so-called cystic fibrosis gene, for instance, is actually a mutated version of the CFTR gene.
- Testing to determine future disease development might not have much value to patients if they have no way to modify their lifestyle or avoid the disease. This is one reason the so-called Alzheimer's disease gene test is of limited value, because the condition has no known cure or effective treatment.
- On the other hand, some tests, like the genetic marker for Alzheimer's disease, might give someone the chance to make preventive choices earlier in life.
- One of the primary benefits of genetic testing is that results often go into a database of information that can be used by researchers in the future to help patients.
- Interpreting test results can be difficult, depending on what your goal is. A trained geneticist is most qualified to analyze tests, but if it is a simple ancestry test, you might not need anyone to help you figure it out.
- Inheritance patterns of some diseases, like rheumatoid arthritis, are not clear. But variations in dozens of genes have been studied as risk

factors. Type 1 diabetes, like rheumatoid arthritis, is considered to be an autoimmune disorder. Certain variants in genes can also be used to alert patients to the potential for developing diabetes.

For more facts and information, consult the NIH's Genetics Home Reference (https://ghr.nim.nih.gov), which offers a fifteen-chapter primer on genetic testing, including costs, benefits, and the length of time it takes to get a test done.

Healthy Habits Can Overcome Genes Linked to Heart Disease

Genetics is not destiny, as the saying goes. Just because you have a genetic predisposition to develop a particular ailment doesn't mean you actually will. This is because lifestyle factors—which you can control—can often offset the unchangeable genetic defect that might put you at greater risk for certain conditions.

If your parent or sibling died young from heart disease, for instance, new research shows that there are effective ways to counteract and even overcome your genetic predisposition through healthy lifestyle modifications.

Scientists with the Center for Human Genetic Research at Massachusetts General Hospital in Boston recently conducted a study showing that people can minimize an inherited risk for heart attack by living right—exercising, eating a healthy diet, staying slim, and quitting smoking.

Even with a little effort in these areas, people can cut their genetic risk of heart disease by more than half, says senior researcher Dr. Sekar Kathiresan.

But the researchers found the opposite also is true. People born with a genetic advantage protecting them against heart disease can ruin their good genetic luck through unhealthy habits.

"For heart attack at least, DNA is not destiny," notes Kathiresan, whose findings were recently presented at an American Heart Association (AHA) annual meeting and published in the *New England Journal of Medicine*. "You have control over your risk for heart attack, even if you've been dealt a bad hand."

For their research, Kathiresan and his colleagues examined the medical records of more than fifty-five thousand participants in four large-scale health studies. They analyzed each person's genetic risk for heart disease using a panel of fifty gene variants associated with elevated heart attack risk and compared them with each person's lifestyle based on four factors: smoking, body weight, diet, and exercise.

The results showed that those who did not smoke, were not obese, exercised at least one day a week, and met even half of the AHA's recommendations for a healthy diet were far less likely to have heart problems. That was true even for people who had high genetic risks for a "coronary event"—heart attack, cardiac arrest, or the need for angioplasty or other procedures to open a blocked artery.

Those with a high genetic risk and a bad lifestyle had a nearly 11 percent chance of having a coronary event over a ten-year period, the study found. But those at high risk who lived well cut the ten-year risk of such a health crisis down to 5 percent.

What's more, those with low genetic risk and a good lifestyle had a 3 percent risk of a coronary event over ten years, but a bad lifestyle would drive their risk up to 5.8 percent.

The study's findings suggest that patients who undergo genetic testing that turns up an increased risk for heart disease can benefit greatly by making healthy lifestyle changes that essentially cut their risk of developing cardiovascular disease and death in half.

Epigenetics: The Wave of the Future in Medicine?

Epigenetics is the study of how to manipulate the expression of our genetic makeup. It is fast becoming the pathway to understanding why dreaded diseases such as cancer occur and developing ways to turn off the gene or genes that cause the disease.

Dr. Jennifer Stagg is a naturopathic physician, founder of the Whole Wellness Center in Connecticut, and author of *Unzip Your Genes: 5 Choices to Reveal a Radically Radiant You*. In the following interview, she explains the finer points of epigenetics and how the field is fundamentally changing the way medicine is practiced.

Q: What is epigenetics, and why is it getting so much attention?

A: About a decade ago, the human genome—our complete set of DNA—was sequenced, allowing a much better understanding of the genetic influence on the development of disease. But it isn't the only factor that determines our health status. It turns out that only a small part of our genome is active at any one time, and even more profound is the concept that genes can get "turned on" and "turned off."

This concept is referred to as epigenetics, and research is showing that we may have far better control over our genome than previously thought. It turns out that while we cannot modify the gene sequence, we can modify how these genes are expressed. This is the science of epigenetics—the intersection of our environment with our DNA—and it is where leading edge research and health care is heading.

Q: What are some examples of how it works?

A: The landmark "Minnesota Twin Family Study" conducted from 1979 to 1999 looked at identical twins separated at birth. The findings definitely supported the role of genetics in health outcomes, but what they also found was that some twins, [despite] having the exact same genetic makeup, had vastly different outcomes.

Our evolving understanding about epigenetics is providing new insight into the debate about nature versus nurture. However, more surprising is the evidence that has emerged that changes in the epigenome, those chemical factors that tell our genes what to do, may be passed along with your genes. Stress from physical traumas, famine, psychological insults (including bullying) and even poverty can be passed through multiple generations.

Q: What are some tools scientists are using to work with genes?

A: The most popular type of testing in the field of genetics is genomic testing for variants in genes referred to as single nucleotide polymorphisms, or SNPs. This type of testing is widely available in medical practice. More advanced testing in epigenetics is the next big thing that has not reached clinicians yet. In research settings, we are testing for alterations in the genome using DNA methylation, where methyl groups are added or subtracted to existing DNA.

The most interesting development is CRISPR technology (short for clustered regularly interspaced short palindromic repeats), which Massachusetts Institute of Technology scientists have developed to turn genes on and off. This technology could result in a world that looks very different—where there are no mosquito-borne illnesses like malaria and the Zika virus. The ability to "edit" DNA could completely cure genetic diseases. And the use of CRISPR in agriculture could eliminate the need for pesticides.

Q: What diseases or medical conditions can we hope to ameliorate or eliminate through epigenetics?

A: The bulk of research on epigenetics in management and treatment of health conditions is in chronic diseases. Currently, there is tremendous evidence in the areas of diabetes and cardiovascular disease. Countless studies have been conducted examining the effects of various plant compounds on genes related to cancer. For example, we know that EGCG [epigallocatechin gallate] found in green tea can increase the expression of genes that suppress tumors.

Also, development of pharmaceutical agents for cancer treatments is very active. We also know that in breast cancer patients, doubling the amount of exercise can reduce the risk of reoccurrence. Other promising conditions include autoimmune diseases, obesity, and mood disorders.

Q: What can we do as individuals right now to change our gene expression for a better outcome?

A: Pay attention to what you eat. The balance of macronutrients in our diet can make a difference to our health in terms of its effect on DNA expression. For example, consuming a Mediterranean-style diet can turn off genes associated with diabetes.

You should make sure your diet is rich in foods that contain compounds that act as beneficial epigenetic modifiers, like green tea, chocolate, garlic, turmeric, coffee, blueberries and other dark berries, apples, cruciferous vegetables, and red wine.

Learn to manage stress. While you may not be able to reduce the stressors in your life, you can change how you respond to those stressors. A regular practice of meditation is most effective, but walks outside in nature and relaxation breathing can also help.

Lastly, stay active. Regular exercise has been shown to turn high genetic risk of disease into low risk. Surprisingly, the effects of exercise can be immediate, with gene expression being altered after a single workout.

Cancer and Genetics: A Primer

Genes are like the quarterbacks of our cells, calling the plays for how they work, grow, and divide. Cancer can develop when something goes awry with one or more of the genes in a cell—a defect that can cause the disease and be passed on to children and grandchildren.

Gene defects can cause healthy cells to grow and divide uncontrollably—the hallmark of cancer. Some defects are inborn; others develop with age and as a result of unhealthy lifestyles (such as smoking) or exposure to carcinogenic substances (such as toxic chemicals or even sunlight, in the case of skin cancer).

Scientists believe that cancers caused by inherited gene defects are far less common (less than 10 percent) than those tied to gene changes due to aging or other factors.

If you are concerned that you might be a risk for a gene-linked cancer—because it runs in the family or a relative was found to have a positive genetic test for it—experts recommend talking to your doctor about the pros and cons of screening.

According to the American Cancer Society (ACS), the best ways to cut your cancer risk (regardless of your genetic makeup) include the following:

- Eat a healthy diet.
- Don't use tobacco.
- Exercise regularly—at least thirty minutes of moderate-intensity activity most days of the week.
- Maintain a healthy weight.
- Avoid excessive exposure to toxic chemicals, pollutants, and sunlight.

Genetics: Headlines and Recent Updates

Google "genetics and health," and you'll come up with more than 93 million hits. (By comparison, "Lady Gaga" retrieves 78.6 million hits.) It goes without saying that the advent of genetics in health care has generated daily headlines for years—a trend that is likely to continue.

Here's a compendium of recent, semirandom reports from the front lines of the genetics revolution. Some represent genuine breakthroughs; others are merely curiosities.

American Attitudes on Genetics

Most Americans think scientific and technological innovations bring positive changes to society but fear some advances do more harm than good when they are used to make people smarter, stronger, or healthier, according to a new Pew Research Center survey.

The nationally representative survey of more than 4,700 US adults found that Americans are roughly evenly divided over the potential use of "gene editing" techniques designed to give babies a lifetime of reduced risk of serious disease.

"Developments in biomedical technologies are accelerating rapidly, raising new societal debates about how we will use these technologies and what uses are appropriate," said lead author Cary Funk, an associate director of research at Pew Research Center. "This study suggests Americans are largely cautious about using emerging technologies in ways that push human capacities beyond what's been possible before."

Among the key findings,

- US adults are split on the question of whether they would want gene editing to prevent diseases for their babies (48 percent would; 50 percent would not).
- The majority say that these enhancements could exacerbate the divide between the haves and have-nots.

- Seven in ten predict that the technology would likely become available before it has been fully tested or understood.
- Many people say that they are not sure whether these interventions are morally acceptable.
- More adults say that the benefits would outweigh the downsides; 36 percent think it will have more benefits than downsides, while 28 percent think it will have more downsides than benefits.
- Opinions are closely divided when it comes to the fundamental question of whether these potential developments are "meddling with nature" and cross a line that should not be crossed or whether they are "no different" from other ways that humans have tried to better themselves over time.
- More religious Americans are, on average, less likely to embrace these potential types of enhancement. More than six in ten of very religious people consider gene editing to be crossing a line that should not be crossed. By contrast, the majority of nonreligious adults say such enhancements would be no different from other ways humans try to better themselves.

Genetic Testing Targets Therapies to Defeat Prostate Cancer

Genetic testing in men with advanced prostate cancer can spot genetic mutations that could point the way to targeting men who would benefit from new precision treatments, new research finds.

Researchers at the Institute of Cancer Research in London found that about 12 percent of men with advanced prostate cancer had inherited gene mutations in genes that normally repair DNA damage. The mutated genes include the breast cancer gene BRCA2, known as the "Angelina Jolie" gene, which might cause one in twenty cases of prostate cancer.

Their discovery could lead to a simple saliva test that could determine the best course of treatment for men as soon as they are diagnosed with the disease.

The researchers examined the DNA code of twenty genes known to be involved in DNA repair in 692 men with advanced prostate cancer. They discovered that about 12 percent had at least one type of gene mutation. The most common defective gene was BRCA2, which was mutated in 5 percent of the men.

The best treatment for these men could be a new type of drug called poly(ADP-ribose) polymerase (PARP) inhibitors. These drugs inhibit the PARP enzyme. Studies have found that blocking PARP kills tumor cells where the ability to repair DNA is impaired.

"Our study has shown that a significant proportion of men with advanced prostate cancer are born with DNA repair mutations—and this could have important implications for patients," said Johann de Bono of the Institute of Cancer Research.

"Genetic testing for these mutations could identify men with advanced prostate cancer who may benefit from precision treatment," he continued. "We could offer these men drugs such as PARP inhibitors, which are effective in patients with certain DNA repair mutations and are showing important antitumor activity in ongoing clinical trials."

The research was published in *The New England Journal of Medicine*.

Alzheimer's Genes Might Be Detectable in Youth: Study

New research shows that genes tied to Alzheimer's disease might be used to predict who will develop the memory-robbing disorder in young adulthood, long before symptoms emerge.

The findings—published online in *Neurology*, the medical journal of the American Academy of Neurology—could lead to a test that could be administered decades before memory loss and other cognitive problems surface, giving doctors a chance to lessen or stave off the disease's impact with medications and other therapies.

"The stage of Alzheimer's before symptoms show up is thought to last over a decade," said Dr. Elizabeth C. Mormino, PhD, at Massachusetts General Hospital, who helped lead the research. "Given that current clinical trials are testing whether therapies can slow memory and thinking decline among people at risk for the disease, it is critical to understand the influence of risk factors before symptoms are present."

For the study, researchers calculated a score based on whether a person has several high-risk Alzheimer's-related gene mutations. The study involved 166 people with dementia and 1,026 without, with an average age of seventy-five years.

The scientists also looked for specific markers of Alzheimer's disease, such as memory loss and thinking decline, clinical progression of the disease, and the size of the hippocampus (the memory center of the brain). They compared the results with those of 1,322 healthy, younger participants between the ages of eighteen and thirty-five.

The study found that older people free of dementia who had a higher risk score tended to have a worse memory and a smaller hippocampus than those who had lower genetic risks.

"Our study was small, and larger numbers of participants will need to be studied to confirm our findings," said Mormino. "The goal of this type of research is to help physicians better identify those at high risk of dementia so that future preventative treatments may be used as early as possible."

The study was funded by the NIH.

Fishing for Longevity Secrets in Sardinia Gene Pool

A British biotech group has bought the genetic data of nearly thirteen thousand Italian residents of a Sardinian province where many people have lived to celebrate their one hundredth birthdays—and beyond.

Tiziana Life Sciences, a British company focused on cancer and diseases of the immune system, said it acquired a "biobank" containing the DNA of residents of the Ogliastra province in Sardinia.

One in every two thousand people in Ogliastra are one hundred years of age or older—five times the rate in most developed countries and second only to the Japanese island of Okinawa.

The biobank includes more than 230,000 samples, including frozen blood from 12,600 Ogliastra residents. The company has also gathered family medical reports and official records such as death certificates dating back more than four hundred years.

Gabriele Cerrone, chief executive of Tiziana, said the company hopes that the trove of data will help researchers identify whether there are any particular genetic traits linked to longevity.

Italian and US researchers are also studying centenarians who live in Acciaroli, a remote fishing village in the south of Italy with two thousand residents—three hundred of whom are one hundred or older.

Hiding Places of Depression Genes Identified

A comprehensive scan of human DNA has turned up what appears to be the hiding places of more than a dozen genes linked to depression.

Lead researcher Ashley Winslow, an author of a paper on the work, told the Associated Press that the findings are not only an important milestone in the development of promising new gene therapies for depression; they also demonstrate the promise of using "data mining" to uncover genetic clues to a range of health problems.

The work by Winslow and others identified fifteen areas of human DNA that show genetic variations that affect the risk of becoming depressed. Winslow was with Pfizer Inc. when she did the work with researchers from Massachusetts General Hospital and the genetic testing company 23andMe. She is now at the University of Pennsylvania. Results were released by the journal *Nature Genetics*.

The new work used data from more than 121,000 customers of 23andMe who indicated that they'd been diagnosed with depression and another 338,000 other customers. They had consented to the use of their data for research.

Those results were combined with information from about 9,000 people diagnosed with the disease and 9,500 others taken from a previous study to find risk genes.

Can Gene Therapy Treat Alzheimer's Disease?

In a finding that could point the way to new gene-based dementia treatments, scientists have prevented the development of Alzheimer's disease in mice by using a modified virus to deliver a specific gene to brain cells.

Researchers from Imperial College London have built on previous studies that found that a gene called PGC1-alpha might prevent the formation of a protein called amyloid-beta peptide in cells in the lab. Amyloid-beta peptide is the main component of amyloid plaques, the sticky clumps of protein found in the brains of people with Alzheimer's that cause memory loss and the death of brain cells.

"Although these findings are very early, they suggest this gene therapy may have potential therapeutic use for patients," said researcher Dr. Magdalena Sastre.

"There are many hurdles to overcome, and at the moment, the only way to deliver the gene is via an injection directly into the brain. However, this proof-of-concept study shows this approach warrants further investigation."

In the new study, the team injected the virus, containing the gene PGC1-alpha, into the brains of mice that had early stages of Alzheimer's-like disease. After four months, the team found that mice who received the gene had very few amyloid plaques compared to the untreated mice. In addition, the treated mice performed better on memory tests.

The study was published in the *Proceedings of the National Academy of Sciences*.

New Ovarian Cancer Drug Corrects Gene Defects

An experimental drug—Tesaro's niraparib—boosted the survival rate of women with recurrent ovarian cancer in a clinical study. The study is the latest to confirm the potential benefits of a closely watched class of new gene-based medicines called PARP inhibitors.

The findings, reported at the annual European Society for Medical Oncology congress in Copenhagen, indicated that the treatment halted the cancer's progress and helped patients live longer. Niraparib and other PARP inhibitors block enzymes involved in repairing damaged DNA, which helps kill cancer cells.

Lead researcher Mansoor Raza Mirza of Copenhagen University told reporters at the congress that he believes the drug can benefit all patients with the condition: "Our conclusion is that all patients have a benefit and all patients must be treated. This is a breakthrough for patients with ovarian cancer. We have never seen such large benefits in progression-free survival (PFS) in recurrent ovarian cancer."

Results of the study were also published online in the *New England Journal of Medicine*.

New Form of Vitamin B Combats DNA Damage

A newly discovered form of vitamin B3 has been found to offer protection against DNA damage, a common factor in cancer and other diseases. In the first controlled clinical trial of nicotinamide riboside (NR), University of Iowa researchers found that the compound safely boosts cellular energy production and helps combat the ravages of stress and DNA damage on the body.

Cellular energy production diminishes as we grow older, which increases the risk for many age-related health conditions, the researchers said. Past studies have shown that reversing this process can combat weight gain, improve control of blood sugar and cholesterol, reduce nerve damage, and lead to a longer lifespan.

The new research, reported in the journal *Nature Communications*, was conducted by Charles Brenner, a professor at the University of Iowa Carver College of Medicine, in collaboration with colleagues at Queen's University Belfast and ChromaDex Corp., which supplied the NR used in the trial.

For the study, six men and six women received single oral doses of 100 mg, 300 mg, or 1,000 mg of NR. The results showed that the compound boosted the study participants' metabolic function and levels of cellular energy without causing serious side effects.

"This trial shows that oral NR safely boosts human [energy production and] metabolism," Brenner said. He also reported that the researchers are "excited" by the findings.

Brenner now plans to test the effects of NR in people with diseases and health conditions, including elevated cholesterol, obesity and diabetes, and people at risk for chemotherapeutic peripheral neuropathy.

The research was funded, in part, by the NIH.

3

STEM CELLS

Breakthrough Therapies That Are Transforming Medicine

For years, stem cell research was controversial because it often involved the use of embryonic tissues. But in late 2014, scientists pioneered a technique that "harvests" stem cells from living patients—providing a new way to use a person's own "master cells" in a variety of therapeutic techniques. Since then, an explosion of advances has led to game-changing new treatments for heart disease, arthritis, spinal cord injuries, leukemia, and other conditions.

New Leading-Edge Treatments Target Stroke, Heart Disease, and Alzheimer's
It's truly the stuff of science fiction: Stroke patients regaining the use of their limbs. Heart patients experiencing a reversal of symptoms. Knee surgery patients "regrowing" their own cartilage. People with Alzheimer's disease recovering lost memories.

It sounds incredible, but in fact, stem cell research is producing such results now—in ways that can only mean good things for the future, medical experts say.

Dr. Joshua Michael Hare, founding director of the Interdisciplinary Stem Cell Institute at the University of Miami Miller School of Medicine, says he is seeing results in patients undergoing such treatments that are nothing short of miraculous.

Hare, whose Miami institute is spearheading some of the most cutting-edge research on stem cells in the nation, is the principal investigator of a new study of stem cell benefits for patients with congestive heart failure. That work is being funded by the National Institutes of Health (NIH) Specialized Center for Cell-Based Therapy.

"We [as doctors] are good at palliating injuries, but we want to regenerate tissues," he explains. "If someone has a heart attack the artery gets blocked, heart muscle dies, and it turns into a scar. In stroke, it is the same thing; part of the brain dies, and the patient loses critical functioning."

But stem cell therapy—which involves treating patients with their own stem cells that have been extracted, engineered to heal such conditions, and then reintroduced to the body through tiny catheters—holds the promise of reversing that damage without posing significant risks.

"Compared to other strategies, it's one of the safest ways to treat people," Hare says. "These cells will work or last for twelve to eighteen months, and then a second injection may help to remove more scar tissue."

Hare has already seen stem cells transform the lives of some of his patients. One—an eighty-year-old heart attack survivor—was given a new lease on life after undergoing stem cell therapy. He'd suffered a serious heart attack and congestive heart failure and could do little more than sit in a chair all day long before undergoing treatment.

"He was able to get out of that chair, go back to work in his garden, and do heavy lifting after stem cell therapy," says Hare. He also had a 40 percent reduction in scar tissue in his heart after he underwent treatment.

"Another young man, who was a cardiac cripple, was able to go back, unencumbered, to break dancing. And eight years later, he is still benefiting."

Therapies Cap Years of Research

Stem cell transplants have been used for years to battle various cancers, with the first therapies emerging thirty years ago.

For instance, stem cell transplants are used in the treatment of leukemia, lymphoma, and myeloma. In some cases, cancer patients receive very high doses of chemotherapy or radiation, which kill tumors but also wipe out stem cells in the bone marrow. Stem cell transplants help regenerate the growth of such cells.

Emerging stem cell research has also shown that it might be promising against diabetes, Parkinson's disease, spinal cord injuries, and other ailments.

It was once believed that embryonic cells, harvested at the earliest stage of life, would have the greatest possibility of success. But the use of such cells was controversial and even banned under President George W. Bush. According to the latest studies, however, adult stem cells have proven to be more promising (and less controversial) than embryonic cells and appear to pose a lower risk of tumor growth.

Hare's own research, which has been ongoing for fifteen years, is exploring new and different ways that adult stem cells can be used to treat cardiovascular disease, among other conditions. He and his colleagues at the Interdisciplinary Stem Cell Institute at University of Miami are participating in two new trials that they hope will lead to US Food and Drug Administration (FDA) approval for wider general use.

"Some scientists are still wondering about cells. Embryonic stem cells have a high risk of tumors and are controversial, but there is no ethical debate over using adult stem cells," Hare notes. "It's still experimental now but may be available to the public in about five years."

How Do Stem Cells Fight Disease?

Stem cells are so promising because they are "master cells" of the body that have the ability to divide and develop into virtually any type of cell. They can be used to repair the body by replenishing cells that are damaged by disease, injury, or normal wear.

When a stem cell divides, each new cell can become another type of cell with a more specialized function, such as a nerve cell, a skin cell, or a red blood cell.

"Stem cells reduce scar tissue and have a proregenerative effect," Hare explains. "Everybody uses the same cell types for many disease areas in cardiology, neuropathy, gastroenterology, and diseases of the lung. Any chronic disease with tissue damage is fair game."

Dr. Dileep Yavagal, an associate professor of neurology and neurosurgery at the University of Miami Miller School of Medicine, has focused his research on stroke recovery.

"My focus has been in delivering bone marrow–derived stem cells into the carotid artery with a catheter," says Yavagal, a faculty member at the Interdisciplinary Stem Cell Institute. "I've been asking, 'If we give stem cells, will they be safe and effective?' There is no surgery, no open incision, as opposed to drilling a hole in the skull."

After getting promising results of stem cell therapies in animals, he launched a clinical trial involving forty-eight stroke patients and found that the treatments were not only safe but very effective.

"I was concerned that these cells could cause a stroke, or they could potentially block arteries," Yavagal says, "but there were no side effects, and that is a big step forward. We can now go on to a larger study."

About 70 percent of the patients who received stem cells demonstrated improvement without suffering negative side effects, researchers found. The study participants were all paralyzed on one side of their bodies, and with the therapy, they regained use of the affected arm. In a comparison group of patients who didn't receive stem cells, only 30 percent improved.

"This is a small trial," Yavagal notes. "Twenty-nine patients got cells and nineteen did not. With that size of a study, the goal is really safety. And indeed, stem cells are very safe." To us, that is exciting. We haven't found any adverse effects or the need for immunosuppressive meds. Stem cells are so primitive that they don't need that. Many other organs have been tested, and cells weren't rejected.

"I'm quite excited about the future. If we had seen side effects, then I would be less optimistic about the future. My hope is that we'll have stem cell therapy as routine treatment."

A Treatment for Alzheimer's?

Stem cell therapy is also being explored as a therapy for Alzheimer's disease, a condition for which there is currently no treatment.

Dr. Bernard S. Baumel, assistant professor of neurology at the Miller School of Medicine, is leading a clinical trial that aims to determine if stem cells can be used to treat Alzheimer's patients. He believes that there is a great deal of hope and promise in the field.

"Medications that are available for Alzheimer's are mediocre at best," Baumel explains, noting available drugs merely ease symptoms or slow progression of the disease. "Some may help improve memory for a few months, but then the disease process continues. Another drug targets behavior problems. There has been no new treatment for Alzheimer's since the behavioral drug was developed in 2002."

For Baumel's study, Alzheimer's patients will receive stem cells through an IV infusion with the hope that they will stimulate the growth of new brain cells to replace those lost to the memory-robbing terminal brain disorder.

"They will go around the body but also to the brain," he explains. "Neurogenesis is the process of the brain making new cells, and the stem cells will accelerate this process."

Prospective participants in this study will include fifty to eighty people with mild symptoms of Alzheimer's disease. "This means [that they are] early in the course of the disease, but [symptoms are] significant enough to be diagnosed," Baumel says. "They should be competent enough to go through testing so we can see if they are getting worse, remaining stable, or getting better with stem cell treatment."

The researchers will use mesenchymal stem cells (MSCs). These particular cells have the ability to develop into many different types of cells and promote the growth of new brain cells in the hippocampus, the memory-forming center of the brain.

In Alzheimer's disease, there is a lot of inflammation in the brain, which is believed to be promoted by a buildup of amyloid protein plaques that cause webs or tangles that block communication between brain cells.

Stem cells are anti-inflammatory and can also promote or accelerate the growth of new brain cells. Baumel's study aims to determine how effectively stem cells encourage that process and whether they can drive the removal of amyloid proteins in the brain, perhaps reversing Alzheimer's.

Baumel expects results will be available within a few years and is optimistic that his research will lead to new an entirely new way to combat Alzheimer's, which strikes five million Americans—a number that is projected to triple by 2050 as the baby boomers grow older.

"There is a lot of frustration out there," he says. "Nothing seems to work so well for these people, and no one else in the country has done any research [on the promise of stem cells to treat Alzheimer's]."

Improving Memory with Stem Cells

Dr. Bernard S. Baumel is recruiting people with mild Alzheimer's disease to participate in a clinical trial designed to assess the benefits of stem cells in treating dementia. He is enrolling patients who meet the following criteria:

- Participants must be between fifty and eighty years old with mild Alzheimer's, meaning they are in early stages of the disease.
- They should have no other serious medical conditions.
- Researchers will use a thirty-point test to select participants. People selected for the study score eighteen to twenty-four.

Enrollment in the clinical trial—"Allogeneic Human Mesenchymal Stem Cell Infusion Versus Placebo in Patients with Alzheimer's Disease"—will continue until 2018. Baumel has signed up some volunteers for the trial but is looking for more people.

For more information about participating, call 305-342-6633 or visit http://www.ummemoryprogram.org.

Banking Your Own Stem Cells

Many companies offer the service of harvesting and banking your own stem cells for possible use later in life. Such cells can be used against illness, injury, or other conditions that develop or as donor cells. Harvesting adult stem cells is not a difficult process.

"We take them from the back of the hip, and it is not really painful," explains Dr. Joshua Michael Hare, founding director of the Interdisciplinary Stem Cell Institute at the University of Miami Miller School of Medicine.

"Having a tooth filled is more uncomfortable. A little sedation, a little lidocaine, sleep through it, and you are on your way."

Stem cells can also come from an umbilical cord, in addition to bone marrow or blood. Many private outfits allow parents to bank a child's umbilical cord cells in case he or she, or someone else in the family, becomes seriously ill in the future.

About 1.7 million cord stem cell samples are now stored in three dozen private banks in the United States, according to the Genetic Literacy Project. Each sample costs about $2,000 to harvest, plus a $125 annual storage fee.

Adult stem cells are so valuable because they have the amazing ability to transform into many different types of cells under the right circumstances. Think of stem cell therapy as a way of growing spare body parts. Stem cells can replace cells that have been harmed by disease, injury, or age.

After they are in place, they renew themselves and continue to divide in a healthy way, explains Alan J. Russell, a professor at Carnegie Mellon University in Pittsburgh.

Another plus is that when stem cells are taken from the patient, there's no risk of the body rejecting them, notes Dipnarine Maharaj, MD, medical director of the South Florida Bone Marrow/Stem Cell Transplant Institute in Boynton Beach, Florida.

"When you consider the mortality and risk associated with other donors, the risk is almost zero with using your own stem cells," he says.

Proactively putting stem cells aside as part of a wellness program enables you to use them as a type of medical insurance, he adds.

"On an annual basis, there are thousands of healthy people who donate stem cells to someone else—that's a very good thing to do—but you can also help yourself and store your own cells in case you need them in the future," says Maharaj.

He adds that people are never too old to bank their own stem cells as long as they're healthy. "If you don't use your own stem cells, you can donate them to a family member," he says. You might save a loved one's life, if not your own.

According to the NIH, the harvesting of cells must follow good manufacturing, freezing, and thawing protocols and use cryoprotectants and animal protein freezing solutions.

The following are a few of the big stem cell banks:

- Sanbio (Sanbio.com)
- Viacord (Viacord.com)
- Celltex (Celltexbank.com)

Stem Cell Therapy: At a Glance

Stem cell therapy typically involves removing the cells from a patient's bone marrow, blood, fat, or—in the case of infants—umbilical cord. The cells are then reintroduced to the patient's body, typically through injection or IV drip.

In the case of stroke recovery, the stem cells are introduced into the heart muscle by a catheter in the groin. They remain inside the blood vessels all the way to the brain. The procedure has low risks because there is no incision, surgery, or a need to drill a hole in the skull. For heart attack patients, stem cells can be injected into the heart muscle.

While some people believe that umbilical stem cells are the best choice, research has shown that these stem cells might cause tumors. Also, banking umbilical stem cells doesn't have much of an advantage—healthy young stem cells harvested from another adult are just as good as those from cord blood in most cases.

Conditions Treated by Stem Cells

Many research studies have found that stem cell therapies hold a great deal of promise in the treatment of a wide variety of ailments, injuries, and health conditions.

In one of the most promising discoveries, scientists from Stanford University School of Medicine have mapped the biological and chemical signals needed to make bone, heart muscle, blood vessels, and ten other cell types from human stem cells within a matter of days.

The findings, reported in the journal *Cell* in June 2016, could enable scientists to repair heart tissue after a heart attack, make cartilage to repair painful joints, or produce bone to help people recover from accidents or other trauma.

Promising research has also been conducted, or is under way, on about seventy different diseases and conditions that might benefit from stem cell therapies. Here are just a few:

Heart disease. Researchers believe that stem cells might one day be able to replace heart tissues damaged by heart attacks and other cardiovascular diseases with healthy cells. Studies involving laboratory animals suggest that when adult stem cells are transplanted into a damaged heart, the cells develop into healthy heart muscle cells. In a heart attack, an artery is blocked, and heart muscle dies and turns into a scar. Stem cells are used to regenerate tissue. This therapy can degrade the scar and help the patient grow new heart muscle.

In one promising study conducted by Japanese researchers, stem cells grown from a single monkey's skin cells revitalized the damaged hearts of five sick macaques. The findings, published in the journal *Nature*, suggest that stem cells have the potential to become a vast and uncontroversial source of rejuvenating cells to transplant into heart attack victims. The Japanese team from

Shinshu University used induced pluripotent stem cells (iPSCs), which are created by stimulating mature cells (such as a skin cell) back into a neutral juvenile state, from which they can develop into any other type of human cell.

Diabetes. In people with type 1 diabetes, the pancreatic cells that would normally produce insulin are destroyed by the sufferer's own immune system. Research has shown that stem cells can be used to generate healthy pancreatic cells capable of producing insulin. The hope is that cells could one day be transplanted into diabetics, removing their need for insulin injection.

Parkinson's disease. This progressive neurological condition causes the destruction of brain cells that produce a neurotransmitter called dopamine. New research has found that transplanted stem cells can be engineered to function and release dopamine, relieving the symptoms of Parkinson's.

Cancer. Many people undergo bone marrow stem cell transplants, which have been used for years to treat cancers such as leukemia. Such procedures allow the marrow to receive healthy cells—to replace those damaged by disease, chemo, or radiation—which multiply and generate the types of blood cells necessary for life. New research aims to overcome the challenges of cell rejection to boost the success rate of bone marrow transplants. Scientists are also studying whether stem cell transplants can be used directly to treat certain cancers, such as multiple myeloma.

Spinal cord injuries. Studies involving laboratory animals have found that stem cell injections can help heal nerve cells damaged by injuries, boosting motility and recovery. Preliminary research suggests that stem cells might one day be used to heal such injuries, perhaps even allowing individuals who use wheelchairs to walk again.

Eye problems. Scientists have been able to direct the growth of "photoreceptor" cells that are necessary for vision from stem cells, introducing them into the retina. This approach might allow individuals who suffer from degenerative retinal diseases to regain their vision or even experience a complete reversal of blindness.

Genetic defects. Preliminary research has suggested that stem cells might be able to address a range of genetic defects that are present from birth by introducing normal, healthy cells that do not have such mutations.

Burns. Burn victims often need donor tissues, but stem cells could be used to produce new and healthy tissues. In burn victims, a small piece of a patient's skin can be progressively grown, allowing doctors to cover a burn. Unfortunately, this skin doesn't have hair follicles or sweat glands, so it isn't a perfect fix, but this therapy makes a difference in life-or-death burn cases.

Osteoporosis. Preliminary experiments conducted by Canadian researchers on mice suggest that osteoporosis, which affects both men and women and causes bones to thin, might one day be reversed with a single injection of stem cells. When the researchers injected MSCs cells from healthy mice into osteoporotic mice, their bones became stronger and more functional.

"We had hoped for a general increase in bone health," said study coauthor John E. Davies of the University of Toronto, "but the huge surprise was to find that the exquisite inner 'coral-like' architecture of the bone structure of the injected animals—which is severely compromised in osteoporosis—was restored to normal." A trial is currently under way in the United States in which elderly patients have been injected with MSCs, and their blood samples will be studied for biological markers of bone growth.

Other conditions. Studies have also been launched to determine the potential use of stem cells to treat Crohn's disease, multiple sclerosis, lupus, Lou Gehrig's disease (ALS), and HIV/AIDS.

For more information, check out the website of Explore Stem Cells, a UK clearinghouse for information and resources on stem cell research: http://www.explorestemcells.co.uk/aboutoursite.html.

Stem Cell Therapy Offers Alternative to Knee Surgery

People who have undergone surgery for painful injuries to the shoulder or knee know how long and difficult recovery can be. But new research in using stem cells is giving new hope for healing that comes naturally without surgery, drugs, or other interventions.

Dr. Kevin Plancher, an orthopedic surgeon and sports medicine expert based in Greenwich, Connecticut, and New York City, is finding that injecting stem cells into painful joints can result in healing and regrowth of cartilage and other tissues.

"It's like the Zamboni on the ice rink," says Plancher, a clinical professor in orthopedics at Albert Einstein College of Medicine in New York. "The stem cells clear the surface, and eventually the placebo effect is gone, but the patients are having fewer symptoms."

Stem cells injected into painful shoulders, knees, and joints can regrow cartilage, heal meniscus tears, and reduce the pain of tennis elbow and Achilles tendons and muscles. They have also shown promise in fixing rotator cuff tears in the shoulder and other injuries resulting from overuse and degenerative conditions.

"Athletes have been getting this treatment for a while," explains Plancher, who founded the Center for Regenerative Medicine at Plancher Orthopedics and lectures globally on issues related to orthopedic procedures and sports injury management. "Kobe Bryant made it famous. He claimed it helped his injured knee. The National Football League's season is short. Those with muscle problems need quick recovery, and this has worked.

"There has been some really valuable research done. We take stem cells from a person's hip or from amniotic fluid. There are billions of cells in amniotic fluid; they are processed, cleansed, and injected into a patient."

He is also using bone marrow, which is not difficult to retrieve from the patient's own hip. "There is minimal discomfort, and we use liposuction to take the cells, process them, and then inject them into the injured areas of the body," adds Plancher.

"I'm anxious for more studies to be done—to show insurance companies that this will save them money in the future. This procedure is not covered by Medicare. It is a personal decision, and we tell patients all we know. That's why we want more studies.

"This procedure is amazing, and I don't believe the turnarounds. One patient was able to move his shoulder again after fourteen months. We believe the stem cells bathe injured tissues in a concentrated slurry of healing cells. After a short period of rest, many patients are able to regain flexible, pain-free movement."

Plancher says that the appeal of new stem cell therapies is that they work with the body—not against it—to heal from within. "It is essentially the body healing itself," he explains. "It works beautifully, and patients recover much quicker than they would from more invasive treatment. It's an option that definitely deserves close consideration."

Beware Unproven Therapies

Because stem cell therapies are so new, experts warn that a variety of web-based outfits are seeking to take advantage of consumers' lack of knowledge about them—marketing unproven, often costly treatments and antiaging services directly to consumers.

A recent study published in the journal *Cell Stem Cell* found that the United States—along with Ireland, Singapore, Australia, Germany, Italy, and Japan—has the most clinics engaging in such marketing.

Lead researcher Dr. John Rasko of the University of Sydney said the marketing of dubious stem cell procedures, especially for antiaging and skin rejuvenation, is a growing industry that is taking in untold numbers of consumers.

The researchers found that direct-to-consumer marketing sites were most common in the United States, with 187 clinics promoting treatments online, followed by India (35), Mexico (28), China (23), Australia (19), and the United Kingdom (16).

The problem is that some nations don't yet have safety regulations in place to govern what's acceptable for such clinics. At best, the services offered might be ineffective. At worst, treatments could be harmful, the researchers warn.

To protect yourself, experts recommend doing the following:

- Consult your doctor before undergoing any stem cell procedure.
- Make sure any stem cell clinic procedure you are considering is provided by a reputable medical center with appropriate regulatory approval.
- Be sure to check a clinic's licensing, registration, and record with your state board of medicine, insurance division, or the FDA. A good place to start is the State Health Insurance Assistance Program (SHIP), a national initiative that offers consumer health information and patient assistance. You can identify your home state's SHIP by visiting https://shiptalk.org and clicking "Find a State SHIP," which will direct you to a page that will allow you to search for SHIP contact information for every state.
- Steer clear of clinics that offer the same treatment for a variety of conditions.
- Avoid clinics that use hard-sell techniques, promise to cure you, or rely on patient testimonials (instead of science-based evidence) to market their treatments on the Internet, through social media, and in newspapers.
- Beware of costly treatments that have not passed through carefully controlled and conducted FDA-approved clinical trials.

For more tips and information, check out the International Society for Stem Cell Research's online guide to "A Closer Look at Stem Cells" (http://www.closerlookatstemcells.org/stem-cells-and-medicine/nine-things-to-know-about-stem-cell-treatments).

4

MENTAL HEALTH

Proven Ways to Stay Mentally Sharp as You Age

Curcumin in Asian curry dishes. Learning to play a musical instrument. Taking up a second language. Maintaining an active social life. Getting regular exercise. Keeping your cholesterol and blood sugar in check. Taking herbal remedies. All have been proven to cut the risk of mental health disorders, including depression and Alzheimer's disease, in the latest cutting-edge research. Here are practical alternative and conventional ways—based on the latest findings from the fields of genetics, neuroscience, and medical technology—to stay young at heart (and mind) as you age.

Drugs: Not the Only Elixir for Alzheimer's and Mental Health
The numbers are nothing short of staggering:

- Millions of Americans with Alzheimer's disease take one of the two types of medications designed to ease symptoms—cholinesterase inhibitors and memantine—but those drugs merely slow the progression of the condition and don't work for everyone.
- Antidepressant drug use has risen 400 percent in the United States since 1988. More than one in six Americans take a psychoactive drug, such as

an antidepressant (Prozac, Paxil, Zoloft, and Celexa), according to a 2016 analysis by the nonprofit Institute for Safe Medication Practices.

- About 11 percent of American children (between the ages of four and seventeen), and smaller numbers of adults, are prescribed medication (such as Ritalin, Adderall, and Concerta) to treat attention deficit hyperactivity disorder (ADHD).

The findings, compiled by the US Centers for Disease Control and Prevention (CDC) and other federal health agencies, make it clear that drugs are the first-line treatment for the range of mental health disorders Americans suffer, leading some to suggest that they are being handed out like candy.

While medication can be a lifesaver for many people with severe mental illness—not only reducing the risk of suicide but also making it easier to cope—drugs don't help everyone, are expensive, and often carry significant negative side effects.

Now for the good news: A variety of natural methods, lifestyle modifications, and psychotherapies have been scientifically proven to be helpful in many cases. Some might even be as good as (or better than) conventional medications.

Here's a primer on drug-free methods for treating psychological issues and staying mentally sharp as you age.

Healthy Habits That Help Stave Off Alzheimer's Disease

Alzheimer's disease is too often thought of as an inevitable part of aging, but in fact, that's a myth, and a handful of lifestyle changes and healthy behaviors can prevent or even reverse it, a top expert says.

"You can accelerate your risk of Alzheimer's disease, delay it, or even make changes that will help reverse it, depending on your behavior," says Dr. Daniel Amen, a renowned psychiatrist and author of several bestsellers, including *Change Your Brain, Change Your Life*. "These behaviors include preventing head injuries, cardiovascular disease, high blood pressure and diabetes, and other factors."

Even people who inherit the genetic mutation that drastically increases the likelihood of developing Alzheimer's disease can forestall it by following these recommendations, says Amen.

Amen bases his findings on more than 120,000 brain scans, from which he can deduce changes that signal brain damage. Working with such scans over three decades has led him to conclude the following: "You are not stuck with the brain you have. You can make it better."

Here are Amen's top seven ways to prevent Alzheimer's disease:

STAY LEAN. Don't become overweight because excess fat isn't innocuous. It produces inflammatory cytokines that damage every organ in your body, including your brain. Two-thirds of Americans are overweight or obese, according to the CDC. This is the biggest brain drain in our country.

ELIMINATE SUGAR. When it comes to the brain, sugar is public enemy number one. Sugar is inflammatory, increases erratic brain cell firings, and is addictive. Avoid it at all costs.

EXERCISE DAILY. Exercise is the best way to increase all your feel-good neurotransmitters, and research also finds that it increases the brain's gray matter as well. No prescription drug has ever been able to grow your brain like exercise does. The secret to increasing exercise is to do what you love, whether it's running, swimming, biking, sports, or even table tennis, which increases hand-eye coordination.

GET PLENTY OF SLEEP. Your brain is the most oxygen-hungry organ in your body. When you stop breathing, it suffocates and kills brain cells. Sleep apnea triples the risk of dementia. So if you snore loudly, get evaluated for sleep apnea and treated.

ELIMINATE OR MINIMIZE ALCOHOL USE. Alcohol kills brain cells. If you do drink, limit your consumption to two or three drinks per week.

TAKE A MULTIVITAMIN DAILY. If we all ate fresh foods every day, we would get all the nutrients we need, but most of us don't. That's why the CDC finds that Americans are dangerously low in many nutrients, including vitamins D and E and magnesium. A multivitamin can fill in those gaps. It's also a good idea to take 1,000–2,000 mg of brain-boosting fish oil daily.

EAT MORE HEALTHY FATS. Of all the solid weight of your brain, 60 percent is fat, and eating fat is essential to brain health—especially foods high in omega-3 fatty acids (salmon, walnuts, avocados, olive oil, and dark chocolate). Eating such foods before taking your vitamins helps your body absorb them better.

Is Alzheimer's Tied to Infections?

Alzheimer's disease is not contagious, but provocative new research suggests that it might result—at least in part—from the brain's natural reaction to infectious pathogens.

Growing evidence shows that infections trigger the buildup of sticky amyloid and tau proteins in the brain that act as a natural defense mechanism to fight off infections. But those webs and tangles can grow out of control, hanging around and breaking down communication between brain cells, leading to memory loss and eventually death.

Chief culprits include the herpes simplex virus (which causes cold sores), chlamydia, and other bacteria, more than one hundred studies have suggested.

While it's scary to think that infections are linked to Alzheimer's, there is also some good news here: new lines of research are examining the effects of treatments that target infections, as well as the benefits of immune-boosting foods, such as good bacteria (in yogurt and other fermented foods), in combatting the brain disorder.

In a recent issue of the *Journal of Alzheimer's Disease*, thirty-one dementia experts call for a significant change in the focus of dementia research—away from the historic emphasis on developing new drugs to treat it and toward investigating the role of microbes.

They argue that it's been a neglected area of research, sidelined by the primary focus on drug development. They noted that pharmaceutical research has been disappointing, with about four hundred unsuccessful clinical trials of experimental drugs and therapies over the past ten years that have proven to be ineffective or unsafe.

As a result, the authors of the new report say enough is enough; it's time to look more closely at microbes.

"We write to express our concern that one particular aspect of the disease has been neglected, even though treatment based on it might slow or arrest Alzheimer's disease progression," the authors declare. "We propose that further research on the role of infectious agents in Alzheimer's disease causation, including prospective trials of antimicrobial therapy, is now justified."

Healing Power of Song: Health Experts Sing Praises of Music's Ability to Combat Alzheimer's

"Where words fail, music speaks."

That famous quote, attributed to Hans Christian Andersen, is gaining a new meaning as a growing body of medical research is finding that music has extraordinary healing powers for dementia sufferers.

A spate of new studies has shown that music can dramatically improve the mood of Alzheimer's patients. Even listening to favorite songs can boost a person's memories and cognitive skills in ways that scientists are just beginning to understand.

"There is relatively strong evidence, with respect with music's ability to affect behavior, such as reducing anxiety and agitation," says Sarah Lock, senior vice president of policy, research, and international affairs at AARP, which recently spotlighted the latest music-therapy findings in the organization's *AARP Bulletin* newsletter.

Lock explains that the most exciting scientific research shows that dementia sufferers who listen to music score better on tests of thinking, memory, and learning. "A study out of Boston University found people can learn things better if they're listening to . . . their favorite songs," she notes. "So if we could understand more about that and apply to it to people in treatment, it would really help."

Mental health specialists say that such findings provide compelling evidence that music offers new hope in the treatment of Alzheimer's; however, scientists don't know why music therapy appears to help these patients. Music might affect the brain in ways that are beyond the normal channels of intellectual processes that are damaged by dementia. It's also possible that the brain processes music in ways that are closely linked to how memories are formed, stored, and recalled—a connection that might somehow allow certain songs to unlock memories.

These theories might explain why some Alzheimer's patients can remember songs they learned as kids, even though they can't remember the names of their own spouses or children.

Lock, who lost both of her parents to Alzheimer's, has seen the benefits of music therapy firsthand in dementia care facilities she's visited and in her personal life. "We don't know exactly why, but people talk about the ability of music to affect the natural rhythms [of the brain]," she says. "My father, who was not musically inclined, could sing the 'Battle Hymn of the Republic' until the very last."

Among the many research projects involving music therapy and Alzheimer's, a handful of studies stand out:

- The Boston University Alzheimer's Disease Center found that dementia patients have an easier time recalling words sung to them—an approach that might help them learn tasks, such as when to take their meds (with instructions encapsulated in songs).
- George Mason University researchers showed that Alzheimer's patients who sang songs like "Over the Rainbow" scored better on cognitive and memory tests.

- Music therapist Connie Tomaino, who founded the Institute for Music and Neurologic Function, has determined that people with dementia respond to songs that are meaningful to them, triggering and strengthening memory.
- Other research has found that pairing music with everyday activities helps patients recall how to do them, singing songs from a person's youth can spark other memories, and up-tempo tunes stimulate both mental and physical activity.

Some states, including Wisconsin and Utah, are incorporating music therapy into their Alzheimer's care facilities and home health care programs. Documentary filmmaker Michael Rossato-Bennett also chronicled the rise of music therapy in his recent film *Alive Inside*, which profiles Music & Memory—a program that is now used in one thousand nursing homes worldwide.

Lock notes that AARP is developing an app to help caregivers find individualized music for Alzheimer's patients. But even burning a CD or creating an iPod playlist of favorite songs for a friend or relative with dementia can have a positive effect on that person's life.

She also predicts that music therapy will gain in popularity in the decades ahead as the number of Americans with Alzheimer's grows. "There are lots of good reasons for that," Lock says. "It's cheap, it's effective, it involves the caregiver in terms of interaction with the patient, and . . . although there is no cure for people with dementia, music can greatly enhance their quality of life."

Curcumin: Nature's Antidepressant

For Dr. Ajay Goel, a medical investigator with Baylor University Medical Center, a single simple question has driven his clinical research in recent years: Can a natural supplement be just as effective as powerful prescription antidepressants taken by millions of Americans?

The surprising answer is a resounding *Yes*.

Goel and his colleagues at Baylor have found that curcumin—a compound in turmeric, the spice used in popular South Asian curry dishes—is nearly as powerful as Prozac in easing depression symptoms. "It was a surprise to us to see that curcumin actually worked as good as the antidepressant," he says. "So this is amazing news."

To reach their conclusions, Goel and his team enlisted three groups of twenty volunteers: One group took 500 mg of curcumin twice a day; the second was given Prozac; and the third received a combination of the two. After six weeks, the team found that the spice compound was as beneficial as Prozac in treating patients' symptoms—including mood swings, suicidal thoughts, insomnia, agitation, anxiety, weight loss, and other factors.

Goel is now conducting larger studies to confirm his results, reported in the journal *Phytotherapy Research*. "But this initial evidence is very encouraging, considering that curcumin is safe, it is nontoxic, and it has many more beneficial effects . . . besides its ability control depression," he notes.

Although eating foods that contain turmeric, such as Indian curry dishes, can increase your curcumin intake, most Americans don't eat enough of it to make a difference. Goel recommends taking a high-potency supplement known as BCM-95 that is ten times more potent than standard curcumin.

"In order to get the benefits of curcumin, you'll need to eat enough turmeric probably multiple times a day—two to three meals loaded with turmeric," he explains. "[So] for people in the Western world . . . I think it would be best to consume curcumin as a health supplement."

Other Promising Natural Remedies

In addition to curcumin, a number of other nondrug alternatives have been shown to combat depression, anxiety, and other mental health conditions. Among them are the following:

ST. JOHN'S WORT. Extracts of this plant contain high levels of a chemical called hypercium, which has been found to be as beneficial as antidepressants and antianxiety medications. In Germany, it is the most commonly prescribed antidepressant.

OMEGA-3 FATTY ACIDS. Having low levels of omega-3 fats, which are found in fish and fish oil, has been shown to significantly increase one's risk of developing depression and anxiety. Taking supplements that include the active components in fish oil—docosapentaenoic acid (DHA) and eicosapentaenoic acid (EPA)—can reduce depression and anxiety symptoms, numerous studies show.

COCONUT OIL. This natural compound has been shown to reduce brain inflammation and combat depression and anxiety.

PHYTOCHEMICALS. A number of plant phytochemicals have antidepressant and antianxiety properties. These include hesperidin, quercetin, ginkgo biloba, resveratrol, berberine, and luteolin.

METHLYCOBALAMIN AND FOLATE. This natural form of vitamin B12 has been shown to reduce depression by combatting inflammation.

ZINC. Several studies have shown that low zinc levels are associated with depression and that supplementation can improve symptoms.

GINKGO BILOBA. This herb has been used in traditional Chinese medicine for almost five thousand years. Supplements that use the plant's leaves boost mental functioning by increasing blood circulation to the brain. A study from the University of Miami Miller School of Medicine found that ginkgo biloba improved the brain's speed in making connections in healthy older adults by 68 percent. Researchers at the University of California, Los Angeles (UCLA) examined the effects of gingko biloba in patients who complained of mild age-related memory loss and found that it improved verbal recall.

ACETYL-L-CARNITINE (ALC OR ALCAR). Several clinical trials indicate that ALC delays the onset of age-related cognitive decline and can increase cognitive function in the elderly. ALC can cross the blood-brain barrier, where it helps produce brain chemicals, keeps mitochondria (the cell's energy powerhouses) from deteriorating, and helps regenerate neurons.

ALPHA-LIPOIC ACID. Some studies have found that this substance can enhance the body's ability to synthesize glutathione, the main antioxidant found in cells. A study published in the *Journal of Neural Transmission* found that alpha-lipoic acid stabilized cognitive function in a small group of Alzheimer's disease patients.

Anxious? Restore Your Peace of Mind with Nondrug Remedies

Anxiety and insomnia are not only major drains on your quality of life; they can also increase your risk of serious conditions such as heart disease and your risk of premature death.

Unfortunately, the most commonly prescribed antianxiety medications are double-edged swords. "They can quickly change brain chemistry to alleviate the symptoms of anxiety," says Mark Stengler, a California-based naturopathic medical doctor (NMD), "but they often do not address the underlying problem for the anxiety so that the root problem or problems are not addressed."

Such underlying problems can include the following:

- Poor stress management, including use of substances such as nicotine, caffeine, alcohol, and street drugs
- Conditions such as food allergies, thyroid problems, adrenal disorders, low blood sugar, and mitral valve prolapse

- Imbalances of brain neurotransmitters
- Exposure to environmental toxins

Doctors rely on three main classes of antianxiety medications:

1. **Antianxiolytics.** These include benzodiazepines such as Xanax (alpra-zolam), Klonopin (clonazepam), and Ativan (lorazepam).
2. **Antidepressants.** These include several different classes, most often selective serotonin reuptake inhibitors (SSRIs) such as Prozac (fluoxe-tine), Zoloft (sertraline), and Paxil (paroxetine).
3. **Beta-blockers.** These include medications such as Tenormin (atenolol) and Inderal (propranolol).

All three classes of antianxiety drugs are associated with adverse side effects that can affect everything from memory, cognition, and speech to gastrointes-tinal and sexual health. For example, recent research suggests a strong link between benzodiazepine use and mild cognitive impairment (MCI) and Alzhei-mer's disease.

If you take benzodiazepines, it's extremely important to work with your doc-tor to slowly wean yourself off these highly addictive drugs. Abrupt withdrawal can cause serious side effects and, in rare cases, death. But if you want to try natural alternatives, here are eleven dietary supplements that have a proven track record for treating anxiety and/or depression:

1. **Calcium:** 250 mg twice daily
2. **Chamomile:** 250 mg three times daily
3. **5-hydroxytryptophan (5-HTP):** 100 mg three times daily, preferably on an empty stomach
4. **GABA (gamma-aminobutyric acid):** 250–500 mg three times daily, preferably on an empty stomach
5. **Inositol:** 6,000 mg taken two to three times daily in divided doses
6. **L-theanine:** 250 mg twice daily, preferably on an empty stomach
7. **Lavender oil:** 20-mg supplements twice daily or smelling lavender essential oil
8. **Magnesium:** 250 mg twice daily
9. **Passionflower:** 250 mg three times daily
10. **St. John's Wort:** 300 mg three times daily
11. **Valerian:** 300 mg two times daily

Healthy Habits Can Ease Anxiety

Many experts recommend other nondrug interventions such as regular exercise, meditation, prayer, neurofeedback, cognitive behavioral therapy (CBT), and improved diet and sleep hygiene to help control anxiety and insomnia.

Here are some worth trying:

TAKE ADAPTOGENS. Scientific research shows that adaptogenic herbs such as ginseng, rhodiola, ashwagandha, and eleuthera root help regulate levels of the stress-triggered hormone cortisol.

TRY AROMATHERAPY. Some essential oils—lavender, rose, frankincense, ylang ylang, bergamot, and vetiver—are known for their calming capabilities.

HEAT THINGS UP. Saunas, steam rooms, Jacuzzis, lying in the sun, or sitting close to a campfire can also melt your cares away.

SEEK OUT NATURE. A stroll through the local park is a great respite from the helter-skelter of modern life, and research shows that it can lower levels of stress hormones.

GUT IT OUT. Studies show that keeping your gut flora robust with the help of probiotics reduces stress and anxiety levels.

GET MOVING. Exercise is one of the simplest, most convenient, and cheapest ways to bust stress.

BREATHE DEEP. There are many therapeutic breathing techniques, but the key is to focus on each breath, which will naturally take your mind off of things that are causing you anxiety.

DON'T OVERREACT. How often do we worry about things that never come to pass? One study puts the figure at 85 percent. And when the participants' fears did come true, a vast majority of them found that the "catastrophe" wasn't as bad as they had imagined.

TAKE YOUR VITAMINS. Many Americans are deficient in vitamins D and B12, which can lead to all sorts of cognitive trouble. Both have profound effects on brain function and mood, and deficiencies have been found to exacerbate symptoms of depression and anxiety and even contribute to memory loss and cognitive decline.

GET IN TUNE. Music can soothe the wild beast—and boost brainpower. Called the "Mozart Effect," listening to classical tunes appears to improve cognitive function. "Musical activity involves nearly every region of the brain that we know about, and nearly every neural subsystem," notes psychologist Daniel J. Levitin in his book *This Is Your Brain on Music*.

LEARN SOMETHING NEW. Seniors who learn new things, such as how to quilt or play a musical instrument, can improve their cognitive abilities, concludes a University of Texas at Dallas study. "It is important to get out and do something that is unfamiliar and mentally challenging," notes lead researcher Denise Park.

DITCH THE REMOTE. Staring at the boob tube for hours can literally be mind-numbing. A long-term study found that sedentary young adults who watched four or more hours of TV a day were twice as likely to suffer from cognitive decline in middle age.

BREAK THE ROUTINE. Run your normal jogging route backward, take a different way home from work, and try new restaurants in your area. Your brain gets lazy when you go to the same places and do the same things all the time.

MAKE NEW FRIENDS. Social connections are good for brain connections. People with rich social networks are mentally sharper and less likely to suffer from dementia.

CHILL OUT. Stress is bad news for your gray matter because it releases the hormone cortisol, which causes brain atrophy. Try practicing stress management daily with things like deep breathing, meditation, yoga, or journaling.

SLEEP WELL. Neurologist Dr. Romie Mushtag says that sleep is the key to mental health: "Sleep is sacred. When we deprive ourselves of sleep, we deprive our minds and bodies of critical rest and healing time. The end result of sleep deprivation is poor focus, declining memory and cognition, depression, imbalanced hormones, and weight gain."

Psychiatry: Book Uncovers Psychiatry's Dirty Little Secrets

Is psychiatry more guesswork than medical science? That's the provocative question posed by psychotherapist Gary Greenberg.

Greenberg, author of *The Book of Woe: The DSM and the Unmaking of Psychiatry*, argues that many basic tenets of psychiatry are based on soft science and the

Diagnostic and Statistical Manual of Mental Disorders (DSM)—the reference book psychiatrists use to guide diagnoses and treatments—is largely a work of fiction.

He also contends that the many psychological disorders the DSM describes have no definitive biological markers, are often diagnosed by hunch, and might not even be real.

What's more, psychiatrists have a financial incentive to use the DSM's diagnostic labels because insurance companies require them to do so before paying for treatment.

The net result is that many people diagnosed with depression, anxiety, bipolar disorder, and other "official" mental health conditions might come to view their problems as biological problems—like heart disease or cancer—and falsely believe the only solution is a drug.

That kind of thinking, Greenberg argues, prevents them from taking active steps to heal, recover, and manage their problems in healthy ways. "By telling somebody they're suffering from a disease, it changes the way people understand themselves and their problems," Greenberg says, arguing that psychiatrists need to stop treating everyday problems like "pathological diseases" with biological roots requiring medical treatment.

"Let's say I'm depressed and I go to my doctor, and my doctor says I have a biochemical imbalance and puts me on Prozac. . . . Instead of thinking about [how to cope with] the problems I have, I think I have a chemical imbalance. In many cases, that explanation guides the way the patient thinks about [his or her] own condition and suffering."

The problem, he says, is that there is little scientific evidence that brain chemistry is at the root of many mental disorders. Drugs don't cure such conditions; they only treat symptoms. He argues that psychiatrists should do more to help troubled individuals see their problems as issues they can address or manage by changing their behaviors and their thinking to cope.

"We have this idea that our lives are our lives to live, that basically we understand our lives are something we are supposed to fashion and make something of," he explains. "And our society depends on the idea that we take responsibility for our lives. And while there are many problems with that idea, there are even more problems when you put it outside of your [power]—when you say: 'There's nothing I can do about my depression but take the pills my doctor gives me.'"

DSM: Science or Science Fiction?

Greenberg's book is the result of two years of research and interviews with many insiders in the psychiatric establishment on the DSM. First published in 1952 and frequently revised, the DSM reflects the official take of modern-day psychiatry on mental illness. But over the years, the book has taken many controversial and even embarrassing positions that were later reversed or overturned.

Homosexuality, for instance, was deemed a mental illness until 1973, and controversies over the book's waffling positions on autism have dogged its authors right through the latest fifth edition. Greenberg and other critics say that the book pushes doctors to diagnose ever more illnesses based on fuzzy definitions of symptoms and prescribe a growing list of powerful, sometimes risky drugs. As a result, sadness over a job loss or divorce can qualify as clinical depression.

Greenberg is not arguing that psychotherapy does not help people. But he contends that the most effective therapy helps patients take control of their lives and focuses on solution-oriented ways to deal with their struggles instead of diagnosing possible biochemical causes, which are often unknown and unknowable.

"Psychotherapy works by the placebo effect, but that doesn't mean it's a scam," he says. "It's based on the relationship between therapist and patient. But a DSM diagnosis doesn't have much to do with that.

"The problem is that we expect a diagnosis of a medical condition to be something that is scientifically ascertained through scientific findings, but that isn't always the case with mental illnesses. . . . Psychiatry doesn't have any biomarkers for mental illnesses, so the DSM's attempts to put mental health into medical language fails. I don't think it's doable."

Greenberg knocks the American Psychiatric Association (APA) and drug companies for turning psychiatry into a money-making enterprise that treats individuals' daily life struggles as illnesses that require medication.

"It has a lot to do with economics and the way health care is funded. We need we have to have a [DSM] diagnosis to attach a payment to service," he says. "So in that respect, economic incentive is behind all of these efforts. The incentive has to do with money and power. If you want to get money to research some kind of mental disorder [from] the National Institutes of Health, you have to tie your research to a specific diagnosis. The rest of the research that is done is done by the pharmaceutical companies, and it's far easier to get your drug approved if you have a specific condition it treats."

Not surprisingly, the *Book of Woe*—like Greenberg's 2010 book, *Manufacturing Depression*—has sparked intense debate in the mental health community. Critics, including some within the APA (which declined a request for comment on the book), have suggested that Greenberg's ideas are irresponsible and could lead some seriously ill patients to stop taking antidepressants and other medications.

Greenberg's response? "I'm not advocating that people on meds stop taking them," he says. "And by the way, some patients' lives have been saved and vastly improved by virtue of treatment of psychiatrists. But psychiatrists do not treat mental disorders; they treat symptoms. It's not only that there's no cure, but the reason for the underlying mechanisms for these disorders is not well understood."

He adds that he is concerned that the debate over his book might lead some suicidal patients to stop taking their medications. "I'm more than vaguely concerned about the precious life of any person," he says. "But I believe the truth is the most important thing. And I'm sure whatever damage my book might do is doing less damage than psychiatric drugs are doing."

5

FOOD AS MEDICINE

Latest Clinical Nutrition Research Confirms You Can Eat Your Way to Good Health

A host of new nutritional research has shown that many superfoods—rich in nutrients, healing compounds, and cancer-fighting ingredients—are as good as (or better than) medication in treating a host of ailments. Compounds in herbs like rosemary have been proven to combat Alzheimer's. Polyphenols in berries, grapes, and red wine have been linked to heart and brain health. Fiber in whole-grain foods can cut heart-damaging cholesterol. Omega-3 fatty acids in oily fish combat diabetes and arthritis pain. Lycopene in tomatoes fights prostate cancer. The Mediterranean diet cuts breast cancer risk. But even the healthiest diet today can't guarantee enough essential nutrients because our soils are depleted, much of the food we eat is processed, and fruits and vegetables are picked before ripening and fully developing all their beneficial nutrients.

Eating Your Way to Top Mental and Physical Health

"Let food be thy medicine and medicine be thy food."

That advice—from Hippocrates, the father of modern medicine—dates to 400 BC. But its wisdom still resonates today. In fact, eating the right foods and avoiding the wrong ones can boost your immune system to fight infections, including cold and flu viruses, and stave off cancer, heart disease, diabetes, Alzheimer's disease, and other chronic conditions.

While conventional doctors have not made diet a primary focus of health and wellness, alternative medicine practitioners have long preached the gospel of food as medicine. Increasingly, hard-line nutritional science is confirming the benefits of eating your way to top mental and physical health. And a growing body of evidence suggests that healthy foods might be as good as—or better than—medications for a range of health conditions.

"What you put in your mouth can have an enormous influence on the digestive tract and the balance of healthy gut flora, which has been scientifically proven to affect all kinds of conditions, from mental health to immune response," says Sophie Manolas, clinical nutritionist and author of *The Essential Edible Pharmacy*. She explains that good nutrition is the "cornerstone of good health," adding, "When you are ill, using medicinal foods [that] have been proven to be effective for millennia should always be the starting point to recovery."

Here's what you need to know.

The End of Dieting?

Dozens of diets have come and gone in the past few decades, and some still linger with question marks from nutritional experts. From Atkins to Zone to South Beach, we've been deluged with eating plans that promise the panacea for our weight loss and health issues.

But research shows that while many of these diets do work in the short term, few are sustainable, let along enjoyable, for life. That's why many nutrition experts believe the concept "of going on a diet" should be abandoned in favor of developing a healthy eating plan that can be maintained over a lifetime.

As just one example, the editors of the famous *Eat This, Not That* books recently teamed up with experts at AARP to bring us a new approach to eating that isn't a diet but a simple strategy that allows you to eat all your favorite foods with a few tweaks.

"Simple switches can have a dramatic impact on one's health," says Dr. Craig Title, a noted weight-loss expert from New York City. "Small changes—such as a 10 percent decrease in your body weight—decrease your risk of heart disease, diabetes, and arthritis, to name a few."

By eating healthier versions of your favorite foods, you can address major health concerns without feeling deprived. Here are a few pointers to get you started.

Combatting Heart Disease

LEAN PROTEIN. Cutting back on fatty red meat in favor of leaner chicken or fish boosts "good" high-density lipoprotein (HDL) cholesterol, which is linked to heart health. People who eat the leanest protein, like fish or chicken, are 20 percent less likely to suffer cardiovascular problems compared to those who eat poorer sources of protein, according to numerous studies. By comparison, the US Statin Diabetes Safety Task Force estimates that cholesterol-lowering statin drugs lower the relative risk of heart attack, stroke, and death by 25 to 30 percent. Plant proteins—in nuts, beans, tofu, quinoa, and certain other grains—are also healthy choices.

TOMATOES. New research shows that tomatoes are good for the heart. The study, published in the journal *Food & Nutrition Research*, found that taking the carotenoid-rich tomato extract supplement known as CardioMato reduced "bad" low-density lipoprotein (LDL) cholesterol associated with heart disease in as little as two weeks. The study, funded by supplement maker Lycored, was carried out by scientists at Naturalpha Clinical Nutrition Center at Hôpital Saint-Vincent-de-Paul and adds to a growing body of research that has found that lycopene—a compound in tomatoes—plays a role in cardiovascular health. The compound has also been linked to a reduced risk of prostate cancer.

FATTY FISH. Studies have shown that eating fatty cold-water fish such as salmon, mackerel, sardines, and tuna—high in omega-3 fatty acids—might decrease triglycerides, lower blood pressure, reduce blood clotting, and boost immunity. Eating one to two servings of fish weekly also appears to reduce the risk of heart disease, particularly sudden cardiac death, which might be related to high levels of stress.

LEAFY GREENS AND CRUCIFEROUS VEGGIES. Both are incredibly high in anti-inflammatory phytonutrients such as vitamins A, C, and E; beta-carotene; lutein; zeaxanthin; and folate. Some, such as collards and kale, are particularly rich in calcium and potassium, both of which are important for blood pressure management and overall heart health.

Controlling Blood Pressure

Cutting down on salt is always a good idea to control blood pressure. According to the latest US Dietary Guidelines, the recommend daily amount is 2,300 mg, or about half a teaspoon. While that seems like a lot if you use the salt shaker, you'd be surprised how many foods contain hidden sources of salt. Check food labels for sodium levels and plan your daily diet accordingly.

The following represents another way to cut down on salt:

EAT WALNUTS, NOT ROASTED, SALTED NUT MIX. A diet rich in walnuts and walnut oil might help your body respond better to stress and can also keep diastolic blood pressure levels down, according to a Pennsylvania study. But while all nuts are naturally healthy, roasting them with salt can ramp up the sodium and calorie count.

Boosting Your Mental Health

Comfort foods that ease the soul are notoriously bad for your body. Mac and cheese, mashed potatoes and gravy, french fries—all can be overly processed or made with oils derived from corn or soy, which are high in omega-6 fatty acids. These fats are linked to depression and inflammation, according to a study published in the journal *Psychosomatic Medicine.*

Instead of choosing such foods, you're better off going with meal items that contain vitamins and nutrients that can change your brain chemistry and boost your mood and overall mental health.

Some examples include the following:

SPINACH. This superfood is an excellent source of folate, a B vitamin that supports the production of serotonin and dopamine, two feel-good brain neurochemicals. It's also rich in magnesium, a mineral linked to lowering depression.

GRASS-FED BEEF. Unlike conventionally raised beef, cows fed a diet of grass produce beef that is rich in conjugated linoleic acid and omega-3 fatty acids—two fats associated with better mood.

PARSNIPS. These heart-healthy vegetables are loaded with complex carbohydrates and minerals that aid in serotonin production, which boosts mood and eases stress.

FRUIT, ESPECIALLY BERRIES. Packed with brain-boosting compounds, blueberries are rated as one of the top foods in antioxidant value. Some studies show that blueberry consumption might help heal oxidative damage in the brain, reducing memory loss and potentially slowing down other types of cognitive decline. All berries—including raspberries, blackberries, cranberries, and strawberries—are high in the phytonutrients that provide protection from inflammation caused by rampant stress.

NUTS AND SEEDS. Both are rich in healthy fats, high in fiber, and easy to incorporate into your diet. Brazil nuts especially contain selenium, which helps reduce oxidative stress that the hormone cortisol creates in the body. It also protects your cells and calms your nerves, say experts, but don't overdo it. One or two Brazil nuts are sufficient. Don't forget about healthy nut butters such as almond butter as a great replacement for peanut butter, which might be higher in toxins and proinflammatory omega-6.

BEANS AND LENTILS. The soluble fiber found in beans and lentils can ameliorate stressful situations such as high blood sugar and unhealthy levels of bad cholesterol and triglycerides. They are also low-glycemic foods, which means that they take longer to break down into usable energy, preventing the blood sugar spikes and crashes that can trigger inflammation and stress.

EGGS. Long considered a nutritional no-no, eggs have become a favorite brain-booster due to their high levels of choline, an essential nutrient that plays a critical role in the normal development of the brain, especially its memory center, the hippocampus. Eggs are rich in protein and B vitamins, and some studies show that they might boost the production of healthy forms of cholesterol. Opt for eggs that are derived from grass-fed, free-range hens—preferably with a diet rich in omega-3—for added benefit.

OLIVE, AVOCADO, AND COCONUT OILS. Olive oil is a staple of the Mediterranean diet. Rich in monounsaturated fat and polyphenols, extra virgin olive oil is an excellent anti-inflammatory dressing for cold dishes. Avocado also reduces inflammation caused by stress. Although coconut oil is high in saturated fat, which increases inflammation when consumed from animal products, it has been shown to decrease inflammatory markers.

FERMENTED FOODS. Linda Illingworth, a dietitian from San Diego, says that these foods are good sources of probiotic bacteria, which are largely responsible for making serotonin, the "feel-good" hormone in our bodies. Yogurt, kefir, kombucha, and sauerkraut are examples of easy-to-find fermented foods.

TEA. This favorite beverage of the Brits has a "secret weapon"—L-theanine, which research shows creates more alpha brain waves. This helps the brain focus while still getting a lift from the lighter caffeine load. Before going to bed, choose herbal teas like chamomile or valerian to provide soothing sleep, which is a profound defense against stress.

Countering Cancer with Diet

Clinical nutritionists note that many foods contain compounds that have anticancer properties. While few mainstream medical experts suggest that they can be used to treat cancer, eating a diet loaded with cancer-fighting nutrients can decrease your odds of developing some types of cancer and boost your natural defenses to fight tumors.

Here are some of the best bets:

CRUCIFEROUS VEGETABLES. Broccoli, cauliflower, arugula, cabbage, and kale contain chemicals called glucosinolates, which create compounds that fight cancer. According to the Linus Pauling Institute, they work by eliminating carcinogens before they can damage DNA. Some also contain specific compounds that have been shown to aid in detoxification and might help eliminate carcinogenic substances from the body.

GRAPES AND RED WINE. Resveratrol, found in grapes and wine, is an extremely powerful antioxidant that inhibits cyclooxygenase-2 (COX-2) production, which is related to cancers and other types of inflammation. COX-2 inhibitors such as resveratrol have been shown to decrease the incidence of cancer and precancerous growths.

SEA VEGETABLES. Nori, arame, kombu, and wakame contain a variety of antioxidant and anti-inflammatory compounds that can prevent and reverse the damage done by foods and other factors that cause inflammation and oxidative stress—two known contributing factors to many types of cancers.

TURMERIC. Curcumin, the ingredient in the Asian spice turmeric, is an extremely powerful antioxidant and anti-inflammatory that reduces the metastases of tumors and might destroy or prevent their growth in the first place. The spice has also been shown to block the formation of new blood vessels in cancer cells—a crucial step in delaying cancer's spread.

GREEN TEA. Green tea contains cancer-destroying plant flavonoids known as catechins. One of these catechins—epigallocatechin gallate (EGCG)—is the most powerful anti-inflammatory and also disrupts the development of cancer cells.

GARLIC. The National Cancer Institute (NCI) says that garlic might reduce the risk of stomach, colon, esophageal, and breast cancer. The Iowa Women's Study revealed that women who consumed the most garlic had a 50 percent lower risk of colon cancer.

GINGER. Certain compounds in ginger make it a powerful anti-inflammatory and antioxidant to reduce oxidative stress. Studies have shown that ginger can reduce cancerous tumors and might be as effective as conventional therapies for certain types of cancers.

TOMATOES. These red fruits and products made from them contain lycopene, a compound known for its ability to destroy cancer cells. Scientific studies show that lycopene helps prevent prostate, lung, and stomach cancers. This powerful antioxidant offers a double whammy, as it also reduces your risk of heart disease by lowering LDL cholesterol and blood pressure.

Fighting a Cold or Flu

ZINC. Ramp up your intake of foods rich in zinc—such as pumpkin seeds, pecans, almonds, beans, and lentils—to increase your intake of this vital nutrient, which research shows can help combat viruses. Zinc has been shown to reduce the duration of a cold or viral infection. Honey (a natural antimicrobial agent), coconut oil (an antiviral), and essential oils like thyme (which promote healing) can also ease congestion and a stuffy nose.

RED PEPPER. Snacking on red peppers boosts your immune system by giving it a megadose of vitamin C as well as carotenoids, fiber, and vitamin E.

GINGER. If you have an upset stomach, ginger might be your best go-to rescue remedy. This powerful spice has been proven to be effective against morning sickness and motion sickness. It contains a potent compound called gingerol, which quells bloating and indigestion. It also keeps bacterial infections at bay.

GREENS AND FRUITS. These healthy foods help maintain optimal levels of vitamins and minerals as well as micronutrients called phytonutrients that boost your immune system and your overall health. Best bets include broccoli, leafy greens, green tea, apples, and berries, which contain anthocyanins that boost immunity and might stave off infections, studies show.

Easing a Headache

WATER. The simplest and most effective remedy for tension headaches is water. Staying hydrated is an important foundation in preventing headaches too, but even at the first sign of a headache coming on, drink a large glass of water.

MAGNESIUM. Eating magnesium-rich foods like nuts—especially almonds, cashews, and Brazil nuts—can offer relief as well.

TURMERIC. This popular Asian spice has potent anti-inflammatory properties that make it a good bet for easing a headache or other types of pain. It has also proven to be nearly as effective in treating depression as Prozac.

Diabetes: Lowering Blood Sugar

FATTY FISH. Salmon, tuna, halibut, cod, and sardines are cold-water fish that are packed with omega-3 fatty acids that reduce your risk of diabetes by naturally lowering blood sugar. A University of Finland study revealed that men with the highest intake of omega-3s had a 33 percent lower risk for type 2 diabetes.

BERRIES. Cranberries, blueberries, and red grapes are rich sources of anthocyanins, which are associated with a lower risk of developing type 2 diabetes. According to a 2012 *American Journal of Clinical Nutrition* study of more than two hundred thousand people, a higher consumption of berries was linked with a much lower risk of high blood sugar.

REGULAR FARE. Other foods that have a track record for reducing blood sugar include cinnamon, nuts, avocado, garlic, tart cherries, blueberries, and apple cider vinegar.

In addition to these foods, the following natural supplements and plant compounds have shown promise in lowering blood glucose levels:

- **Berberine.** This compound found in goldenseal, Oregon grape, philodendron, and tree turmeric lowers blood sugar by activating a protein that helps regulate metabolism.
- **Gymnema.** This climbing plant grows in India and has been used to treat diabetes for more than two thousand years. It kills a person's ability to taste sweetness but is thought to reduce blood sugar by stimulating the pancreas to produce insulin.
- **Malabar gourd.** An extract from the seeds of this plant in the cucumber family have been shown to revive pancreatic cells and boost their insulin-producing capabilities, lowering the risk of type 2 diabetes.
- **Neem leaf.** Another native of India that's long been used in traditional medicine, neem leaf works by improving insulin sensitivity, allowing the body to better regulate sugar.
- **Fenugreek.** The small brown seeds from this plant, used as a medicine since ancient Egypt, are high in fiber, amino acids, and other compounds that slow digestion and the body's absorption of sugar and promote insulin production.

Medical Foods: They're Not Drugs, but They Can Help Manage Diseases

While it is certainly true that good food is good medicine, some foods take that concept to an extreme—and that's a very good thing.

These foods are called "medical foods," which aren't regular healthy foods, ordinary supplements, or drugs. Medical foods are specially formulated products composed of combinations of vitamins, minerals, fatty acids, specialized proteins, soy derivatives, and/or botanicals.

They are specifically designed to treat various nutrient deficiencies that are associated with particular diseases and can affect the progression of those conditions.

Although they've been around since the 1960s, they are becoming increasingly available—for Alzheimer's disease, osteoporosis, osteoarthritis, chronic pain, attention deficit hyperactivity disorder (ADHD), and other conditions.

"Medical foods live in between supplements, which are meant for healthy people, and prescription medications, which are used to *treat* a disease," explains Dr. James E. Galvin, a professor and associate dean for clinical research at the Charles E. Schmidt College of Medicine at Florida Atlantic University in Boca Raton. "A medical food is designed to treat some form of deficit that's associated with a disease—to provide replacement of some kind."

Food Components as Medicine

Unlike naturally occurring foods, medical foods are specifically formulated and processed products that are taken orally by patients who have unique nutrient needs that result from a specific disease or condition such as asthma, digestive disorders, or chronic pain.

As with dietary supplements, medical foods haven't been evaluated for safety or efficacy, and they are not required to gain approval by the Food and Drug Administration (FDA) before entering the market.

But that doesn't mean they don't have to pass muster with federal regulators, experts note. "The ingredients of a medical food must have GRAS—generally recognized as safe—status as designated by the FDA or independent review," explains Dr. Kantha Shelke, PhD, a food scientist in Chicago and a member of the Institute of Food Technologists.

While they can be purchased at a store or online, sometimes without a prescription, medical foods are intended to be used under a physician's supervision because they either have drug-like capabilities or are used as an adjunct to conventional medications.

What Medical Foods Actually Do

Many nutrient-rich foods offer health-promoting properties. For example, calcium helps increase bone mineral density. Folic acid can help prevent certain birth defects during pregnancy. And antioxidants, polyphenols, and other natural disease-fighting components in many foods—berries, tomatoes, fish, olive oil, wine, herbs, and spices—have been shown to help combat diabetes, cardiovascular disease, certain forms of cancer, and other physical and psychological conditions.

But medical foods are a different category entirely. They are designed to provide specific physiological benefits that can't be obtained from naturally occurring foods. "They're all involved in metabolic processes, so they're affecting hormones, enzymes, or levels of inflammatory proteins," explains Mary Franz, MS, RD, a research nutritionist at the Harvard School of Public Health.

An abundance of recent medical research has confirmed the health benefits of medical foods. For example,

- **Cholesterol.** A 2011 study at the University of Connecticut found that medical foods had a significant positive impact on cholesterol.

   Researchers found that women with metabolic syndrome (a cluster of conditions that increases the risk of heart disease, stroke, and type 2 diabetes) who followed a Mediterranean-style diet *and* took a medical food (containing phytosterols, soy protein, and extracts from hops and acacia) experienced greater reductions in harmful cholesterol and homocysteine levels than those who simply followed the healthy diet. Benefits were evident after just twelve weeks.

- **Omega-3 fatty acid levels.** A 2014 study at the University of Toronto found that taking a medical food can correct low blood levels of long-chain omega-3 fatty acids and lower the risk for cardiovascular disease.

   Researchers found that when people who were deficient in docosapentaenoic acid (DHA) and eicosapentaenoic acid (EPA) took oral capsules with these omega-3 fatty acids daily, their blood levels of these heart-healthy compounds increased significantly, and their lipid levels (including their triglycerides) improved considerably after eight weeks.

- **Memory.** A 2010 study from the Netherlands found that medical foods might boost memory in people with dementia.

   Researchers found that people with mild Alzheimer's disease who drank a nutritional beverage called Souverain (which contains uridine monophosphate, choline, omega-3 fatty acids, phospholipids, vitamins C and E, selenium, and several B vitamins) experienced significant improvements in memory (particularly their delayed verbal recall). The study participants consumed the beverage daily for twelve weeks and were compared with a similar group of Alzheimer's sufferers who consumed a placebo beverage.

- **Asthma.** A 2008 study from the University of Moncton in Canada suggests that medical foods might help fight asthma and other allergic conditions, perhaps by having a positive impact on the immune system.

Researchers found that when adults with mild to moderate asthma took a medical food containing EPA and gamma linolenic acid (GLA)—omega-3 and omega-6 and fatty acids, respectively—daily, they experienced an improvement in their quality of life and a decrease in their use of rescue medication after four weeks.

- **Pain.** A 2014 study in the *American Journal of Therapeutics* found that a medical food might improve chronic back pain and reduce inflammation.

Researchers found that when adults between the ages of eighteen and seventy-five with chronic back pain took Theramine, a blend of amino acids that are precursors to neurotransmitters (brain chemicals), they experienced a 42 percent improvement in their disability level and a 50 percent improvement in their pain level. Interestingly, those who took Theramine *and* ibuprofen saw their disability and pain levels improve even more, while those who just took ibuprofen experienced a slight worsening of their disability and pain scores.

So while medical foods don't treat the underlying pathology of a medical condition, they often can improve symptoms and functionality.

The Great Medical Food–Condition Matchup

Here's a look at some of the primary medical foods available in the United States that improve the symptoms of various medical conditions:

Osteoporosis. Fosteum Plus; Osteoben (both are oral capsules).

Cardiovascular disease. Vascazen (oral capsules for those with omega-3 deficiency); Lovaza (oral capsules for high triglycerides).

Osteoarthritis. Limbrel (oral capsules).

Alzheimer's. Axona (a vanilla flavored powder that's mixed with liquid); CerefolinNAC (oral caplets).

GI disorders. EnteraGam; UltraGI Replenish (both are powders that are mixed into liquids or soft foods).

Pain. Metanx; Theramine (both are oral capsules).

Metabolic syndrome. UltraMeal® Plus 360° (a chocolate-flavored powder that's mixed into a liquid).

The Depleted Diet: Are You Suffering from a Nutrient Deficiency?

Even the healthiest diet can't guarantee enough essential nutrients because soils are depleted, much of our food is processed, and fruits and vegetables are picked before ripening and fully developing all their beneficial nutrients.

And as we get older, the problem intensifies. "It becomes more difficult to absorb and assimilate many of the vitamins and minerals that are absolutely critical for our health and well-being," says Dr. Tieraona Low Dog, an internationally recognized expert in the field of integrative medicine and author of *Fortify Your Life: Your Guide to Vitamins, Minerals, and More.*

Lack of vital nutrients contributes to heart disease, diabetes, poor memory, creaky joints, fatigue, and other symptoms we sometimes think are simply a part of growing older. "Supplements can make sure that any of those symptoms that you're feeling are not due to some deficiency in a vitamin," she explains.

As a rule, she recommends taking a good-quality multivitamin—without iron for men and postmenopausal women. For anyone over age fifty, the following sections discuss the most important shortfalls to avoid.

Deficiency: Vitamin B12

PREVALENCE. Up to 30 percent of Americans over age fifty don't get enough of this vitamin.

CAUSE. Decreased production of stomach acid reduces B12 absorption.

WHAT IT DOES. Vitamin B12 is essential for physical and mental energy, and a shortage can lead to memory loss, dementia, and Alzheimer's and Parkinson's diseases. Symptoms can include tiredness, shortness of breath, heart palpitations, weakness, depression, and paranoia. Because a deficiency can damage nerves—irreversibly, if not caught early enough—tingling in the hands and feet is another possible sign.

"It's really impossible to get it without supplementation after fifty," says Low Dog. Even eating B12-rich foods such as beef, seafood, poultry, eggs, and dairy products isn't likely to deliver enough for optimum health because low levels of stomach acid impair its absorption.

Metformin, commonly prescribed for diabetes, increases the risk of deficiency. An analysis of twenty-nine studies, with more than eight thousand patients, found that the risk of B12 deficiency was 245 percent higher among people taking the drug. Low B12 is also a side effect of proton pump inhibitors (PPIs) for heartburn.

REMEDIES. Get 25–50 mcg daily in a supplement of the methylcobalamin form, the most absorbable type. Some multivitamins contain this amount. For anyone with signs of dementia, the American Academy of Neurology recommends a blood test to check for B12 deficiency, and depending on results, higher doses might be needed.

Deficiency: Vitamin D

PREVALENCE. About ninety million Americans suffer from this deficiency.

CAUSE. Too little sun exposure or an inability to synthesize the vitamin from sunlight leads to low vitamin D.

WHAT IT DOES. Vitamin D affects more than one thousand genes and more than thirty tissues in the body. It's necessary for healthy bones, for resisting viral and bacterial infections, for healthy breathing, for protecting against diabetes, for maintaining normal heart function and healthy blood pressure levels, and for muscle strength, which helps prevent falls and fractures.

Our bodies synthesize vitamin D when we're exposed to the sun, without sunscreen, during warm months. But as we age, our skin becomes thinner and less able to synthesize the vitamin, so food and supplements become vital sources.

Although it's considered a silent deficiency, meaning it has no obvious symptoms, Low Dog has seen tangible signs of low vitamin D.

"Many older people who are deficient have a harder time getting up out of a seat, their muscles feel weaker in their thighs, their lower back hurts, [and] they have hip pain," she says. "So be careful not to write all that off as arthritis or just getting old—make sure that your vitamin D levels are checked."

Small amounts of vitamin D are added to milk and some cereals and juices. Other food sources include herring, wild salmon, and sardines but are not likely to provide sufficient amounts.

REMEDIES. Take 1,000–2,000 IU daily of vitamin D3 (the absorbable form), an amount found in some multivitamins. But ideally, get vitamin D levels checked with a blood test and supplement as needed to get to 40 ng/ml or 100 nmol/l—these are two different measurement systems used by doctors. Many people need higher doses to reach an optimum level initially and then a lower maintenance dose. Sun exposure doesn't require getting a burn; for very light-skinned people, as little as ten minutes a few times a week is usually sufficient, while people with darker skin usually require more.

Deficiency: Magnesium

PREVALENCE. This deficiency occurs in at least one in two Americans.

CAUSES. Poor absorption, too much calcium and salt, and heartburn drugs lead to low magnesium.

WHAT IT DOES. Low levels of magnesium are linked to high blood pressure, diabetes, heart attacks and other heart problems, migraines, muscle cramps, depression, anxiety, asthma, osteoporosis, and colon cancer. Among its key functions, says Low Dog, "magnesium is necessary for keeping our heart rate normal and for keeping our blood pressure normal." And it helps reduce chronic inflammation and the risk for diabetes. Taken at bedtime, magnesium improves sleep and helps prevent leg cramps.

The odds of a deficiency increase with age for several reasons: (1) the digestive system becomes less efficient at absorbing the mineral and some foods can interfere, (2) high levels of calcium in fortified foods and supplements, sodium, and fiber reduce absorption, and (3) lack of protein—less than 30 grams daily, equivalent to 3 ounces of red meat or 1 cup of cooked beans—also reduce absorption of magnesium.

Signs of deficiency can include cramps, irregular heartbeat, muscle spasms, anxiety, fatigue, tingling in the arms and legs, and even seizures. Popular heartburn drugs, known as PPIs, increase the risk of deficiency by 75 percent, and the FDA advises that magnesium blood levels should be checked in people taking these drugs.

REMEDIES. Take 300–400 mg daily in a supplement or more if needed as per blood tests of your personal levels. This amount will not be in a multivitamin. Magnesium supplements come in capsules, tablets, and powders that can be mixed with water or juice. People with poor kidney function should talk to their doctor before taking more than about 200 mg daily.

Deficiency: Omega-3 Fatty Acids

PREVALENCE. Most Americans do not get enough of these fatty acids, causing ninety-six thousand deaths annually.

CAUSE. Not eating the right kind of fish leads to this particular deficiency.

WHAT IT DOES. The omega-3 fats in fish protect the human body against the most prevalent chronic diseases and premature aging by reducing harmful chronic inflammation. Low-grade, silent inflammation fuels heart disease, diabetes, arthritis pain, neurological problems, and even skin conditions. Stress, obesity, lack of physical activity, and poor sleep all add to inflammation and disease.

"If people don't eat fish regularly—which many older people don't for cost, taste, or other reasons—they should take a fish oil supplement," says Low Dog. But there's a catch: the most common fast-food and casual-restaurant fish is cod, which has very low levels of omega-3s and is usually deep fried, making it more of a liability than a healthy food.

To be beneficial, fish should be high in omega-3s and low in mercury. The top fish that fit the bill are wild salmon, herring, and sardines and should be grilled or broiled without batter, a lot of added fat, or sauces. At least two servings per week, the size of the palm of your hand, would be a beneficial amount.

REMEDIES. Take a daily fish oil supplement with 200–300 mg of DHA and 500–600 mg of EPA. These two key components of fish oil are the active ingredients and are listed in the supplement facts section of the label. Some fish oils are more concentrated, so fewer pills deliver a higher quantity of DHA and EPA. Liquid fish oils are another option; good-quality products are usually flavored and will not have a fishy smell or taste.

Cereal Pitfalls to Avoid

Fortified cereals are a common source of extra nutrients, but they have downsides. Although B vitamins, vitamin C, and calcium in these can be helpful, iron is another commonly added nutrient.

Men and postmenopausal women should not consume extra iron in supplements or fortified foods, as these can cause an overload. Most supermarket cereals also contain chemical preservatives and pesticides and come from genetically modified grains.

Whole-grain organic cereals are a healthier option, as they don't contain chemical additives or genetically modified organisms (GMOs). However, they might not be fortified with vitamins or minerals, or if they are, they might contain added iron.

Green Tea: Nature's Health

For the past ten years, hundreds of studies have been published touting the health benefits of tea, especially green tea. The health-boosting elements in green tea are powerful antioxidants—specifically, a compound known as EGCG—and studies have shown its health advantages benefit the body from head to toe, including a 90 percent reduced risk of prostate cancer.

Adding green tea to your diet has shown benefits in the following areas:

BONES. Tea might be the key to strong bones, says Australian research published in the *American Journal of Clinical Nutrition.* A ten-year study of elderly women whose average age was eighty found that those who drank at least 3 cups of tea a day lowered their risk of fractures by almost a third when compared to those who rarely or never drank tea. Researchers believe that flavonoids in black and green tea speed the building of new bone while slowing the breakdown of existing bone.

EYES. Researchers from the University of Scranton found that tea, both black and green, reduced glucose levels in the eye lens of rats and cut their risk of cataracts in half. In addition, Chinese researchers found that catechins, powerful antioxidants found in green tea, protect eyes from glaucoma. The study, which was published in the American Chemical Society's *Journal of Agricultural and Food Chemistry,* found that the effects of a single cup of green tea last for up to twenty hours.

ALZHEIMER'S. In Alzheimer's patients, amyloid protein in the brain forms into clumps and fastens onto nerves in brain cells, causing them to die. EGCG, which is found in green tea, is a potent antioxidant, as is resveratrol, another antioxidant that is found in wine.

Scientists at Britain's University of Leeds found that treating the proteins with extracts of green tea and resveratrol disrupted the ability of amyloid to clump. "While these early stage results should not be a signal for people to stock up on green tea and red wine, they could provide an important new lead in the search for new and effective treatments," said lead researcher Nigel Hooper.

CANCER. Men who took three 200-mg capsules of green tea daily for a year slashed their risk of developing prostate cancer by 90 percent when compared to men taking a placebo, according to an Italian study conducted at the University of Parma. Researchers at Louisiana State University found that when men scheduled for radical surgery took four capsules containing Polyphenol E, an active ingredient in tea that was the equivalent to 12 cups of green tea—their prostate-specific antigen (PSA) levels dropped as much as 30 percent.

A Taiwanese study found that drinking green tea daily reduced the risk of developing lung cancer by 66 percent, while smokers who didn't drink green tea increased their risk thirteen-fold. Other studies link green tea to a lower risk of numerous other cancers, including breast, stomach, skin, oral, esophageal, uterine, pancreatic, and colorectal, as well as leukemia.

STROKE RISK. Drinking at least 4 cups of black tea a day can cut the risk of having a stroke by 21 percent, say scientists at Sweden's Karolinska Institute. The records of almost seventy-five thousand men and women were studied for ten years, and during that time, four thousand suffered a stroke. Those who drank 4 or more cups a day were a fifth less likely to be stricken, but drinking fewer cups didn't provide any protective effects.

Researchers at Japan's Okayama University discovered that when compared to people who drank less than 1 cup of green tea each day, those who drank 7 cups or more lowered their risk of dying from cardiovascular disease by an average of 76 percent. Men lowered their risk by 70 percent, and women lowered their risk by a whopping 82 percent.

ALLERGIES. A Japanese study published in the *Journal of Agricultural and Food Chemistry* found that the antioxidant EGCG in green tea blocks the production of histamine and also cuts the production of immunoglobulin E, both of which trigger allergy symptoms. "If you have allergies, you should consider drinking it," said study leader Hirofumi Tachibana, an associate professor of chemistry at Kyushu University.

DIABETES. Green tea helps regulate blood sugar, the function impaired by diabetes. A Dutch study found that drinking 3 cups of green tea daily helped keep glucose levels in check, reducing the risk of developing type 2 diabetes by 40 percent.

The authors of a study published in the *Journal of Agricultural and Food Chemistry* wrote that "tea may be a simple, inexpensive means of preventing or retarding human diabetes." Some experts recommend 2–3 cups of green tea each day. Skip the milk, though. Another study found that adding milk decreases tea's ability to stimulate the production of insulin.

DOWN SYNDROME. EGCG significantly improved the cognitive function of people with Down syndrome, according to Spanish researchers. A supplement containing 45 percent EGCG steadily improved brain functions, such as verbal recall and the ability to remember patterns, throughout the yearlong testing period, and progress remained six months after the study ended. The researchers noted that this was the first time any treatment had been found to be effective in treating Down syndrome.

How to Use MyPlate

The MyPlate Daily Checklist Calculator, one of the online tools on the US Department of Agriculture (USDA) website (http://www.choosemyplate.gov), enables you to anonymously input a few facts about yourself (height, weight, age, gender, level of physical activity) and get a daily eating checklist.

It isn't a menu but gives amounts of different types of foods to eat per day based on your daily calorie requirement. Some of the information might be difficult to translate into real life, but here are some ways to make it practical:

Daily limit for added sugars. The amount is expressed in grams, so you have to check amounts in foods and beverages you might consume. As an example, for someone who needs 1,600 daily calories, the added sugar limit is 40 grams; for some perspective, one 12-ounce can of Pepsi contains 41 grams. Since sugar is added to many foods, it's quite likely that drinking one can of soda will exceed the limit for most people.

Hidden sugar. When sugar is found naturally in a food, such as plain milk, and is also added—in flavored milk, for example—the two types of sugar are not listed separately on a food label (although they will be in 2018). You could compare plain milk to flavored milk and calculate the difference, but in some cases, it's impossible to determine.

Daily saturated fat limit. Again, the amount is expressed in grams. Packaged foods will list amounts, but for freshly prepared foods, there isn't any handy reference from MyPlate. You can search at http://www.nutrition.gov/whats-food.

The Case for Organic Food

There's no doubt that organic food is more expensive than its conventional counterpart—by an average of 47 percent, according to *Consumer Reports*. But is it more nutritious or safer to eat, and thus worth the added cost?

Marion Nestle, a professor in the department of nutrition, food studies, and public health at New York University, is one of many experts who believe that the answer is an unqualified *yes*. The reason being, organic food is certified to be produced without the use of synthetic pesticides, chemical fertilizers, growth hormones, antibiotics, or genetic engineering.

"Organics are about production values, less use of chemicals, [and] better treatment of soil," says Nestle, author of *What to Eat*. "I think those values are important."

Not all experts agree. In 2012, Stanford University researchers performed a meta-analysis of more than 200 previous studies and concluded that organic food was no more nutritious or healthy than conventional products.

But two years later, researchers who scrutinized 343 studies found that organic produce is indeed higher in healthy antioxidants while also containing fewer pesticides and cadmium, a heavy metal and known carcinogen.

"This shows clearly that organically grown fruits, vegetables, and grains deliver tangible nutrition and food safety benefits," declares study coauthor Charles Benbrook, a research professor at Washington State University's Center for Sustaining Agriculture and Natural Resources.

While the debate about nutrition rages on, most experts agree that the chemicals, antibiotics, and hormones used to produce conventional foods pose potential health threats.

Here's a guide to help you decide when to splash the extra cash to go organic:

PRODUCE. As a rule of thumb, says New York–based dietician and author Tanya Zuckerbrot, "if you're going to eat the skin, consider organics. But if you can peel the fruit or vegetable, you're going to strip away a lot of the residues anyway—so it's not really worth the extra money." Typically, apples, peaches, berries, grapes, celery, and lettuce are among the produce most contaminated with pesticides. On the other end of the scale, you're probably all right buying conventional onions, bananas, avocados, pineapples, cabbage, and broccoli. For a more comprehensive list, check out the Environmental Working Group's "Guide to Pesticides in Produce" (https://www.ewg.org/foodnews/list.php).

MEAT. Studies show that organic, grass-fed beef has a better ratio of healthy omega-3 fatty acids to the artery-clogging omega-6 type than conventional animals, which are typically fattened up on grain in feedlots. Grass-fed beef is also lower in calories and contains more vitamins A and E, higher levels of antioxidants, and up to seven times more beta-carotene. Meanwhile, conventional beef is more likely to carry antibiotic-resistant "superbugs," and the growth hormones often used to speed up their fattening for the slaughter have been linked to endocrine disruption in the humans who consume them.

CHICKEN. Nutritionally, there doesn't appear to be much difference between organic and conventional chicken. The main difference is that buying organic ensures that you are not eating chickens that were given growth hormones and antibiotics.

DAIRY. Organic milk from grass-fed cows offers many of the same benefits as grass-fed beef, but the omega-3 advantage is mostly neutralized if you drink low- or non-fat milk. The same holds true for cheese and butter. Organic eggs come from hens that were fed certified-organic feed free from the arsenic, antibiotics, pesticides, animal by-products, and GMOs that conventional-egg hens might eat. There is also a reduced risk of salmonella contamination.

"Whether organics are worth the price difference depends on whether you think it's important to have food raised with fewer pesticides and no antibiotics," says Nestle. "I do."

6

THE EXERCISE CURE

Working Out Beats Drugs for a Host of Ailments, Including Arthritis, Heart Disease, and Diabetes

Groundbreaking scientific research has proven what fitness experts have argued for decades: regular exercise can combat a host of mental and physical ailments at least as effectively as conventional medication. The so-called exercise cure has been shown to fight everything from diabetes to high blood pressure, high cholesterol, heart disease, Alzheimer's, and depression. Maybe Jack LaLanne, who lived to celebrate his ninety-sixth birthday, was on to something all those years ago.

Exercise Cuts Risk of Five Leading Causes of Death

If you could take a pill that dramatically cuts your risk of dying from five leading causes of death—without causing any negative side effects—would you do so?

If your answer is *yes*, a groundbreaking 2016 study by French researchers offers both good and bad news.

First, the bad news: no such pill exists today.

Now for the good news: getting just ten to fifteen minutes of exercise each day can greatly reduce your risk of developing one of the five leading causes of death—namely, breast cancer, colon cancer, diabetes, heart disease, and stroke.

The research, published in the *British Medical Journal* (*BMJ*), is the first meta-analysis to quantify the dose-response association between physical activity and the risk of these five diseases. The results suggest that total physical activity needs to be several times higher than the current minimum recommended by the World Health Organization (WHO).

But people who engage in regular activity—being more physically active at work or at home (through housework and gardening) and/or engaging in active exercise (such as walking and cycling)—are far less likely to die from these conditions.

The WHO, citing many studies showing the health benefits of exercise, recommends a minimum total physical activity level of 600 metabolic equivalent (MET) minutes a week—a measure of the intensity of exercise. (METs measure the amount of oxygen you consume and the number of calories you burn at rest.)

For the new study, a team of researchers based in the United States and Australia analyzed 174 studies published between 1980 and 2016 examining the associations between total physical activity and at least one of five chronic diseases—breast cancer, colon cancer, diabetes, ischemic heart disease, and ischemic stroke.

They found that a higher level of physical activity was associated with a lower risk of all five conditions. Most health gains were seen at activity levels of 3,000–4,000 MET minutes a week.

The researchers said individuals can achieve 3,000 MET minutes a week by incorporating different types of physical activity into their daily routine. Among them,

- climbing stairs for ten minutes
- vacuuming for fifteen minutes
- gardening for twenty minutes
- running for twenty minutes
- walking or cycling for twenty-five minutes

"With population aging, and an increasing number of cardiovascular and diabetes deaths since 1990, greater attention and investments in interventions to promote physical activity in the general public is required," the researchers say. "More studies using the detailed quantification of total physical activity will help to find a more precise estimate for different levels of physical activity."

Working Out Beats Drugs for Many Conditions

As the French study suggests, exercise beats medication when it comes to combatting many common illnesses.

Of course, working out is not a cure-all, notes Dr. Kevin D. Plancher, an orthopedic surgeon and sports medicine expert based in Greenwich, Connecticut, and New York City. But there is virtually no downside to building moderate physical activity into your daily routine, even if you take medication for a chronic disease. In fact, exercise can boost the effectiveness of many medications.

"Movement of the human body is good," notes Plancher. "The combination of necessary medications with some exercise is important." Exercise helps improve some of the following conditions:

HEART DISEASE, HIGH BLOOD PRESSURE. Heart disease is perhaps the best example of a health condition that can be dramatically improved with exercise. Working out not only builds heart muscle and blood vessel strength but also lowers hypertension. In fact, some people have been able to get off hypertension drugs with consistent exercise.

HIGH CHOLESTEROL. Statins are the go-to therapy for lowering "bad" low-density lipoprotein (LDL) cholesterol, but weight loss (through exercise and dietary modification) also can effectively reduce the risk of future heart problems, a new evidence review reports. Researchers with Brigham and Women's Hospital in Boston reported in the *Journal of the American Medical Association* that nonstatin therapies reduce the risk of heart problems by 25 percent—about the same as the 23 percent reduction seen with statins like atorvastatin (Lipitor) and simvastatin (Zocor).

DIABETES. Exercise can also virtually cure patients with type 2 diabetes if it leads to significant weight loss. For those who are overweight or have extra fat cells, working out can mitigate the disease to the point where medication is no longer needed to manage it. An analysis of 133 exercise studies by Australia's Bond University, published in the *Canadian Medical Association Journal*, found strong evidence that exercise can cut the risk of diabetes as much as medication, but many doctors don't know enough about it to recommend it to patients. The best options include aerobic exercise, progressive resistance training, or a combination of the two.

ARTHRITIS. People with rheumatoid arthritis often avoid exercise because their condition is very painful. But surprisingly, exercise can both ease the discomfort and stiffness that comes with arthritis and reduce the need for pain medication and other drugs. This is because exercise increases the release of endorphins, natural "feel-good" chemicals that ease pain. Studies show that supervised resistance training can ease symptoms of osteoarthritis in the hips and knees, reducing pain and improving function. Osteoarthritis isn't a wear-and-tear disease, and any discomfort or pain during exercise doesn't indicate further damage to joints, experts note.

DIGESTIVE DISORDERS. Perhaps there's a reason that a morning or evening "constitutional"—typically a brisk stroll after breakfast or dinner—has been a cultural experience going back centuries. Regular activity aids in digestion and can even improve such digestive disorders as irritable bowel syndrome (IBS), constipation, or irregularity, studies show. You can do something as simple as taking a walk after dinner to improve your digestion.

LUNG CONDITIONS. Exercise can also help patients with chronic obstructive pulmonary disease (COPD), which affects a patient's lung capacity. COPD is a catchall term describing lung conditions that include emphysema, bronchitis, asthma, and bronchiectasis. Although it can make breathing difficult, light or moderate activity can alleviate symptoms and boost pulmonary function, as long as it doesn't overtax sufferers. You might not be able to sprint or jog with COPD, but swimming, a nongravity sport, would help improve lung function.

CHRONIC BACK OR JOINT PAIN. It might seem counterintuitive to exercise if you're experiencing joint or back pain; however, the latest research suggests it's actually a very good idea. Recent studies have shown that increased activity helps physical functioning in people with back and joint pain, as well as arthritis, ankylosing spondylitis, and low-back pain caused by disc problems, pinched nerves, and other conditions.

For people suffering from low-back pain in particular, supervised exercises have been shown to strengthen trunk muscles and overcome physical impairments that can cause back pain.

CHRONIC FATIGUE SYNDROME (CFS). Exercise programs have been successful in combating CFS, as well as fibromyalgia, by gradually reengaging the person in physical activity, which boosts energy levels.

PARKINSON'S DISEASE, MULTIPLE SCLEROSIS. For people with diseases that cause rigidity, such as Parkinson's disease and multiple sclerosis, exercise can help with mobility, and the benefits of endorphins from exercise might ease symptoms.

How Much Exercise Do You Need?

How much exercise you need depends on your overall health status and your goals. But the consensus opinion of sports scientists is that most Americans generally don't get enough. The standard level recommended by the American College of Sports Medicine (ACSM) and federal health officials to control or prevent disease is

30 minutes of moderate to vigorous activity most days of the week or 150 minutes of exercise each week.

That's enough to raise your heart rate to 80 percent of its capacity. For most people, that means doing some form of aerobic activity that doesn't stress you so much that you can't carry on a conversation while doing it but is vigorous enough that you wouldn't have enough breath to carry a tune.

In addition to cardiovascular activities—such as walking, jogging, dancing, swimming, or playing tennis or other sports—you should also aim to do some type of weight lifting or resistance training three to four times a week to boost muscle and strengthen your bones.

There's even evidence that building muscle can lower your body weight, because muscle burns more calories at rest than fat.

Most people associate the benefits of exercise with improved cardiovascular health and stronger bones and muscles. But exercise benefits just about every system in the body. The immune system of a fit person works better to fight both chronic and acute diseases. And numerous studies show that regular physical activity helps the body work better in general.

Another side benefit of exercise is that people who spend hours working out each week tend to have healthier habits overall. They eat healthier diets, tend to sleep better, and are less likely to engage in unhealthy activities, such as smoking or drinking too much.

"It's all about being more healthy overall," says Joel Anderson, an exercise physiologist with the Western Connecticut Health Network. "People who exercise eat well and tend to be healthier than those who don't."

A Few Caveats for Beginners

If you're just starting a new exercise program and have been inactive for a long time, the American Heart Association (AHA) recommends taking a few precautions.

First, you should talk to your doctor about your plans. Second, don't overdo it at first, which can cause injury or put you at risk. Here are a few more pointers:

- If you have been inactive, start slowly and build up your stamina gradually as you work your way up to a more vigorous workout regimen.
- Find something you enjoy doing, which will increase the odds that you'll stick with it. Swimming, tennis, and dancing are good bets.
- Consider starting with doing little things that the AHA recommends, like housework, mowing your lawn, walking or biking to the store, or standing up while talking on the phone.

- Moderate-intensity exercise might be easier than you think. Walking briskly or bicycling can get your heart rate up to between 110 and 140 beats per minute, which is high enough for most people.
- Never go off medications without consulting your doctor first.

Fit *and* Fat? A Guide to Better Health Tests than BMI

If your weight is above average for your height, it doesn't necessarily mean that you're overweight or unhealthy. In fact, obesity experts now say the once-vaunted body mass index (BMI)—used for decades as a measure of healthy weight—is about as outmoded as the 8-track tape player and VHS recorder.

In what is being regarded as the death knell for the BMI, new research out of the University of California, Santa Barbara (UCSB) suggests that millions of Americans are healthy and fit, despite the fact that they are considered over-weight by BMI guidelines.

In an new analysis published in the *International Journal of Obesity*, UCSB psychologist Jeffrey Hunger and colleagues project that nearly 35 million Americans labeled overweight or obese based on their BMI are actually in very good health—as are 19.8 million others who are considered obese.

"In the overweight BMI category, 47 percent are perfectly healthy," says Hunger, arguing that BMI is a deeply flawed measure of health and should be abandoned. "So to be using BMI as a health proxy—particularly for everyone within that category—is simply incorrect. Our study should be the final nail in the coffin for BMI."

The BMI—calculated by dividing a person's weight in kilograms by the square of the person's height in meters—was developed by Adolphe Quetelet, a Belgian mathematician and scientist born in 1796. Quetelet studied population groups globally, designing BMI to aid his research.

Generally, a BMI of twenty-five and above indicates that a person is over-weight, while thirty and above indicates obesity. Someone who is five feet nine inches tall would hit that obesity threshold at 203 pounds. But health researchers note that the BMI was originally designed to measure and compare societies, not individuals. As a result, many experts now suggest that basing a person's health status on weight and height alone doesn't make much sense.

For one thing, the index doesn't accurately measure body fat content or highlight critical health factors, such as fat distribution and proportion of muscle to fat. Nor does the BMI take into account gender, age, and racial differences in body composition. Where fat occurs on a person's body is every bit as important to health as how much he or she weighs. Abdominal fat is more closely linked to a greater risk for diabetes and heart disease than other types of fat, many studies have found.

The BMI also treats body weight the same, no matter what it's composed of—fat, muscle, bone, or other tissues. But many people who are very muscular can be falsely labeled overweight by the BMI because muscle weighs more than fat. Conversely, individuals who fall within BMI's weight parameters might be skinny but unfit and have high levels of body-fat content, which puts them at risk.

What's more, BMI doesn't take into account other critical health factors, such as cholesterol or blood sugar levels, blood pressure, or heart rate. So what alternatives can be used in place of BMI to more accurately measure health and obesity? Here are a few health markers that experts recommend that provide a broader picture of a person's overall health than BMI:

Body-fat content devices. Instruments such as dual-energy X-ray absorptiometry (DEXA) scanners—widely available at health clubs and clinics—provide a highly accurate measurement of body fat, lean mass distribution, and bone health.

Waist measurements. Simply taking a tape measure to check your waist size can provide a clue as to whether you need to lose weight. Generally, a waist size over thirty-five inches in women and forty inches in men indicates that weight loss is warranted.

Vital signs and health numbers. Blood tests that check for cholesterol levels, blood glucose, and hypertension are more reliable ways to gauge your overall health than the BMI, along with measures of your heart rate and pulse. For some individuals, measurements of hormone levels, heart function, and cardiovascular fitness are also helpful.

"We need to move away from trying to find a single metric on which to penalize or incentivize people and instead focus on finding effective ways to improve behaviors known to have positive outcomes over time," Hunger says.

How Much Exercise Is Needed to Burn the Calories You Consume?

How much time do you need to spend at the gym to work off that burger you had for lunch or last night's pizza dinner? New research suggests that labeling food with the precise amount of exercise needed to burn off dietary calories would boost weight-loss efforts.

The article, published in the *BMJ*, suggests that "activity equivalent" calorie information posted on food products would alert consumers to how much they'd have to exercise to burn them off and would combat the nation's growing obesity epidemic.

"Most people don't have a reference point for calories," explains Dr. Charles Platkin, director of the New York City Food Policy Center and distinguished lecturer at Hunter College, City University of New York.

Platkin, a nationally syndicated health columnist known as the "Diet Detective," says that understanding the "cost" of a food in terms of calories consumed can help people control their diets. His own recent research suggests that people with knowledge of exercise equivalents tend to order and eat foods with fewer calories than those who have no information. There is not a significant amount of data on this topic, but it is possible that if food were labeled consistently, people might make better food choices.

"If you have a food budget of two thousand calories, for instance," he says, "then after you've exceeded the budget, the exercise equivalent comes in."

Platkin's book *The Diet Detective Countdown* offers the exercise equivalent of eight thousand different foods—detailing what it would take to burn off the calories of each item. "You have to decide if something is splurge worthy," he says. "Is a rich piece of pizza worth two hours of walking? You might say yes, but knowing the exercise equivalent creates an ability to negotiate with yourself.

"If you are talking about widgets, with no reference point, it is meaningless. Exercise creates a reference point for those calories. People can look at the calories and compare with the equivalent amount of exercise. This is an element for people to use, to give them guidance."

Examples from Platkin's research give easy-to-remember activity equivalent calorie information for the following foods:

- **Nachos.** If you eat a half order of fast-food nachos (500 calories), you need to play an hour of tennis to burn it off. A lower-calorie alternative: eat an 84-calorie shrimp cocktail and play ten minutes of tennis.
- **Cookies.** Three oatmeal raisin cookies contain 660 calories—the amount you'd burn off in several hours of cart-free golfing. A lower-calorie alternative: eat 94 calories of cantaloupe (about half of a cantaloupe)—the equivalent to seventeen minutes of golfing.
- **Fried chicken.** A fast-food, fried, extracrispy chicken breast (585 calories) would require about one hour of swimming. A lower-calorie alternative: a 4.6-ounce chicken breast dressed with veggies and herbs (160 calories) would require just a twenty-minute swim.

- **Potato chips.** A 6-ounce snack bag of potato chips (900 calories) would require about two and a half hours of stair climbing. A lower-calorie alternative: eat 2 cups of plain popcorn (62 calories)—requiring seven minutes of stair climbing.
- **Muffins.** To burn off the 630 calories in a chocolate chip muffin, you'd need to do three and a half hours of housecleaning. A lower-calorie alternative: eat a 154-calorie cup of low-fat plain yogurt with berries—requiring fifty-one minutes of housecleaning.
- **Pancakes.** A breakfast of flapjacks adds up to a whopping 1,457 calories, requiring seven hours of walking to burn off. A lower-calorie alternative: a 210-calorie bowl of cereal requires one hour of walking.
- **Pizza.** A single slice of pizza (600 calories) would require one hour and twenty minutes of bike riding. A lower-calorie alternative: a bowl of chicken noodle soup (180 calories) could be burned off in a twenty-five-minute bike ride.
- **Ice cream.** A 1,200-calorie ice cream sundae would require six hours of walking. A lower-calorie alternative: a 110-calorie fruit bowl requires a thirty-minute walk.

7

NATURAL REMEDIES

What Works and What Doesn't When It Comes to Alternative Healing Practices

Why do the Amish live longer than the average American, despite eschewing modern medicine? How is it that residents of remote third-world villages in Asia and South America have lower rates of certain diseases than their first-world counterparts? What can ancient Chinese healing practices teach us about how to improve twenty-first-century medicine? These are just a few of the questions modern-day scientists are attempting to answer in exploring the medicinal value of herbal, botanical, and natural compounds that have been used for centuries by traditional healers. What lessons do these cultures and practices have to teach the rest of us?

"Medicine Hunter" Travels the World to Find Natural Cures

Chris Kilham is the Indiana Jones of natural medicine. Instead of hunting for archeological treasures or adventure, Kilham has spent a lifetime traveling the world in search of medicinal plants that can treat everything from depression to heart disease to diabetes.

Kilham, an ethnobotanist and author of more than a dozen books on natural medicine, has identified a number of healing compounds that have long been used in traditional healing practices that modern-day scientists have validated in clinical studies. Garlic, ginseng, turmeric, and other more exotic botanicals all contain substances that offer health benefits.

His take is that Mother Nature's medicine chest holds the key to boosting health and longevity in ways that twenty-first-century scientists are just beginning to understand. "We have gotten our treatments from the earth for all of history—up until about 1940," he explains. "We have thousands of medicinal plants that are lifesavers that are the basis of modern pharmacy that are used widely in hospitals all over the world. [And] I'm totally in favor of keeping that trend going."

Kilham has spent a lifetime working with companies and health groups to develop, popularize, and market plant-based food and medicinal products. He has also written extensively about new treatments, therapies, and health-boosting foods derived from herbs, plants, and trees that he argues are less-risky alternatives to synthetic drugs, most of which carry potentially dangerous side effects.

"Plants are safer medicines," he says. "Every year, about two hundred thousand or more Americans die from the proper use of over-the-counter and prescription drugs. Most years, not one American dies from herbs. They have a longer history of use, and they have as many scientific papers [supporting their effectiveness] published as drugs do.

"We've coevolved with plants, so we metabolize their compounds. We know how to take them into our bodies and utilize them. [Humans] and plants are virtually inseparable on this planet."

Big Pharma Taking Note

Increasingly, even the world's pharmaceutical companies are recognizing the enormous potential of plant-based treatments. For instance, the National Institutes of Health (NIH) reports that about 140 new drugs have been developed from Chinese medicinal plants alone in recent decades—including new treatments for leukemia, hepatitis, dementia, and malaria.

In many cases, plant-based drugs take less time—and cost dramatically less—to develop and bring to market than medicines derived from other sources or synthesized entirely in the lab.

Noted health and wellness expert Dr. Erika Schwartz explains that many drugs are derived from plants, including bioidentical hormones, which (unlike synthetic chemical hormones) are derived from yams and soy.

"All our pharmaceuticals have evolved from plants," she says, adding that drug companies are "still using plants, only they use [them] in the lab ways in which they just change a little bit of a molecule, even though it's from a plant, so they can get a patent on it, and then they can sell it for a few billion dollars for the drug companies. They're not helping you and me; they're helping themselves."

Kilham notes that a handful of key natural remedies are common staples in many kitchens. Among them are the following:

GARLIC. A natural antibiotic, garlic has also been shown to boost cardiovascular health. "Very good for thinning the blood, reducing triglycerides [dangerous blood fats], reducing the risk of atherosclerosis—hardening of the arteries," Kilham notes, adding with a smile, "[It's] excellent for keeping away vampires, of course. There are a lot of studies that show benefits of garlic including reducing high blood pressure."

TURMERIC. Several studies have shown that this common Asian spice can boost brainpower, ease depression, and even improve the memory of people who are in the very early stages of Alzheimer's and at risk for dementia. Antioxidant compounds in the spice—long used in traditional curry dishes—could halt the progression of dementia or reduce its impact, according to the latest research out of the Monash Asia Institute in Taiwan.

GINGER ROOT. Used in traditional medicine for several thousand years, ginger root is effective in treating motion sickness and some viruses and is available in virtually every supermarket. "In human clinical studies, it proves to be every bit as effective for motion sickness as Dramamine but more effective when you're sea sick," Kilham says. "It's good for treating colds. It kills the rhinovirus that causes colds [and treats] nausea [and] indigestion. You can grate it, and you can drink a tea out of it. You can also get ginger chews, which are these kind of pleasant candies that are superinfused with ginger extract."

SANGRE DE GRADO. This exotic elixir, derived from the sap of a tree, is used to treat skin problems in South America. It is harder to find than garlic, ginger root, and turmeric, but it is available in some specialty ethnic and health food stories. "This stuff is the number-one remedy for skin problems in the Amazon," Kilham notes. "This is antibacterial, antiviral, antifungal, anti-inflammatory . . . so it kills the bad stuff in a cut, in a wound. It makes a little latex bandage over it to protect the skin. It's a rapid skin-healing agent . . . [used to treat] a burn, a bite, a sting, a cut, [or] an abrasion."

Schwartz adds that conventional doctors are trained to treat individual health conditions—such as diabetes, heart disease, cancer, and depression—with pills and medicines. But alternative practitioners using natural medicines often take a more holistic approach, boosting general health and wellness while also addressing specific ailments.

"The problem is that . . . conventional doctors [are] trained that you have to give somebody a pill for a particular problem," she says. "The reality is, if you're taking an herb or a supplement, it's going to affect everything . . . and they probably do it a lot gentler, a lot better, and a lot safer."

Health Secrets of the Amish

The Amish defy much of today's conventional wisdom about health. Most doctors would say that their diet is terrible because it is high in fat, salt, sugar, and calories. They eat relatively few vegetables. They spend much of their time working in the cancer-causing sun. And the Amish often don't partake in modern, high-tech medical diagnostics and treatment.

Yet somehow, Amish men live longer than other Americans. Amish men and women have lower rates of heart disease, cancer, and diabetes. As they age, they experience better health than the rest of us, often remaining able to do hard physical labor long into old age.

How do they do it? Researchers have studied the "Amish paradox" and have uncovered at least a partial explanation. Their findings hold lessons that we all can use to improve our health and extend our lives.

"The good health of the Amish is clearly influenced by both lifestyle and genes. Indeed, the two interact in ways that are inseparable," says Dr. Alan Shuldiner, who has led more than a dozen studies of the Amish in Pennsylvania at the University of Maryland School of Medicine. But surprisingly, Amish genes are not wholly positive when it comes to health.

Lifestyle versus Genes

"Some Amish have genes that cause increased cholesterol," Shuldiner says. "And the effect of this gene is large, so that lifestyle cannot easily overcome it."

Others have a gene that increases risk for obesity. But he adds, "It seems that the effect of that gene is weaker and that high levels of physical activity can overcome—at least in part—the Amish genetic propensity for being overweight."

Both high cholesterol and excess weight in the Amish should—but doesn't—increase their odds of developing type 2 diabetes, which would triple the risk for heart disease. Studies have found that while American Amish are just as overweight as the rest of the country, incidence of type 2 diabetes among them is only half the national norm, and rates of heart disease are even lower. "Some Amish have a variation in a gene that actually protects from heart disease," says Shuldiner.

In a study of Pennsylvania Amish, his research team found that one in twenty has a genetic mutation that stops the rise of triglycerides, blood fats that increase risk for diabetes and heart disease when elevated. In comparison, one in one hundred fifty non-Amish Americans has this type of genetic mutation.

In the end, with both positives and negatives, Amish health genetics might be about a wash. This means that lifestyle is likely the reason for their longevity and higher fitness levels.

Physical Activity Is Key

In several studies, researchers have measured physical activity with a pedometer, which tracks movement. The Amish are much more physically active than their non-Amish rural neighbors or average Americans. For example, a study at Ohio State University logged the number of steps taken daily by population groups.

Amish men were found to take an average of 11,447 steps a day, compared to only 7,605 steps for their non-Amish male neighbors. The differences are slightly less dramatic among women: Amish women were found to take 7,750 steps a day compared to 6,547 for non-Amish females.

As a reference point, experts consider less than 5,000 steps per day a sedentary lifestyle. However, many Americans don't take more than 1,000 or 2,000 steps daily. Taking 2,000 steps, on average, equals walking one mile, and 200 steps generally equals one city block.

Because they often don't use modern conveniences, the Amish are forced to be much more physically active than their neighbors.

Diabetes Prevention

Although body weight among Amish adults doesn't typically differ from that of other Americans, Amish children are significantly leaner. A University of Tennessee study of Amish youth, ages six to eighteen, found that only 1.4 percent were obese and 7.2 percent were overweight.

Being lean early in life reduces the chances of type 2 diabetes, even if the individual gains weight down the road. Although Amish children are less likely to participate in the typical competitive sports, physical activity is woven into their lives. For example, they are much more likely than non-Amish to walk to school, do household chores, care for farm animals, and engage in physical play instead of watching TV or using a computer.

Low Cancer Rates

When Ohio State University researchers began studying cancer among the Amish, they expected higher incidence because intermarriage within these close-knit communities is likely to increase cancer-related gene mutations. They found the opposite.

Among Amish adults, the incidence of tobacco-related cancers was only 37 percent of the rate for Ohio adults. The incidence of non-tobacco-related cancers was only 72 percent of other Ohio adults.

Lifestyle, the researchers concluded, was at the root of these positive statistics. Specifically, cancer rates are reduced because the Amish smoke and drink less, are less sexually promiscuous, are exposed to fewer chemicals and processed foods, and lead very physically active lives.

In the case of skin cancer, it seems that the Amish should suffer much higher rates than the rest of us due to their sun exposure from outdoor labor. Instead, their risk is actually lower. Researchers cite their use of traditional wide-brimmed hats and long-sleeved clothing that protects them from UV rays.

Lessons for the Rest of Us

Most of us are not likely to give up electricity, cars, televisions, and computers, but it's quite realistic to build more physical activity into our lives, such as gardening, walking the golf course instead of riding in a cart, or adopting the often recommended strategies of using stairs instead of elevators or parking at the far end of the lot. It all adds up.

The Amish show that you don't need fancy gyms, weight equipment, or personal trainers to get the benefit of exercise; all you need to do is to walk more or do some other kind of physical activity consistently every day. In addition, Ohio State University studies found some other Amish lifestyle traits that can be incorporated, at least to some extent, into anyone's daily routines.

Compared to the American norm, the Amish eat more freshly prepared food, including meat raised in a traditional, rather than a factory-farm, way. Although their food isn't organically certified, it isn't likely to contain the same levels of antibiotics, toxins, and additives as conventional food.

Most of the milk they drink is produced by cows that are not treated with hormones and antibiotics. Much of it is unpasteurized.

Compared to other Americans, the Amish take more vitamins, minerals, and other natural supplements. And they often use herbs to treat maladies instead of modern drugs.

The degree to which a traditional lifestyle is followed varies from one Amish community to another.

Shuldiner considers daily physical activity to be the most important lifestyle trait that improves Amish health.

"While they tend to eat 'natural,' the Amish do still purchase some processed foods from supermarkets and the like, just like us," he says, "and they also do eat fast food, albeit probably less often on average than non-Amish."

ABCs of Antioxidants

Antioxidant has been a buzzword for health. And you've probably seen the latest health headlines on studies linking nutritious foods containing them to health:

- Blueberries might help prevent heart disease.
- Carrots boost eyesight.
- Tomatoes can stave off prostate cancer.

Antioxidants are natural compounds believed to combat what are called "free radicals" in the body, which can cause unhealthy changes in cells and tissues that lead to disease.

"We've known about antioxidants for a very long time but were not always aware of their healthy properties," says Claudia Fajardo-Lira, a professor of food science at California State University, Northridge. "With more recent scientific discoveries, we were able to understand all of the good things they do for us."

But there's been a lot of misinformation spread about these amazing compounds in the past few years, in part because food manufacturers started boasting about the antioxidant content in processed products, ranging from cereals to health bars to fruit juices. Even bottled water got into the act.

"When people began hearing about antioxidants, some food companies thought it would be a good marketing tool to start advertising that their products were very high in them," Fajardo-Lira says. "The truth is, you can get enough antioxidants from eating a balanced diet that includes plenty of fruits and vegetables."

The US Food and Drug Administration (FDA) eventually clamped down on the food manufacturers' claims. Still, there's a lot of confusion about what antioxidants are and how they affect health. So here's a primer on what you need to know about these superhealthy substances.

What Are Antioxidants?

As the name implies, these compounds primarily found in fruits and vegetables fight against oxidation, a chemical process that damages cells. Although our bodies need oxygen to survive, the metabolism of it creates free radicals. These are unstable molecules that steal electrons from other molecules, damaging them in the process.

A healthy body can deal with naturally occurring free radicals, but toxins from the environment and processed foods can create an overload of free radicals, which in turn accelerates the aging process and has been linked to many chronic ailments. Antioxidants stabilize free radicals by giving them the missing electrons.

"The production of free radicals starts a chain reaction that creates more free radicals and more oxidation," says Fajardo-Lira, a member of the Institute of Food Technologists. "So if a person is able to consume a healthy diet including a lot of different foods that contain these antioxidants, they can protect their cells from this damage."

What Are the Different Types of Antioxidants?

There are thousands of antioxidants, but they fall into two major categories: water-soluble and fat-soluble. Both are needed because free radicals attack cell membranes, which are made of fat, as well as the fluid inside the cells, which is water-based.

"Water-based antioxidants are found in many fruits and vegetables—things like broccoli, green beans, [and] pomegranates," says Fajardo-Lira. "The fat-based ones are found in foods higher in fat, such as avocados and nuts, and those with a rich orange color, like sweet potatoes and carrots. You need both types to help protect your body."

Which Foods Are Highest in Antioxidants?

The oxygen radical absorption capacity (ORAC) score developed by the US Department of Agriculture (USDA) rates different foods by their power to neutralize free radicals. Topping the list is dragon's blood, the bright-red sap from a South American tree. Experts say more common antioxidant powerhouses include berries, dark leafy greens, beans, cruciferous veggies, bell peppers, dark chocolate, tomatoes, artichokes, nuts, cherries, plums, melons, and peaches.

"In general, the more intense the color of the food, the higher the amount of antioxidants," notes Fajardo-Lira. "For example, kale, with its dark-green color, has more antioxidants than potatoes. But there are some notable exceptions, such as onions, garlic, and cauliflower. They have antioxidant phytochemicals without the intense pigments."

Which Antioxidants Are Most Beneficial?

Antioxidants include some vitamins (such as vitamins C and E), minerals (such as selenium), and flavonoids found in plants. The best sources of antioxidants are fruits and vegetables but they are also in red wine and tea and available in supplements.

The jury is still out about whether any one antioxidant is better than any other, according to Fajardo-Lira. "The best advice is to eat a variety of foods to get all different types of antioxidants in enough quantities," she suggests.

What about Supplements?

Naturally occurring antioxidants work synergistically with each other, so experts say separating one from the rest, like you might find in a resveratrol supplement, could handicap its effectiveness.

"Supplements are a tricky area," says Fajardo-Lira. "They tend to have only one type, so you have to question if they are useful. Also, some studies show there may be certain health risks from getting too many antioxidants."

Can They Really Prevent Diseases?

Antioxidants might play a role in the management or prevention of some medical conditions, such as heart disease, some cancers, macular degeneration, Alzheimer's disease, and some arthritis-related conditions.

According to the NIH, studies have shown that antioxidants might prevent the types of free radical damage that has been associated with cancer and other health conditions. One of the most encouraging antioxidant studies tracked men participating in the long-running Health Professionals Follow-Up Study and found that those whose diets included lots of tomato products had a reduced risk of developing prostate cancer—the likely reason being high levels of lycopene, a carotenoid from tomatoes. The researchers concluded, "Frequent consumption of tomato products is associated with a lower risk of prostate cancer."

Another major study—the Age-Related Eye Disease Study (AREDS)—found a beneficial effect of antioxidant supplements on vision. This study, led by the National Eye Institute and cosponsored by the NIH, showed that a combination of antioxidants—vitamin C, vitamin E, beta-carotene (in carrots), and zinc—reduced the risk of developing the advanced stage of age-related macular degeneration by 25 percent in people with the disease, a leading cause of blindness. A follow-up study, AREDS2, found that adding lutein and zeaxanthin (two carotenoids) improved the supplement's effectiveness.

A third study—the Linxian General Population Nutrition Intervention Trial—found that Chinese men and women taking selenium daily, along with beta-carotene and alpha-tocopherol, had a lower risk of death from gastric cancer.

Another large trial—the SU.VI.MAX Study—found that French men taking daily multivitamin supplements containing vitamin C, vitamin E, beta-carotene, and the minerals selenium and zinc for more than seven years had lower risk of cancer and death from all causes.

But with all these studies, there is a caveat: antioxidants alone are not a cure-all. "Scientists believe that, by themselves, antioxidants won't prevent any disease," explains Fajardo-Lira. "But if you include them in a healthy lifestyle, they will help your body stay in a balanced state, and that may reduce the risk of cancer as well as memory loss, gut problems, cardiovascular disease, diabetes, arthritis, and other diseases. And maintaining the body's oxidative balance is one way to deal with aging.

"When asked about nutrition, I stress that variety and balance is key. You always want to eat a number of different foods in moderation to stay as healthy as you can."

Inflammation: Hidden Cause of Many Health Disorders

Inflammation is a double-edged sword when it comes to health.

On one side of the blade, inflammation is a beneficial part of the body's immune response to illness and injury—such as when you bang your knee or suffer a bug bite, and the swelling and redness in the area signals that your body is attempting to heal itself or fight infection.

On the other side, inflammation can sometimes lead to more serious problems, particularly when it persists over time. In fact, chronic inflammation is the driving factor in the nation's number-one killer, heart disease.

But this is a good-news, bad-news story. The good news is that a host of supplements, natural products, and healthy habits—including making simple changes in your diet—can help combat the ravages of runaway inflammation.

What Is Inflammation?

The word *inflammation* comes from the Latin word *inflammo*, meaning "I ignite." Doctors in medical school learn that inflammation is beneficial—to a degree. Redness, swelling, pain, and limited range of motion are important defense mechanisms and play a major role in the healing process. But you can get too much of a good thing. When inflammation persists over time, it can wreak havoc on the body and brain.

Research shows that while inflammation can be caused by lifestyle factors—including high-sugar diets, lack of exercise, obesity, and other bad habits—it appears to be more common in some people for reasons that are genetic.

Scientists from Stanford University have linked twenty-five genetic factors to coronary artery disease and found that people with this common heart condition are most likely predisposed to the disease because they have gene variants linked to inflammation.

Two physiological processes play a major role in inflammation: the immune system and the prostaglandin system.

They interact with each other and either enhance inflammation or reduce it, Blaylock says. There is growing evidence that one or both of these systems stops functioning correctly in many people and gets stuck in the inflammation mode. A process meant to speed recovery in fact goes into overdrive, potentially causing far greater problems.

Here are the key players that influence this process:

- toxins
- infections
- injury
- heredity
- diet

Diagnosing the Problem

If you suffer from a chronic disease like cancer, colitis, arthritis, or lupus, chances are you already have a systemic inflammation problem and need to address it as soon as possible. But many of us might be harboring inflammation that hasn't openly manifested itself.

So how do you know if you have it? Common warning signs are hypertension, high blood sugar, allergies, asthma, joint pain, skin problems, or just general lethargy. If you have any of these symptoms, you should see a doctor who will review your health history and test your blood for inflammation's telltale markers, such as C-reactive protein (CRP).

In one study of generally healthy seniors, those with the highest levels of CRP and another inflammation marker called interleukin-6 were 2.6 times more likely to die within the next four years than those with low levels.

Inflammation can spark different health woes depending on what's causing it along with your own body's unique chemistry. The following are some of the most serious problems and what experts say you can do to reduce your risk of suffering from them.

Heart Disease

Cardiac arteries clogged with fat cause heart attacks, right? Well, not exactly, say researchers. In fact, inflammation is now a leading suspect. That's because blood vessels suffer damage through the years from things like hypertension, cigarette smoke, and high blood sugar, and they get scarring that encourages cholesterol to stick to their interior walls. This creates plaque, which is basically a foreign element that attracts an immune response.

Antibodies called macrophages flock to the site to gobble up the plaque, a process that inflames the walls of the vessel, potentially destabilizing the plaque and eventually causing it to rupture. That can trigger a major clot, blocking blood flow and causing a heart attack.

"Our entire understanding of what causes coronary atherosclerosis is changing right before our eyes," says Harvard Medical School professor Dr. Paul Ridker.

That shift in focus has prompted cardiologists to more regularly test patients' C-reactive protein (CRP) levels in determining heart attack risk.

"Once we started looking for [inflammation], we couldn't get over how frequent it was," notes Cleveland Clinic cardiologist Dr. Eric Topol.

One way to fight the kind of systemic inflammation that contributes to heart disease is to take statins. These drugs are designed to lower cholesterol but also have anti-inflammatory effects that researchers believe might be the real reason they reduce heart attack risk. Other anti-inflammatories, including aspirin, ibuprofen, naproxen, and arthritis medications like Celebrex might also work, but they all have potentially serious side effects when used long term.

Instead, you can help yourself by eating a Mediterranean-style diet—heavy on olive oil, nuts, fish, and greens—exercising regularly, reducing stress, minimizing exposure to toxins, and getting between seven and nine hours of sleep every night.

Diabesity

Obesity and type 2 diabetes are so closely related that the term *diabesity* has been coined to represent our nation's epidemic of the two conditions. They are intertwined not only with each other but also with inflammation, which is both a cause and effect of diabesity.

"Two-thirds of Americans are overweight, which is a cause of inflammation," explains Dr. Kenneth Woliner, an integrative physician based in Boca Raton, Florida. "But it's a chicken and egg type of thing. People who are inflamed become overweight, and people who are overweight become inflamed."

Inflammation in the brain and gut can also come into play. It causes a resistance to the appetite-controlling hormone leptin, which makes people eat more, even when they should be feeling full.

"Once obesity and/or insulin resistance have been established, each can further stimulate the production of inflammatory cytokines, forming a vicious cycle of inflammation and diabesity," notes alternative medicine practitioner Chris Kresser. "It follows, then, that the key to preventing and treating diabesity is reducing inflammation."

The way to do that should be obvious—lose weight.

"I tell people to plan ahead, so you know you're going to have sardines and avocado for lunch and do some exercise, hopefully high-intensity interval training, after work," says Woliner. "Taking some supplements, especially folic acid, vitamins B12 and D, omega-3 fatty acids, and magnesium may also help."

Cancer

German pathologist Rudolf Virchow discovered a link between inflammation and cancer way back in 1863, and numerous studies since then have confirmed that people with chronic inflammation are predisposed to cancer.

Once again, it appears to be a case of an overactive immune system backfiring. Immune cells not only destroy foreign invaders but also facilitate the healing process by promoting cell division and the growth of tissue. Once the area is healed, the inflammation subsides.

But chronic inflammation can feed a tumor, helping the aberrant cells reproduce and even establish a network of blood vessels to nourish its growth. It can also facilitate metastasis, the spread of the cancer to other parts of the body.

Furthermore, chronic inflammation in itself can cause the kind of DNA damage that leads to cancer. That's why people with inflammatory bowel diseases such as Crohn's or ulcerative colitis are more prone to colon cancer.

To reduce the risk of inflammation-spawned cancer, experts say to eat a healthy diet of organically grown fruits and veggies, fish rich in healthy omega-3 fats, and whole grains while avoiding sugar-laden food and drinks. Identify and treat any lingering infection and try some anti-inflammatory herbs such as ginger root, milk thistle, boswellia, cat's claw, resveratrol, and turmeric.

Alzheimer's

The same type of inflammation-spawned atherosclerosis that contributes to heart disease has been linked to Alzheimer's.

Dr. Thomas Beach, who runs the Sun Health Research Institute brain bank in Sun City, Arizona, says that Alzheimer's patients are twice as likely to have hardening of the arteries than others. "We don't understand the mechanism by which atherosclerosis influences Alzheimer's disease," he adds. "Inflammation may be behind both."

A study published in the medical journal *Brain* earlier this year suggests that "inflammation could be the cause" of Alzheimer's "rather than the result of it."

Working with both human and mice brains, the researchers discovered that when levels of inflammatory immune cells called microglia were kept in check, brain cells communicated better. Alzheimer's patients lack that kind of communication, which causes their cognitive problems.

This study leads to hope for a drug that can modulate the microglia and thus eliminate a contributor to the mind-wasting disease.

Still, a "cure" for Alzheimer's remains elusive. In the meantime, experts at the Dana Foundation, a philanthropic organization that supports brain research, suggest several natural ways to reduce the kind of inflammation that raises the risk of developing Alzheimer's. Lose weight, eat a healthy diet, get some regular exercise, keep your vitamin D levels up, find ways to ease stress and depression, and avoid head injuries. They also say to avoid cooking foods at high temperatures—such as grilling, broiling, and roasting—because they create compounds that "promote inflammation and Alzheimer's."

Easing Inflammation

Conventional doctors have long used painkillers called nonsteroidal anti-inflammatory drugs (NSAIDs) to ease inflammation—such as ibuprofen, naproxen, and aspirin—as well as steroid hormones. But these drugs carry well-known side effects and are generally not a good long-term solution.

Alternative medicine practitioners have long turned to herbs and natural substances that have anti-inflammatory properties. Among them are the following:

Vitamin C. Adequate dietary intake of this antioxidant vitamin knocks down disease-causing substances in the body known as free radicals, which have inflammatory effects. Studies have found that vitamin C might help protect against coronary heart disease and gout.

Apigenin (chamomile extract). This is a nontoxic natural flavonoid present in many fruits and vegetables and has potent anti-inflammatory properties. Research shows that it might combat atherosclerosis, diabetes, sepsis, various liver diseases, and other metabolic diseases.

Hesperidin. A natural flavonoid, hesperidin might help blood vessels function better, improving overall cardiovascular health and offering protection for the brain and other body organs.

Vinpocetine. This powerful antioxidant might play a key role in neuroprotection and reducing neural inflammation, studies have suggested. It increases blood flow to the brain, dilates the blood vessels, and reduces blood clotting, offering better circulation.

Luteolin. Recent studies show that luteolin reduces age-related inflammation in the brain and can boost memory.

Bromelain. Preliminary clinical trials have found the anti-inflammatory and analgesic properties of bromelain might reduce symptoms of osteo- and rheumatoid arthritis.

Resveratrol. This well-known component of red wine and grapes has been shown to have potent anticancer and anti-inflammatory properties in a host of studies.

Quercetin. Another strong antioxidant and a major dietary flavonoid, quercetin has been proven to protect against cardiovascular disease and might even combat insulin resistance—a hallmark of diabetes.

Green tea. Many studies have found that polyphenols in green tea—particularly epigallocatechin gallate (EGCG)—have strong anticancer properties.

Other substances. A variety of other herbs and natural substances have also been shown to be powerful inflammation fighters, including ginger, turmeric (curcumin), tart cherries, fish oil (omega-3 fatty acids), and even cannabis.

Avoiding Inflammation Promoters

In addition to using nontoxic approaches to treat inflammation, it's equally important to avoid common causes of inflammation in the foods we eat and our environment. This is particularly important as we grow older. Among the most common inflammation promoters are mercury, aluminum, cadmium, lead, pesticides, herbicides, and industrial chemicals.

Nonconventional Cancer Treatments: A Primer

The diagnosis of cancer can strike terror into your heart, sending the stress response into overdrive. And when you're under stress, harmful hormones like cortisol attack the immune system, making the illness and its side effects even worse. This is one area where alternative medicine techniques can help—namely, by lowering stress and boosting the immune system to fight cancer.

"Complementary therapies can support the body's natural healing abilities and help people manage their illness and the side effects of treatment as well as their ability to cope with the emotional devastation of this dreaded disease," says Dr. Delia Chiaramonte, an assistant professor and director of education at the University of Maryland School of Medicine Center for Integrative Medicine.

"When we feel frightened or worried about something, our body activates the 'stress response,' which creates changes in our cardiovascular system—such as elevated pulse and blood pressure, secretion of stress hormones—and impacts other systems as well, such as the gastrointestinal system, the endocrine system, and more," she says. "This can create a feedback loop where anxiety itself creates symptoms such as a racing heart, which then creates even stronger feelings of anxiety. Mind-body techniques create the 'relaxation response,' which is essentially the opposite response, infusing a feeling of well-being and other significant, healthy physiological changes in the body.

"There is good evidence that mind-body techniques such as diaphragmatic breathing, guided imagery, and hypnosis are effective tools in treating anxiety and helping patients cope with cancer."

Here are some examples:

Meditation. This ancient relaxation technique calms the mind and combats worrisome thoughts that can lead to anxiety over a cancer diagnosis, treatment, and costs for care.

Meditation, the state of deep concentration, helps you focus your mind on more positive thoughts. It helps people with cancer by relieving anxiety and stress. You might also incorporate deep, diaphragmatic breathing exercises while meditating to further enhance the benefits.

Acupuncture. Studies have shown that acupuncture helps control nausea caused by chemotherapy. It might also relieve pain in patients, according to the Mayo Clinic. Make sure that the treatment is performed by a licensed practitioner.

Exercise. Research has shown that exercise not only helps prevent cancer but is essential in aiding patients with the disease manage fatigue, insomnia, and stress during treatment.

"It may seem hard to believe that exercise helps fight fatigue when resting seems to be the best thing to do, but exercise is actually better," says Chiaramonte. "The Mayo Clinic cites evidence that exercise may also help people with cancer live longer and improve their overall quality of life." Always check with your doctor before starting any exercise program.

Hypnosis. In a deep state of concentration during hypnotherapy sessions, you can take charge of your physical and emotional reactions to the disease, says

Shirly Gilad, founder of Integrative Hypnotherapy in Boca Raton, Florida. "It can help reduce postsurgery pain," she says. "It can also reduce the fear and anxiety of the disease as well as help the patient cope with the side effects of cancer treatment, finding inner peace within the chaos."

Massage. A carefully planned massage treatment can be helpful in relieving pain, fatigue, and stress, says Chiaramonte. "Many cancer centers have a massage therapist on staff who is knowledgeable and regularly works with people who have cancer," she says.

Relaxation techniques. Visualization exercises, deep breathing, and progressive muscle relaxation are techniques that might be useful in relieving anxiety and stress. They can also help patients sleep better.

Music therapy. As the often repeated quote goes, "Music hath charms to soothe the savage breast." While the author was referring more to healing a broken heart, music can also help calm the ravages of cancer. In a medical musical therapy session, you might listen to music, play instruments, sing songs, or write lyrics.

"It's a wonderfully safe way to alleviate pain and help control nausea and vomiting," says Chiaramonte. Many medical centers have certified music therapists on staff.

Tips for Finding an Alternative Practitioner

Choosing an alternative medicine practitioner—or a conventional doctor, for that matter—can be a challenge. How can you tell if a particular doctor is right for you?

Here are some tips and suggestions:

ASK YOUR DOCTOR. Your primary-care physician might be in the best position to recommend an alternative specialist who is licensed, trained, and knowledgeable. Many conventional doctors are expanding their networks of specialists, including alternative practitioners, nutritionists, and other wellness specialists.

CHECK YOUR LOCAL HOSPITAL. Many hospital networks have complementary or integrative health departments that can make referrals to local practitioners.

CONTACT HEALTH ORGANIZATIONS. Clinical nutritionists, chiropractors, acupuncturists, and other alternative medicine practitioners have professional organizations that can be good sources for finding a specialist. They can also provide important information about training, education, and licensing requirements.

CHECK WITH YOUR INSURER. Insurance companies are increasingly offering some coverage for alternative medicine, including chiropractic, massage therapy, and acupuncture. Your insurer might have also have a list of in-network practitioners.

QUESTIONS TO ASK. Once you've identified a practitioner, it's a good idea to ask some questions about his or her qualifications and treatment approach. Among the questions you should ask are the following:

- What kind of specialized training, education, and license do you have?
- What's your area of specialty?
- Do you work with conventional doctors?
- What research informs your treatment approach? (Is it based on solid clinical science or just a "hunch" or anecdotal evidence—in which case, you should be careful.)
- Do you accept gifts or funding from any organization or company with a financial stake in the medicine you practice?
- How long before I can expect to see the results of your care?

Curcumin: One Remedy for Many Ills

In the past few years, curcumin has skyrocketed in popularity, becoming the top-selling herb in health foods stores and natural supermarkets among certain consumers.

- Athletes use it to reduce inflammation and soreness after hard workouts or competitions.
- People with chronic or recurring pain, such as arthritis, take it to reduce or replace medications.
- Others take it to prevent cancer or relieve many other conditions, from acne to atherosclerosis.

"The reason curcumin is so effective is that it can act on more than one hundred different pathways in the body," says Holly Lucille, a naturopathic doctor and educator based in Los Angeles. "Drugs only work on one."

For example, a widely used class of anti-inflammatory drugs for arthritis pain, cyclooxygenase-2 (COX-2) inhibitors such as Celebrex, inhibit one pathway: the

COX-2 enzyme. Side effects include increased risk for heart attacks, strokes, and death.

By contrast, curcumin multitasks, influencing many enzymes, substances, and mechanisms in the human body.

"Its ability to influence these pathways across the board creates more of a synergistic result," Lucille says.

This synergistic action is believed to be the reason the herb, unlike drugs, can be therapeutic without dangerous side effects.

Reducing Drug Damage

Curcumin is an extract of turmeric, the bright-yellow curry spice in Asian dishes. Technically speaking, it's a group of three substances (curcumin, demethoxy-curcumin, and bisdemethoxycurcumin) collectively called "curcuminoids," which work on multiple levels.

In cancer treatment, studies have found that curcumin improves the effects of chemotherapy and radiation and reduces their side effects. And it helps protect healthy people against cancer.

Among pain relievers, acetaminophen (Tylenol) is popular but toxic. Found in more than six hundred other over-the-counter (OTC) and prescription drugs, acetaminophen is the top cause of acute liver failure in the United States, says Lucille.

Studies show that curcumin protects the liver against acetaminophen damage. The herb also improves the effects of antiviral drugs used to treat hepatitis B. And it fights nonalcoholic fatty liver, the most common liver disease today.

In the case of diabetes, studies reveal several beneficial actions of the herb:

- It lowers blood sugar levels, even with a high-fat diet, and improves the natural function of insulin.
- It blocks deposition of fat in the liver, which contributes to both diabetes and liver disease.
- It reduces levels of chronic inflammation, which underlies diabetes, heart disease, arthritis, and most other ills that are not infectious diseases.

Growing Scientific Support

Although curcumin has been widely used in Eastern medicine for thousands of years, it's only during the last half century that Western scientists have been studying it, but the research is growing fast. So far, more than eight thousand scientific articles have been published about the herb, and many more studies are ongoing.

Lucille points out that with any ailment, there are many factors at play, including our diet, lifestyle, and level of stress. "With curcumin," she says, "you've got the beauty of it being able to target many different things."

Who Can Benefit?

In studies and clinical experience, Lucille has seen curcumin be effective in preventing, treating, or improving a long list of conditions. Some examples include the following:

- acne
- Alzheimer's disease
- asthma
- atherosclerosis
- breast cancer
- chemotherapy (reducing side effects)
- chronic lymphocytic leukemia
- colon cancer
- cystic fibrosis
- depression
- diabetes
- epilepsy
- hepatitis B and C
- HIV and AIDS
- human papillomavirus (HPV)
- inflammatory bowel disease
- liver diseases such as nonalcoholic fatty liver disease
- major depression
- melanoma
- multiple sclerosis
- osteoarthritis
- osteoporosis
- pain
- pancreatic cancer
- Parkinson's disease
- post-traumatic stress disorder
- prostate cancer
- psoriasis

- rheumatoid arthritis
- ulcerative colitis

Doses. In studies, doses have most often varied from 500 to 1,000 mg of curcuminoids daily, but higher doses have also been used.

Side effects. Although not common, nausea and diarrhea have been reported. Reducing the dosage should eliminate these side effects.

Nature's Best Weapon against Cancer?

Curcumin is also proving to be something of a natural powerhouse when it comes to combatting cancer.

A recent study found that it reduces the spread of cancer cells and increases the effectiveness of chemotherapy in advanced colorectal cancer, the third most common cancer diagnosed in both men and women in the United States. It might not only prevent this aggressive cancer but work with chemotherapy to shrink existing tumors, the researchers say.

Dr. Ajay Goel—director of epigenetics, cancer prevention, and genomics at Baylor University Medical Center in Dallas—has spent twenty years researching the prevention of gastrointestinal cancers and has come to the conclusion that curcumin might be as close as we can come to finding a "magic bullet" in the war on cancer.

"Colorectal cancer is especially devastating because of its high recurrence rate," he says. "Cancer stem cells exist in very small numbers in a tumor and can hide from chemotherapy. While they are very small in number, they do survive and cause cancer to reoccur.

"But in our studies, we discovered that curcumin impeded cancer growth and production by signaling proteins and blocking tumor cell promotion. The beauty of curcumin is its ability to balance gene expression and positively influence anticancer pathways."

Goel, author of the recently published book *Curcumin: Nature's Answer to Cancer and Other Chronic Diseases*, says that curcumin has been the subject of more than nine thousand published, peer-reviewed studies. Almost all have touted its ability to treat not only colorectal cancers but breast, cervical, and prostate cancers as well.

"Is there a reason why people in Africa and India do not die from cancer at the alarming rate of North Americans and Europeans?" he asks. "If you check the color of a typical Indian meal, it is yellow. The Chinese and the Indians use spices such as turmeric to enhance not only the flavor of their food but the health benefits as well."

Goel notes that curcumin is a powerful anti-inflammatory and, as a result, holds promise against many chronic diseases that are caused by inflammation. "Curcumin is not only effective in fighting cancer, but I have hundreds of testimonials on it efficacy in helping arthritis and even Alzheimer's patients," he says. "Inflammation and oxidative stress are the root causes of all diseases, and this is one way to prevent getting sick, and in the case of cancer, downgrading its stage if you already have it.

"Curcumin has also been proven to fight depression as efficiently as prescription medication like Prozac in head-to-head studies."

Goel stresses that early detection and screening are also keys strategies to knock out cancer: "The earlier you detect cancer, the better your chances of survival."

He notes that while curcumin and turmeric supplements abound, he only recommends BCM-95 curcumin, which is available in many different brands because of its unique specification. "Curcumin needs to have fat in order to be highly absorbed, and this formula blends curcumin with its own turmeric oils, which makes it a superior product," he says.

For cancer prevention, Goel recommends 300–500 mg of BCM-95 curcumin in whatever brand you prefer and up to 1–2 grams for cancer patients to shrink tumors. "Since there is no toxicity, it is a perfectly safe and effective product to prevent and treat chronic disease including cancer," he says. "So why [would] anyone not want to disease-proof their bodies with this scientifically proven treatment?"

Mind-Body Medicine Eases Modern-Day Mental Ailments

If you suffer from aches, pains, and chronic illnesses—or if you are just getting older and find most exercise programs too strenuous—try Tai Chi.

Tai Chi (pronounced "tie-gee") grew from Chinese martial arts and is a gentle but effective form of exercise that increases the flow of vital energy throughout the body.

"In China, there are more than three hundred different known martial arts styles," says stress management expert Darrin Zeer, an American relaxation professional. "They are characterized as either internal or external martial arts systems. Tai Chi is an internal system."

In the United States, Tai Chi is taught as a series of slow rhythmic stretching movements. "Some experts have called Tai Chi the ultimate low-impact exercise," Zeer explains. "It can be done by almost anyone."

According to Zeer, as Tai Chi entered the modern age, clinical studies began to verify its beneficial effects on health. A recent analysis of thirty-three studies published in the *British Journal of Sports Medicine* found that Tai Chi is especially suitable for people who suffer from chronic medical conditions such as heart failure and chronic obstructive pulmonary disease (COPD) that might prevent them from participating in more strenuous forms of exercise.

Another recent study conducted by the University of South Florida and China's Fudan University demonstrated that practicing Tai Chi just three times a week over a period of eight months increased brain volume and boosted thinking and memory skills of seniors. Those in a placebo group did worse on cognitive tests and showed brain shrinkage consistent with people in their sixties and seventies.

Studies have found that Tai Chi also improves the following:

Heart function. A study published in the *European Journal of Preventive Cardiology* found that the large and small arteries of people in their seventies who regularly practiced Tai Chi were more than 40 percent more flexible than nonpractitioners.

Balance, strength, and flexibility. Stanford University researchers discovered that after twelve weeks of Tai Chi exercise, senior citizens saw significant improvements in balance, strength, and flexibility. The researchers called Tai Chi a "potent intervention" that could reduce disability from chronic health conditions. A Japanese study, also lasting twelve weeks, found a 30 percent increase in lower body strength as well as a 25 percent improvement in arm strength—almost as much as resistance training.

Blood pressure. A twelve-week Taiwanese study of patients with high blood pressure showed moderate drops in blood pressure along with lower levels of "bad" low-density lipoprotein (LDL) cholesterol and higher levels of "good" high-density lipoprotein (HDL) cholesterol. In fact, a review of studies published in *Preventive Cardiology* found that Tai Chi reduced high blood pressure in twenty-two of twenty-six studies.

Immunity. After being vaccinated with the shingles shot, elderly practitioners of Tai Chi had immunity levels against the virus normally seen in people almost half their age. The randomized, controlled trial, which was published in the *Journal of the American Geriatrics Society*, divided volunteers into two groups—one practiced Tai Chi, while the other participated in a health education class before being vaccinated. Those practicing Tai Chi had twice the immune response of the second group.

Depression. Older adults who remained depressed after being treated with the drug Lexapro were enrolled in a study conducted by the University of California. One group practiced Tai Chi, and a second group participated in a health education class that also included ten minutes of stretching exercises. After ten weeks, 94 percent of the Tai Chi group showed significant improvement in measures of depression compared to 77 percent in the education group, a result researchers called "dramatic."

Pain. The *New England Journal of Medicine* reported a study at Boston's Tufts Medical Center that found that Tai Chi reduced pain and fatigue in patients suffering from fibromyalgia, a condition that's notoriously difficult to treat. Another Tufts study, which was published in the journal *Arthritis Care & Research*, found that patients with arthritis of the knee had less pain and were able to move more easily after practicing Tai Chi for twelve weeks.

Want to try Tai Chi? "Classes are available in most communities, but online classes are becoming more popular," says Zeer. "Do a search on YouTube to find a teaching style that is helpful for your body and mobility. Classes tend to last an hour, but when you first start, even a few minutes can provide benefits. Our modern lives are so sedentary that the slow, flowing movements of Tai Chi will provide health benefits including deep relief from tightness and tension."

Medicine Chest Makeover: How to Switch Out
Risky Drugs with Natural Alternatives

Having a fully stocked medicine cabinet to treat infections, aches, pains, and certain chronic conditions might seem like a good idea. But health experts say that the plethora of prescription and OTC drugs not only is costly but can carry the risk of potentially dangerous side effects. In fact, adverse effects from medications are a leading cause of emergency room visits, says Sherry Torkos, an award-winning pharmacist and author of *The Canadian Encyclopedia of Natural Medicine*.

Torkos notes that some products can be hard on the liver or kidneys, while others can cause bleeding in the stomach, racing heart, insomnia, and anxiety. Many OTC drugs are not safe or recommended for young children because the risks can outweigh their potential benefits.

"Don't be lulled into thinking that just because a drug is readily available over-the-counter it should be used in a flippant manner," says Dr. Ellen Kamhi, author of *The Natural Medicine Chest*. "Pharmaceutical drugs can be lifesaving when used appropriately but often carry risks of illnesses far worse that what the drug was taken for in the first place!"

To keep your family safe and healthy, consider some natural remedies in your medicine cabinet makeover, Torkos says. "Many natural alternatives to OTC drugs can safely and effectively manage minor ailments for the whole family."

Aches and Pains

Whether it's arthritis, sports injuries, or backache, pain drives millions of Americans to use OTC drugs such as ibuprofen, aspirin, and acetaminophen for relief. But these drugs can cause serious side effects, such as liver and kidney damage, ringing in the ears, stomach bleeding, and rebound headaches. Natural options for managing joint pain and inflammation include curcumin, omega-3 fatty acids (in fish oil and tablets), and products that contain natural eggshell membrane (NEM). For headaches, try a few drops of lavender on your temples or a supplement that contains butterbur, such as Petadolex by Enzymatic Therapy.

Bruises and Muscle Strains

Keep ice packs in your freezer to provide relief for minor injuries. Apply the ice pack to the affected area—ten minutes on followed by ten minutes off. Ice relieves pain and reduces swelling. Follow with a cream that contains arnica, which can improve healing and reduce bruising.

Cold and Flu

OTC drugs for managing symptoms like congestion and runny nose can cause a range of side effects such as racing heart, insomnia, drowsiness, and upset stomach. Instead of reaching for an OTC medication, try using a vaporizer with eucalyptus oil to improve breathing. To clear congestion and mucus, try Similasan Cold and Mucus Relief; it contains gentle ingredients that relieve symptoms of sneezing, runny nose, and head and chest congestion. It is also free of dye, gluten, and alcohol and is safe for children as young as two years old. Using a neti pot or saline nasal drops or spray can also hydrate the sinus passages and clear mucus. To speed healing—and shorten the duration of a viral infection—try zinc lozenges or Sambucol black elderberry extract.

Cough and Sore Throat

Buckwheat honey can calm a cough and soothe a sore throat, and it also contains antioxidants and nutrients that help speed healing. Buckwheat honey can be given to children ages one year and older. You can also make a soothing tea with warm water, lemon, and honey.

Cuts and Scrapes

Tea tree oil is an effective natural antiseptic with antibacterial and antiviral properties. Try it for minor cuts and skin irritations.

Digestive Distress

Gas, bloating, diarrhea, and constipation are common and distressing problems. Probiotic supplements can aid digestion by improving levels of good bacteria in the gut. Probiotics also improve nutrient absorption and support immune health. Try Kyo-Dophilus probiotics, which are stable at room temperature and available in both capsules and chewable tablets for children. Soluble fiber supplements can compensate for a lack of dietary fiber and help both constipation and diarrhea. Look for Sunfiber, a clear, tasteless fiber that can easily be added to any fluid or recipe.

Dry Eyes

When the furnace is running in winter months, the air inside our homes, workplaces, and schools becomes drier, which can lead to dryness, burning, and irritation of the eyes and increased risks for cold and flu infections. To lubricate the eyes and relieve symptoms of dry eyes, try Similasan Dry Eye Relief. It is free of harsh chemicals and safe to use every day.

Dry Skin and Eczema

Colder outdoor weather combined with dry indoor air can be harsh on the skin. To sooth dry, itchy skin, add 2 cups of ground colloidal oatmeal (not breakfast oatmeal) to a tub of warm water. Avoid hot water because it can further dry and irritate skin. You can make your own colloidal oatmeal by grinding whole oats in a coffee grinder. After bathing, apply a moisturizer with soothing and hydrating ingredients like vitamin E.

Insomnia

Most OTC sleep aids contain antihistamines, which make you drowsy but can also cause dry eyes and mouth and next-day sleepiness. Instead, try a supplement that contains Suntheanine (L-theanine). This amino acid promotes relaxation and improves sleep quality without causing any drowsiness or dry mouth the next day. Melatonin is also helpful for getting to sleep and supporting restful sleep.

Motion Sickness

To prevent and manage motion sickness, try ginger root. Ginger contains potent anti-inflammatory compounds called gingerols. Research has found that it can relieve motion sickness, dizziness, nausea, and gas and soothe the intestinal tract. A few options to consider are Solaray Ginger Trips (a chewable formula that can be taken by children), Traditional Medicinal Ginger Aid tea, and Sea Band ginger gum.

Storing Medicine Safely

The NIH offers the following recommendations for using and storing medicines safely:

- Store all medications in a cool, dry place. Heat, air, light, and moisture can damage your medicine, so choose a location that's not in the bathroom or kitchen—unless it's far away from the stove, sink, or hot appliances. Never store in the refrigerator.
- Always keep medications in their original containers and pull the cotton ball out of the medicine bottle. The ball pulls moisture into the container.
- Check expiration dates and reviews dosages. Read the warning labels, and if you have concerns, check with your health care practitioner or pharmacist.
- Do not flush expired or damaged medicine down the toilet. Instead, mix with a product that ruins it, such as coffee grinds or kitty litter, or return to the pharmacy.
- Always store medicine out of reach and out of sight of children and make sure you use a child latch or lock.

OTC Medications: By the Numbers

- One in thirty Americans who suffer from chronic pain turn to OTC pain relievers.
- There are fifty thousand estimated deaths from heart attacks, strokes, bleeding ulcers, and other conditions tied to ibuprofen-related medicines called NSAIDs.

- Annual hospitalizations linked to acetaminophen products, such as Tylenol, amount to twenty-six thousand. Such pain relievers are also tied to one hundred thousand calls to poison control centers, fifty thousand emergency room visits, and four hundred fifty deaths from liver failure.

Homeopathy 101: What's behind the Hype Surrounding This Natural Medicine Alternative?

You've probably heard of homeopathy and maybe even perused the endless aisles of homeopathic medicines at the health food store or supermarket.

In fact, there's a good chance you've contributed to the estimated $2.9 billion spent on such remedies and $170 million spent on appointments with homeopathic practitioners in this country.

But despite the dollars dished out each year, many Americans don't actually know what homeopathy is, how it works, and what's behind all the hype.

In essence, homeopathy is a natural form of healing that originated in Europe centuries ago and is used to treat adults, children, and yes, even pets.

"Homeopathy is a system of medicine that uses natural substances to stimulate the body's own immune system to heal disease," explains Dr. Susanne Saltzman of Hartsdale Homeopathy in New York, who specializes in homeopathic and functional medicine in adults and children.

Practitioners say that the substances that are used cause mild symptoms of an illness in a healthy person but can actually alleviate that ailment in someone who is already experiencing it.

For example, while cutting up an onion, a person might experience watery, burning eyes and a runny nose. Since these very same symptoms can appear in someone experiencing allergies, an allergy sufferer can be completely cured with a very diluted and specially prepared homeopathic form of the onion called allium cepa. This concept applies to many other homeopathic treatments.

"Like Cures Like"

Dr. Samuel Hahnemann, the doctor who first formulated the basic principles of homeopathy around 1800, called the healing concept behind it "like cures like." In fact, the term *homeopathy* literally means "similar [homeo] suffering [pathos]."

The active ingredients in homeopathic preparations are typically derived from botanical, mineral, or biological substances in highly diluted amounts. Proponents of this complementary and alternative medicine say that it can treat a large array of health issues.

According to the *Journal of the Royal Society of Medicine*, asthma, depression, middle ear infections, hay fever, headaches and migraines, neurotic disorders, allergies, dermatitis, arthritis, and hypertension are the top ailments treated by homeopaths today.

Another unique aspect of this field is that practitioners look at the whole person—their life as well as their ailment—in making a diagnosis and treating whatever set of symptoms they might have. "I can have five people with the same 'disease' and give them five completely different homeopathic remedies," explains Saltzman. "In homeopathy, the mental/emotional symptoms are just as important as the physical symptoms in finding the correct 'constitutional' homeopathic remedy."

This more natural approach to health care is appealing to many of us, but not everyone is sold on the concept. Skeptics of homeopathy have raised several concerns, including questions about the safety and efficacy of treatments.

Traditional medications have to be evaluated for both these things by the FDA. But this isn't the case with homeopathic remedies, even though the FDA classifies them as drugs.

Homeopathic remedies are simply required to list their ingredients, which must be found in a database called the Homeopathic Pharmacopoeia of the United States. The FDA considers this an "official compendium" that details standards for the composition and preparation of homeopathic drugs. They also need to include usage directions and describe the medical condition they claim to treat.

Another concern is that the packaging of OTC homeopathic remedies can appear to be similar to conventional OTC medications. When stores put the two together on their shelves, it might be confusing for consumers.

In addition, potentially dangerous natural ingredients might get mixed in with the beneficial ones, or the dose of some of these natural ingredients could potentially be dangerous. Even though one of the basic principles of homeopathy is that active ingredients are highly diluted, this is not always the case. For example, in 2012, the FDA recalled a product called Hyland's Teething Tablets because they had inconsistent amounts of their active ingredient, belladonna. This was of concern because this is a plant that can be toxic at high doses.

Part of the controversy between traditional medicine and this more alternative form comes down to scientific proof and the fact that conventionally trained doctors tend to take a dim view of alternative medicine approaches. Others note that conventional scientific studies aren't well suited to evaluating the benefits of homeopathic remedies in the same way clinical trials can determine whether a drug is safe and effective.

But many practitioners and patients swear by the homeopathic remedies they take, which might account for growing interest in them. Some have also pointed to substantial evidence that such therapies have been effective in treating animals and children.

Some studies suggest that the placebo effect might be at work in those who reap benefits from this form of health care, while others say that it might indeed treat a handful of ailments like the flu and allergies but not all the others that it claims to.

A review of 176 studies on homeopathy by Australia's National Health and Medical Research Council (NHMRC) in 2015 concluded that "there are no health conditions for which there is reliable evidence that homeopathy is effective."

But the lack of strong scientific evidence of homeopathy's benefits doesn't necessarily mean it doesn't work. Listen to the anecdotal evidence from an array of patients who have found relief, if not a cure, for their symptoms via homeopathy when conventional medicine didn't work and you might be convinced.

"For years, I suffered with painful headaches that traditional over-the-counter medication didn't alleviate," explains Melissa Raab, forty-six, a teacher in Long Island, New York, "but it was a homeopath who cured them. It was truly life changing."

History of Homeopathy

This ancient form of medicine was founded in Europe in 1796 by Dr. Samuel Hahnemann, a German medical doctor and chemist. As the story goes, Dr. Hahnemann was a thirty-year-old doctor who was dissatisfied with the conventional medical practices of the time because he viewed them as too aggressive. (These practices included leeching, bloodletting, and using toxic substances to "purge" sick people.)

His search for a gentler form of healing led him to discover homeopathy, which used extremely small and diluted doses of natural substances to treat various conditions. "Any substance that can produce a totality of symptoms in a healthy human being can cure that totality of symptoms in a sick human being," he said.

Although Dr. Hahnemann's discovery was controversial at the time, the practice of homeopathy gained popularity and spread not only through Europe but to the United States. According to the National Center for Homeopathy, it is a little known fact that "at the turn of the last century . . . the majority of medical schools in the United States at that time were originally homeopathic medical schools."

This didn't last, and conventional medicine took over, making homeopathy a thing of the past. It wasn't until the 1970s, when the trend toward natural health emerged, that this complementary and alternative medicine regained a following.

In 2002, the use of homeopathic remedies was estimated to have increased 500 percent compared to just seven years earlier. Today, it's as popular as ever, with Americans spending an estimated $2.9 billion on homeopathic remedies and $170 million on appointments with homeopathic practitioners annually.

For More Information

Want help from a homeopath? Find one in your area by searching the National Center for Homeopathy database at http://www.homeopathycenter .org/find-homeopath.

8

HIDDEN TOXINS

Common Contaminants That Threaten Your Health

Chemical and biological toxins are a fact of modern living—in the food we eat, the air we breathe, the clothes we wear, the household products we use, and the furnishings and building materials that make up our homes and workplaces. In fact, indoor air contaminants pose a greater threat to our health than outdoor pollutants, according to the US Environmental Protection Agency (EPA) and World Health Organization (WHO). The good news, however, is that you can reduce your risk by making simple lifestyle changes that can rid the body of lead, heavy metals, volatile organic compounds, and other toxins.

Home Toxic Home: Hidden Dangers in Your Home

For many Americans, "home sweet home" is also "home toxic home." Common household products—as well as those in your car, workplace, and other indoor environments—contain or emit harmful compounds that can harm your health immediately or after extended exposure.

Key culprits are volatile organic compounds (VOCs), which can cause a range of health disorders, from nausea to cancer and organ damage.

"They are emitted from a slew of everyday items, so there's a pretty good chance that your home, your new car, and even that shiny new airplane you took your last business trip in are bathing you in a chemical cocktail," says Dr. Ellen Kamhi, an expert in natural health solutions who is based in Oyster Bay, New York.

The EPA says that concentrations of VOCs are consistently up to ten times higher indoors than outdoors. That's one reason the agency ranks indoor air pollution as the top environmental health risk—ahead of outdoor air contaminants, tainted water, and hazardous waste sites that garner billions of dollars in mitigation costs.

But air pollution isn't the only indoor hazard you might face. Here's a primer on hidden indoor toxins that can put your health at risk.

VOCs: Where Do They Come From?

New materials, such as those used in new homes and cars, tend to "off-gas" more VOCs than older materials because the gases decrease over time. "In fact, it is the heavy mixture of VOCs that gives new vehicles the characteristic new-car smell," says Kamhi, adding that the automakers now try to limit the most potent VOC-emitting items, which means recent models might not have that smell consumers love.

This is "good for your health but potentially bad for business," says Kamhi.

Anne Steinemann, a professor of civil engineering and public affairs at the University of Washington, Seattle, tested twenty-five scented air fresheners, laundry detergents, soaps, and other common household items and found that even products labeled "green," "natural," or "organic" sometimes emit as many hazardous chemicals as standard ones.

Some of those chemical are even classified as toxic by federal laws. Unfortunately, the Consumer Product Safety Commission, which regulates cleaning supplies, air fresheners, and laundry products, currently does not require manufacturers to disclose any ingredients on the labels, including fragrances. The same is true for fragrances in personal care items, which are overseen by the US Food and Drug Administration (FDA).

What's more, health officials spend far more time and money regulating outdoor air pollutants than indoor contaminants, even though the EPA's own studies consider indoor toxins to be a far greater public health risk than those outside.

Those risks increase during winter months, when many people shut their houses up tight to keep out cold weather—inadvertently shutting in and increasing concentrations of indoor contaminants. That's one reason cold and flu season occurs during winter months; cold and flu viruses are more easily transmitted indoors, where ventilation is limited.

VOCs Tied to Many Health Problems

The health risks associated with exposure to VOCs—or any other chemical—depend on how much is in the air and how long and how frequently a person breathes it in, notes Dan Tranter, a supervisor with the Indoor Air Unit at the Minnesota Department of Health. "The health risks can vary from person to person, although several studies have shown that people who have asthma or who are chemically sensitive can have more severe reactions," he says.

The short-term health risks tied to high levels of VOCs include eye, nose, and throat irritation; headaches; vomiting; dizziness; and worsening of asthma symptoms. The long-term health risks include cancer, liver and kidney damage, and damage to the central nervous system.

"The first VOC to gain attention historically was formaldehyde, back in the 1960s," Tranter says. "Before that, we used solid wood and plaster for construction. When we moved to particle board and pressed wood, we used more glue and adhesives. Today's building materials contain far less formaldehyde as a result of public awareness, but they still pose health hazards."

Tranter says that the best time to do any household renovation is in early spring or late fall, when you can open the windows and ventilate the home. "I get calls from people who have just laid down carpeting midwinter and complain about the smell; they say they don't feel well. But that's after the fact, and although you can use air cleaners, they don't do a perfect job of eliminating the VOCs."

"It's important that, as a consumer, you ask questions about the levels of VOCs in the products you are using and try to get the answers from a third party, such as the EPA or [the US Centers for Disease Control and Prevention] and not the manufacturer," he adds.

Here are some of the most common sources of VOCs:

- paints
- paint supplies
- wood preservatives
- aerosol sprays
- cleansers and disinfectants
- moth repellents
- air fresheners
- scented candles
- stored fuels and automotive products
- hobby supplies
- dry-cleaned clothes
- cosmetics
- varnishes
- pressed-wood furniture
- vinyl flooring

- carpets
- upholstery fabric
- vehicle exhaust
- tobacco smoke

For more information, visit http://www.epa.gov/iaq/voc.html or http://www.cdc.gov/niosh/toipcs/indoorenv/ChemicalsOdors.html.

Tips to Keep You Safe from Household Chemicals

Source control. Remove or limit the number of products in y our home that give off VOCs. Choose less toxic natural products.

Ventilation. Increase ventilation by opening doors and windows, using ceiling fans, and maximizing fresh air brought in from outside.

Go green to clean. Use only natural cleaning supplies in your home or make your own.

Buy eco-friendly products. Choose new home products that contain low or no VOCs. Check for environmentally friendly products certified by the US General Services administration (http://www.gsa.gov/portal/category/27119).

Change your HVAC filter regularly. Make sure to filter your home's air with a high-quality air filter and change it out regularly.

Don't use chemical dry cleaners. Go with an environmentally friendly dry cleaner that doesn't use perchlorethylene, a chemical that has been shown to cause cancer in animals.

A Word about Radon

Progress made since the 1970s to boost energy efficiency in many US homes has had an unintended negative side effect: sealing up buildings to conserve fuel has also trapped more radon inside, leading to a higher risk of lung cancer.

The EPA estimates that radon—a radioactive gas produced from naturally occurring uranium in soil and water—contributes to about twenty-one thousand lung cancer deaths each year.

It is present in many homes in varying amounts, and energy-efficiency measures—like putting draft strips along doorframes—reduce air ventilation, which causes radon levels to rise indoors. According to the EPA, states in the Midwest and New England have the highest radon levels.

So what can you do to reduce your risks?

- Test your home for radon using an inexpensive do-it-yourself kit (available at most hardware or housewares stores).
- If your home tests high for radon, contact a professional for how address it. Remediation efforts can range from a few hundred to a few thousand dollars.
- Make sure your mechanical ventilation and heating system is working properly to ensure appropriate ventilation.
- Go easy on the weather stripping and other energy-conservation measures in your home that can reduce ventilation and allow radon and other indoor contaminants to build up.
- Open your windows to allow fresh air to circulate.

Six Plants That Naturally Purify the Air in Your Home

Energy-efficient homes could be putting your health at risk. A wide variety of toxic chemicals can build up in tightly sealed indoor environments and affect your health, research shows.

But you can take steps to minimize the chemicals in your home by simply bringing green plants indoors. A NASA study revealed that certain houseplants can bring a breath of fresh air to indoor environments and detoxify our homes without the use of pricey—and noisy—air purifiers.

Dr. Bill Wolverton, scientist and author of *How to Grow Fresh Air*, has confirmed in multiple studies that houseplants can purify and revitalize the air.

"Plants clean the air in our homes, allowing us to breathe easier," says Anita S. Neal, district extension supervisor at the University of Florida and an expert on the power of plants. "They have the ability to take impurities out of the air through respiration. They also pull air down through the soil, where the roots can absorb impurities. We use many chemicals in our homes, from cleaners to products made from harsh ingredients.

"One plant per five hundred square feet will improve the air quality within your home. Almost all plants utilize photosynthesis to produce their food, and a few are really good at cleaning the air. NASA's study helped identify the best choices."

Here are the top six:

Boston fern. These attractive plants remove more formaldehyde than any other plant. They are also highly efficient at removing other indoor air pollutants, such as benzene and xylene—components of gasoline exhaust that can migrate indoors if you have an attached garage. They can be finicky, so make sure you mist or water them daily and feed them seasonally.

Peace lily. The NASA study revealed that these blooming indoor plants are efficient in absorbing benzene, formaldehyde, trichloroethylene, and more. The peace lily thrives in both low and bright light. Keep the soil moist and feed monthly during the spring and summer months with an all-purpose liquid fertilizer. Keep the foliage dust-free for maximum cleaning efficiency.

Dracaena. These diverse houseplants are extremely attractive in the home and help eliminate formaldehyde, xylene, benzene, toluene, and trichloroethylene. Keep the soil damp but not soggy. Feed this plant monthly during spring and summer.

Golden pothos. This virtually indestructible plant is considered to be one of the most effective indoor purifiers of the plant world. You can hang it in a basket or set it beside a tall indoor tree—like the Dracaena corn plant—to cascade over the pot's edge. They help remove formaldehyde, xylene, toluene, benzene, carbon monoxide, and more. These hearty plants grow in any light except direct sunlight. Water when the soil becomes dry to the touch. Trim the long tendrils when the plant becomes too large.

English ivy. This evergreen is a climbing plant that adapts well to indoor conditions. It can be easily grown as a houseplant or in hanging baskets and thrives in low-light conditions. English ivy is recommended for removing allergens such as mold and bacteria. The green-leaved varieties will grow in bright indirect light and low-light situations. The pale, variegated forms need brighter indirect sun to thrive. Water generously during the growing period and keep the soil moist but not waterlogged. Apply a balanced liquid fertilizer monthly.

Areca palm. This is a small cluster-forming palm from Madagascar. It's a graceful addition to any home and, according to the Associated Landscape Contractor of America, one of the most efficient air-purifying plants and an excellent home humidifier. It helps eliminate benzene, carbon monoxide, formaldehyde, xylene, and more. Grow in bright filtered light with shade from the hot sun.

Water frequently during the growth period but reduce watering in winter. Fertilize monthly.

A word of warning for pet owners: some plants are toxic to pets, so be sure to check with your vet about which varieties to avoid before adding greenery to your home.

Chelation Gaining Popularity as a Balm for a Toxic World

Chelation therapy is a controversial treatment that removes toxic metals from the body. Although it is approved by the FDA to treat lead poisoning, it has long been ignored by mainstream medicine as a remedy for other conditions.

Advocates believe it can treat neurological conditions—such as Alzheimer's and autism—and cardiovascular disease by cleansing the body of environmental toxins. But conventional doctors have historically dismissed chelation as quackery or fringe medicine.

But that view is changing, as landmark scientific research has validated its use in treating heart disease and possibly other conditions. An eye-opening study funded by the NIH has found that chelation provides remarkable benefits to people with heart problems.

The new research—led by Dr. Gervasio Lamas, chief cardiologist with the Columbia University Division of Cardiology at Mount Sinai Medical Center in Miami—showed that chelation, when combined with high-dose vitamins, can provide a huge health boost to heart attack survivors that rivals the benefits of standard treatments.

The clinical trial, which was funded by the NIH and published in the *American Heart Journal*, found that the combination treatment cut the death risk for some heart patients by half and is particularly beneficial to those with diabetes. Lamas said that the results came as a complete surprise to the researchers.

"I would say that I was one of the biggest skeptics . . . I thought the issue would be settled with a negative chelation trial—one showing that chelation failed—and that chelation therapy would fade away as a result," the Harvard-trained heart specialist says. "But I didn't find that at all; in fact, we found quite the opposite."

How Does Chelation Work?

Chelation was first used during World War I as an antidote against arsenic-based chemical weapons and to treat sailors suffering from lead poisoning from paints used on navy vessels.

Since then, alternative doctors have used it to treat heart disease, Parkinson's, Alzheimer's, cancer, vision problems, and autism.

More than 110,000 Americans undergo the treatment each year, according to the National Center for Health Statistics. Its popularity has skyrocketed over the last decade, even though it is time-consuming and expensive—$5,000 is the average cost—and not covered by insurance.

"The first publication showing chelation was good for heart disease was back in 1956," says Lamas. But before follow-up studies could be conducted to convince the medical community that chelation worked, drugs and surgical techniques developed to treat coronary disease moved into the mainstream, muscling out other alternatives.

"They turned away with a vengeance, essentially calling anyone who practiced chelation a quack and persecuting them," says Lamas. "That persecution has cost us decades in being able to do a proper scientific investigation.

"In the following decades, a lot of information came out that people who had more lead in their blood were more likely to have a heart attack, hypertension, stroke, and to die, but it was ignored by me and my colleagues. People with more cadmium, arsenic, mercury, and other metals were also found to have more coronary heart disease."

The body does not metabolize heavy metals. They accumulate over time and are associated with numerous health problems, including heart disease, attention deficit hyperactivity disorder (ADHD), Alzheimer's, autism, and gastrointestinal disorders. But chelation can remove those contaminants in the same way that statins scavenge the blood of dangerous cholesterol. Chelation comes from the Greek word *chele* and means "to bind."

In chelation therapy, intravenous infusions of a synthetic solution called ethylenediaminetetraacetic acid (EDTA) are injected into the bloodstream, where it binds to toxic metals and minerals such as lead, arsenic, cadmium, aluminum, copper, and mercury, which are then excreted from the body.

"The chelating solution is a molecule that has a pocket similar to a catcher's mitt with a magnet inside," says Lamas. "Once the metal is trapped inside, the mitt closes over it. Not only is it harmless when covered; it can be excreted from the body in urine."

Skeptic Turned Believer

Lamas began looking into chelation's potential heart benefits in 2002, initially to prove that the technique was a sham: "I became interested in chelation when a patient asked me if he should receive chelation therapy. I said, 'Of course not, that's quackery.' Then decided I should look into it and realized I didn't have any evidence to suggest whether he should or should not undergo chelation therapy."

He launched the first NIH-sponsored chelation study involving more than 1,700 heart attack survivors at 134 research sites across the United States and Canada, including such prestigious facilities as Johns Hopkins and the Mayo Clinic.

Over a seven-year period, the study participants were randomly assigned to receive either forty injections of a chelation solution (known as "infusions") or an inactive placebo. Patients also received either an oral vitamin and mineral regimen or an oral placebo.

Lamas says he expected the study—known as the "Trial to Assess Chelation Therapy" (TACT)—to show that chelation provided no benefits to patients. But in fact, when the trial ended in 2012, the results showed that those who received chelation therapy plus vitamin supplements had a 26 percent lower risk of heart complications (such as a second heart attack, stroke, or bypass surgery) compared to those given placebos.

In diabetic patients, the findings were even more dramatic, with the combination therapy tied to a 49 percent lower risk of heart complications. Chelation (with or without vitamins) was also found to cut the risk of death among diabetics by half over the course of the study.

"There is nothing like this for diabetes care," Lamas said when the study findings were published in the *American Heart Journal* in 2014. "There just isn't."

In follow-up meetings with the FDA, Lamas pressed for a follow-up study of chelation therapy as an approved treatment for heart patients. In 2015, the NIH's National Center for Complementary and Integrative Health (NCCIH) awarded Mount Sinai and Duke $800,000 to allow the research team to design a definitive follow-up study to prove that chelation is not a sham treatment for cardiovascular disease, the nation's number-one killer.

With that earlier grant, Lamas's team met twenty specific milestones for conducting the new study. A year later, the NIH granted Lamas a $37 million grant for the next leg of his research. The study will involve 100 medical facilities and enroll 1,200 patients in the United States and Canada, who will be treated and tracked for five years.

"If this study is positive, as the last one was, we will move to chelation of toxic metals as frontline therapy for heart disease," Lamas says, noting he expects results by 2021.

He explains that the new study—TACT2—will involve 1,200 patients and is being conducted with the Duke Clinical Research Institute and other leading medical institutions around the nation. The new research aims to examine the use of intravenous chelation treatments in combination with oral vitamins in diabetic patients with a prior heart attack. The goal is to determine if chelation can prevent recurrent heart episodes—such as heart attacks, stroke, death, and others—by removing toxins from the blood.

"If TACT2 is positive, it will forever change the way we treat heart attack patients and view toxic metals in the environment," says Lamas. "Therefore, with NIH support and in collaboration with the Duke Clinical Research Institute, Columbia University, New York University, Mount Sinai [Miami], and hundreds of physicians and nurses throughout the United States and Canada, we are moving forward with TACT2."

Lamas hopes that the new research will provide a definitive answer on chelation therapy and lead to "the recognition that environmentally acquired toxic metals are a reversible risk factor for heart disease. This realization will have clinical and public health implications."

Lamas says he hopes his research will convince other cardiologists to embrace chelation but acknowledges it still faces deep skepticism in conventional medical circles. "My colleagues thought I was nutty," he notes, referring to the reaction of other heart specialists to his chelation research. "But I had a lot of scientific credibility, so they thought I was wacked out, but they were nice about it."

And the truth is that views of chelation are starting to change, even among the most stalwart mainstream cardiologists. "They talk about chelation therapy now without looking like they need to put garlic and wolf's bane around their necks," Lamas jokes. "They realized their previous beliefs weren't based on fact."

He adds that this is how the most exciting scientific research works, with new studies disproving previously held conventional beliefs. "When you do research and you get the findings that you expect, they are always less interesting than when you do research and you get findings you don't expect," Lamas says. "That's where you learn—that's where you have to be able to go to the next step, where you can really help patients."

TACT2 Is Recruiting Patients for Participation in Study

- Study participants must be at least fifty years of age.
- Candidates must have diabetes and experienced a prior heart attack.
- Those interested in participating can contact researchers through http://www.tact2.org, by calling 305-674-2260, or by contacting Lamas directly at lamas@tact2.cc.

Replace Toxic Household Cleaners with Natural Alternatives

Antibacterial soaps. Caustic floor cleaners. Chemical disinfectants. Most Americans use household cleaning products loaded with chemicals that would be quite at home in a hazardous waste dumpsite.

Many commercial products include ammonia, formaldehyde, hydrochloric acid, lye, paradichlorobenzenes, butyl cellosolve, ethanol, or triclosan. All have been linked to health problems, including skin conditions and irritation, reproductive problems, and even cancer.

But Melissa K. Norris, a consumer health advocate from the Pacific Northwest, says that natural alternatives made from nontoxic ingredients offer a safer, less costly, but equally effective alternative. What's more, you can make your own from readily available natural materials you probably have around the house.

In her book *The Made-from-Scratch Life*, Norris provides simple recipes for such products that are easier to make than you might think.

"Many of today's cleaning products, from what we use to clean our homes to our bodies, contain dangerous chemicals," she notes. "We shouldn't have to worry about what we're using to clean things as much as the items we're cleaning."

Norris says that two natural ingredients most of us have can be used to clean just about every surface of our homes: vinegar and baking soda. "These two have become a staple in my home and cleaning closet," she states. "For cleaning, I usually use white vinegar, but I always have raw apple cider vinegar on hand for cooking and health reasons. Whichever you happen to have can be used."

Using these and other common household staples, Norris has devised the following recipes for made-from-scratch cleaners that can be used in place of toxic chemical products:

All-purpose citrus cleanser. Ditch your commercial home cleanser and make your own with a combination of citrus peels (four to five) and 3 cups of white vinegar.

1. Place your lemon or orange peels in a quart-size jar.
2. Pour white vinegar over the peels until they are completely submerged.
3. Cover with a lid and set in a dark cupboard for two weeks, shaking the jar every few days.
4. Pour the vinegar through a strainer or cheesecloth.
5. Dilute with two parts water to one part lemon vinegar.

"Use [this] on windows, countertops, mirrors, and as a general multipurpose cleaner," Norris says. "You can use any citrus fruit or add some herbs for your own unique custom blend. If you don't have any citrus peels, you can add ten drops of your favorite lemon or orange essential oil."

Window cleaner. To make an effective solution to clean windows, fill a spray bottle a quarter of the way with vinegar and then top it off with water. "I've used this cleaner with paper towels and washable rags, and it cleans my sliding glass door, the mirrors, and all the windows without a single streak," Norris says.

Laundry detergent. Instead of using chlorine bleach, try adding ¼ cup of vinegar to your laundry to keep your whites clean. "It will kill odor-causing bacteria and clean your washing machine with no discoloring," Norris notes. "I toss mine into the liquid softener dispenser."

Floor, carpet cleaner. For an effective way to keep your floors and carpets clean, add 1 cup or so of vinegar to a bucket or sink full of water—no soap. Use the solution to mop your hardwood, laminate, tile, or linoleum floor or spot-clean carpets with a rag. "If you have little ones or pets, you won't have to worry about harsh chemicals where they play," Norris says.

Drain declogger. Vinegar is good way to unclog drains. Pour ⅛–¼ cup of baking soda down your drain, follow it with a chaser of vinegar, and let it sit for ten to fifteen minutes before finally pouring in 1 cup of boiling water. "For an especially clogged drain, repeat," Norris advises. "I do this every other month or so to keep pipes clear."

Dishwashing solution. If you have baked-on food stuck on your pots, pans, and dishes, liberally sprinkle on baking soda and scrub it away, rinsing with water. "I've found this works best with a dry pan and no added water," Norris says.

Oven degreaser. To clean your oven of grease stains, liberally sprinkle baking soda on them and scrub with a dry rag. The dry baking soda absorbs the grease, and the grit lifts it off. "This method works extremely well and requires a small amount of elbow grease," Norris notes. "Especially soiled spots may need another dousing of baking soda."

Bathroom cleanser. Baking soda is an effective alternative to chemical cleansers for showers, bathtubs, sinks, and toilets. For faucets, dampen a towel in vinegar, wrap it around the faucet and handles, and let it sit for a half hour before wiping clean to remove hard-water stains and gunk. For the toilet seat, handle, and base, use with the homemade all-purpose citrus cleaner and wipe clean.

In devising these recipes, Norris says she did some historical research into cleaning products used by American pioneers in the days before industrial chemicals became commonplace. "The pioneers didn't have aisles of cleaning and personal care products to choose from. They used simple ingredients to meet all of their cleaning needs," she explains. "I began looking into natural cleaners. I knew my great-great grandparents hadn't browsed the aisles at the general store for their favorite brand of cleaner. What had they used?"

9

LIFE STAGES GUIDELINES

Tests and Procedures That Can Save Your Life

When should you have your first cholesterol test or heart checkup? When's the right age to be checked for diabetes? Is a prostate-specific antigen (PSA) screening or mammogram right for you? The debates and arguments over health screenings are so confusing, many Americans simply throw their hands in the air and don't bother. But the truth is that some health tests are critical, some are useful for only some people, and others are entirely useless. Knowing the difference can not only boost your health but add years to your life.

Must-Have Health Screenings for Baby Boomers
We take our cars for regular tune-ups according to the manufacturer's maintenance manual to keep their motors humming. Our bodies, just like any other machine, also need periodic checkups to make adjustments for the changes caused by normal aging.

Regular health screenings should be a key part of your routine health-maintenance schedule. They can gauge your overall health and detect the earliest, most treatable stages of chronic conditions such as diabetes, heart disease, and cancer. The sooner you address such conditions, the more likely you are to enjoy a long and healthy life and the less likely you are to incur potentially ruinous expenses.

If you're an aging baby boomer—one of the seventy-seven million Americans born between 1946 and 1964—it's especially important to have certain health screenings. But sadly, only a minority of older Americans is up to date on their screenings. That includes fewer than 25 percent of those ages fifty to sixty-four and just 50 percent of those ages sixty-five and older.

One reason for this is that many boomers are confused about which tests to have—and when—in part because expert recommendations on health checks are confusing and ever changing. In addition, many health screenings are not a one-size-fits-all proposition but should be done in consultation with your doctor to determine which tests you should—and shouldn't—have, says Dr. John Meigs, a family physician in Centreville, Alabama, and president of the American Academy of Family Physicians (AAFP). "That's why we don't screen everybody for everything with every known test," Meigs says. "You really ought to have a conversation with your family doctor and ask, 'What are my risk factors? What do I need and what do I not need?'"

Meigs says it's "very likely" that many baby boomers are not getting the health tests they should. He is especially distressed that only about four in ten Americans over fifty with health insurance have undergone colonoscopy, which has the highest rate of success of all cancer screenings.

To help you sort out the recommendations, here is a primer on health screenings—both necessary and not.

Health Tests Everyone Should Have

HEART CHECKUP. Acclaimed actor Alan Thicke's sudden death in December 2016 from a fatal heart attack at the age of sixty-nine spotlighted the importance of a simple cardiac screening that can evaluate fitness levels and identify potential risks. The American Heart Association (AHA) issued a scientific statement suggesting that aerobic fitness should be considered a vital sign of health routinely checked by doctors—just as body temperature, blood pressure, and breathing rates are now.

Risk factors for heart disease also include smoking, being male, high cholesterol, diabetes, high blood pressure, and obesity. The AHA explains that aerobic, or cardiorespiratory, fitness is a measure of how well your body can deliver oxygen to tissues. Because this is a pervasive and essential function, it is also a "reflection of overall physiological health and function, especially of the cardiovascular system," according to the report.

The authors noted that while treadmill tests might still be prescribed for those at high risk for heart disease based on other factors, physicians could calculate a person's cardiorespiratory fitness based on simple equations and a few keystrokes, making it a practical test as well as a vital one for patients.

DYSLIPIDEMIA (ELEVATED CHOLESTEROL). The AHA recommends that adults over age twenty with no history of heart disease get their cholesterol levels checked every four to six years. Those with risk factors for heart disease—such as high blood pressure, obesity, diabetes, or a strong family history of high cholesterol or cardiovascular problems—need more frequent screenings. When ordering cholesterol tests, many doctors also ask labs to assess liver enzymes and proteins. An abnormal liver function panel might indicate an infection and/or damage.

HYPERTENSION. Blood pressure checks are extremely important. One in five adults has high blood pressure, known as hypertension, which increases the risk of heart disease and stroke. A painless physical reading using an arm cuff can measure your blood pressure. Most experts agree that 120/80 is normal.

COLORECTAL CANCER. The US Preventive Services Task Force (USPSTF) recommends that adults ages fifty to seventy-five undergo a fecal occult blood test every year; flexible sigmoidoscopy every five years, along with a fecal occult blood test; or colonoscopy every ten years. Tests should be done more often if you have risk factors such as inflammatory bowel disease, a personal or family history of colorectal cancer, or a history of large growths called adenomas.

LUNG CANCER. The USPSTF recommends annual lung cancer screenings with low-dose computed tomography (CT) for anyone aged fifty-five to eighty who has at least a thirty-pack-year smoking history and currently smokes or has quit within the past fifteen years. A thirty-pack-year history is the equivalent of one pack of cigarettes a day for thirty years.

SKIN CANCER. Screening for melanoma and other forms of skin cancer has become a sign of the times, with the incidence of the disease skyrocketing since the 1970s. It is the number-one cancer diagnosed for Americans, and men are at higher risk than women. An annual check is a good idea.

ESOPHAGEAL CANCER. The US Department of Health and Human Services (HHS) recommends that adults ages fifty and up undergo an endoscopy to detect Barrett's esophagus, a condition that increases the risk of esophageal cancer.

DIABETES. According to the American Diabetes Association, adults ages forty-five to sixty-four should have an initial blood sugar screening. One way to detect how readily your body digests sugar is to test blood drawn after you have drunk a sugary beverage on an empty stomach. If the results are abnormal, a hemoglobin A1C test can confirm a diabetes diagnosis. A1C tests can be repeated several times a year to assess the effectiveness of a diabetes treatment plan. Adults ages sixty-five and older should be screened every three years. Diabetes screenings are crucial because, today, the disease is rampant—affecting 25.8 million American adults and children.

OBESITY. The AAFP recommends that all adults be screened for obesity, which is defined as a body mass index (BMI) of thirty or higher. If you're obese, talk to your doctor about counseling and programs that can help you lose weight.

DEPRESSION. The USPSTF recommends screening adults for depression—but only when staff-assisted depression care supports are in place to ensure accurate diagnosis, effective treatment, and follow-up.

HEPATITIS C. Baby boomers account for 75 percent of hepatitis C cases, partly because many of them experimented with injection drugs in their youth. Because most people infected with the hepatitis C virus don't know it, in 2012, the US Centers for Disease Control and Prevention (CDC) recommended that all baby boomers undergo a one-time hepatitis C test. The CDC estimates that this could identify an additional eight hundred thousand cases of the infection, which is now curable.

CHRONIC OBSTRUCTIVE PULMONARY DISEASE (COPD). The HHS recommends that all adults over fifty undergo a spirometry test to detect COPD, a group of lung diseases that includes emphysema, chronic bronchitis, and (in some cases) asthma. This test is especially important for current and former smokers.

HIV/AIDS. The CDC recommends that all adolescents and adults get tested for HIV at least once. Those at higher risk—such as injection drug users, men who have sex with men, and women who are partners of bisexual men—should get tested more frequently.

VACCINE-PREVENTABLE DISEASES. The CDC recommends boomers receive a flu shot every year, as well as the following vaccines:

- Shots for tetanus and whooping cough. Get a tetanus booster if it has been more than ten years since your last shot.
- A shingles vaccine if you are age sixty or older.
- A pneumonia inoculation if you are age sixty-five or older.

- Any other vaccinations your doctor might advise you to have, depending on your personal health history.

TOBACCO AND ALCOHOL USE. The AAFP recommends screening and counseling, if needed, to help patients quit tobacco use and/or limit alcohol use.

VITAMIN D DEFICIENCY. An estimated 75 percent of Americans have a vitamin D deficiency, which can harm bones and muscles and increase the risk of heart disease, cancer, and impaired immunity. It's also associated with an increased risk of falls, especially in older adults. Ask your doctor for a 25-hydroxy vitamin D blood test to assess your vitamin D status.

VISION TESTING. Eye exams do more than measure how near or far you can see. Proper screening can check the overall health of your eyes. The American Academy Ophthalmology says that by the year 2020, forty-three million Americans will have some type of degenerative eye disease.

HEARING CHECKS. Audiograms or hearing tests are important because 14 percent of adults between the ages of forty-five and sixty-four have hearing loss. Men have the highest risk for all types of noise-induced hearing loss, the most common type.

DENTAL SCREENING. A visit to the dentist can help rule out oral cancer, one of the six most common cancers among American adults, and also detect gum disease and tooth decay, which women are especially prone to develop. Regular dental checks can also improve overall health, since gum disease and other oral health problems have been linked to increased risks for heart disease, Alzheimer's, and other disorders.

Tests Women Should Undergo

BREAST CANCER. The American Cancer Society (ACS) recommends that women ages forty-five to fifty-four get mammograms every year. Women ages fifty-five to seventy-four can opt to continue yearly screenings or get them every two years. Although the ACS guidelines state that routine mammograms can be stopped at age seventy-five in women at average risk for breast cancer, some experts believe that screenings should continue as long as a woman is in good health and has a life expectancy of at least ten years. If you have a strong family history of breast, ovarian, or peritoneal cancer, talk to your doctor about getting tested for the BRCA1 and 2 genes.

CERVICAL CANCER. The ACS recommends that women undergo a Pap test every three years or a Pap test coupled with an HPV test for the viruses associated with cervical cancer every five years. Although the ACS states that Pap tests are no longer needed after age sixty-five in women who have had normal results for the previous ten years, some experts believe that screening should continue until age seventy.

OSTEOPOROSIS. The National Osteoporosis Foundation recommends bone density testing using dual-energy X-ray absorptiometry (DEXA) scanners for all women ages sixty-five and older, in those over age fifty who have broken a bone, and in younger women with risk factors such as smoking, oral steroid use, and a previous facture. This crippling bone disease affects nearly ten million Americans, 80 percent of whom are women.

SEXUALLY TRANSMITTED INFECTIONS. The USPSTF recommends sexually active older women be screened for chlamydia and gonorrhea if they're at increased risk of infection. These include women who are not in a mutually monogamous relationship and those who have started a new sexual relationship.

THYROID DISEASE. If you're a woman over age sixty, you should be screened for hypothyroidism (underactive thyroid) if you experience symptoms such as fatigue, dry skin, constipation, weight gain, and increased sensitivity to cold. Get tested for hyperthyroidism (overactive thyroid) if you experience symptoms such as rapid pulse, nervousness, tremor, and increased perspiration.

Tests Men Should Undergo

ABDOMINAL AORTIC ANEURYSM (AAA). The USPSTF recommends a one-time ultrasound screening for AAA in all men ages sixty-five to seventy-five who have *ever* smoked. If an AAA is detected early, it can be repaired before it causes any problems. An untreated AAA can rupture and cause fatal internal bleeding. If you've ever smoked, talk to your doctor about getting this test.

PSA TESTING. The USPSTF no longer recommends regular PSA testing for most men, but many cancer specialists and doctors say that the test—which can flag the presence of prostate cancer—is a good idea for those at risk of the disease because of family history or other factors. Just be aware that a high PSA does not always indicate cancer; it can also be caused by infection or enlarged prostate.

Health experts recommend that men over fifty discuss the pros and cons, and risks and benefits, of PSA testing with their personal physician or a urologist to determine what's right for them.

TESTICULAR CANCER. This disease is more common in younger men but should be part of a regular annual checkup. It is easily cured when detected early.

Health Screenings That Might Be Unnecessary

Each year, the US health care system squanders hundreds of billions of dollars, according to the influential Institute of Medicine. Unnecessary health tests, services, and procedures account for a sizeable portion of that. That's why governmental agencies such as the USPSTF and professional organizations such as the multidisciplinary Choosing Wisely campaign have made an effort to educate doctors and patients about which screenings should not be routinely performed on asymptomatic patients who are not at risk for certain conditions.

These include one of the nation's most widely performed tests: the PSA test for prostate cancer. Research has not shown that the potential benefits of PSA testing outweigh the harms of further testing and treatment for most men who are not at risk of developing the cancer. These harms include pain and infection from prostate biopsies and impotence and incontinence from overly aggressive treatment of low-risk prostate cancers—including surgery, radiation, and chemotherapy—that would not likely develop into life-threatening conditions.

Older men are likely to develop nonaggressive, slow-growing tumors that don't need treatment. In many cases, they're likely to die from some other cause long before the prostate cancer becomes symptomatic. Experts also caution against routine screenings for pancreatic cancer, ovarian cancer, skin cancer, and testicular cancer.

Although an estimated thirty million baby boomers will develop Alzheimer's disease, the USPSTF recommends against routine testing for any type of dementia because there are no effective treatments. The Alzheimer's Association, however, is pushing for more rigorous cognitive assessments so older adults can participate in clinical trials and arrange their finances.

Other screenings that baby boomers might not need include the following:

- C-reactive protein (CRP) testing for heart disease
- exercise stress testing for heart disease
- kidney function tests for chronic kidney disease (CKD)

"The baby boomers are just entering this demographic where they're starting to look to the future and think about their health care over the next one or two decades," says Dr. Ariel Green of the division of geriatrics at Johns Hopkins University. "As people age, we want them to think less of these screening tests as something to check off in a checkbox and more as something to engage with their doctor in a discussion about whether it's still right for them."

Green helped draft the American Geriatrics Society's position for the Choosing Wisely campaign, which recommended against routine screenings for breast, colon, prostate, and lung cancer in patients with limited functional status and life expectancy. "If someone is seventy years old and very active and healthy, [screenings] may certainly make sense for them," she says. "But if someone is seventy years old and has a lot of health problems that may shorten their life expectancy, then they may decide with their doctor that screening is no longer right for them."

Supplements to Take in Your Fifties, Sixties, Seventies, and Beyond

In an ideal world, we could get all our nutrients we need from the foods we eat.

Unfortunately, soil depletion in agriculture and overprocessing of foods strips many natural nutrients from American dietary staples. That's why millions of Americans turn to supplements as an insurance policy for our nutrition and overall well-being.

Studies show that they can help combat the pathological processes of aging in our fifties, sixties, and seventies, when we begin to suffer from chronic inflammation, elevated cortisol levels, insulin sensitively, pain, and hormone imbalances tied to chronic mental and physical health conditions.

Taking certain supplements can support the cells most active in our bodies and combat age-related conditions. Here's a roundup of some of the most important supplements to consider by age.

In Your Fifties

Coenzyme Q10 (CoQ10). CoQ10 helps combat the impacts of environmental toxins on the body, which can accumulate over time, and also boosts heart health. It is particularly important for individuals taking cholesterol-lowering statins, which deplete CoQ10. Most experts recommend taking 100–200 mg daily.

Vitamin D and calcium. Bone loss accelerates in your fifties, especially for women. Take 600 IU of vitamin D plus 1,000 mg of calcium for men and 1,200 mg for women, split into two daily doses.

Omega-3 fatty acids. These heart-healthy compounds in fish and fish oil pills are important to reduce inflammation. They also reduce plaque buildup in the arteries. Take 1,000 mg of docosapentaenoic acid (DHA) and eicosapentaenoic acid (EPA) omega-3s daily.

Probiotics. As we age, our digestive systems are more vulnerable to unhealthy bacteria. Nutritional experts recommend taking top-quality probiotics daily that contain between one billion and ten billion colony-forming units (CFU) of healthy bacteria.

In Your Sixties

Vitamin B12. Deficiency in this important vitamin can lead to dementia, according to a study published in the *Journal of the American Geriatrics Society*. Check your levels and supplement with 2.4 mcg daily if necessary.

Omega-3s. Good brain health requires lots of DHA, the most abundant fatty acid found in the cell membranes. As we age, we lose the ability to absorb DHA in the brain, starving the mind and compromising both brain function and memory. Take 1,000 mg of DHA and EPA daily.

Vitamin D. New research shows the importance of vitamin D in reducing chronic pain, guarding against heart disease, and even warding off certain cancers. The ideal source is sunlight, but we lose our ability to synthesize vitamin D from the sun as we get older. Take 600 IU daily and make sure the supplement contains vitamin D3 for maximum benefit.

In Your Seventies and Beyond

Vitamin B12. This vitamin becomes harder absorbed as we age. The Institute of Medicine advises most adults over the age of fifty to take supplements to compensate. You might find sublingual B12 easier to absorb. Take 2.4 mcg daily.

Vitamin D. This is essential to protect against illness and infection, says Smith. The International Osteoporosis Foundation urges all older folks to take vitamin D for bone strength to prevent falls and fractures. They recommend 1,000 IU daily for this age group.

Protein. We lose crucial muscle mass as we age, and by the time we hit seventy, this can cause many health problems and also damage the immune system. Unfortunately, many elderly also lose their appetite, so they don't eat enough protein to sustain muscle mass. Supplementing with protein powders can increase lean body mass. Mix 20–30 grams of whey protein into a daily shake.

Antiaging Workouts for All Ages

When it comes to healthy living at any age, diet and nutrition are only part of the equation. Daily exercise is at least as important because it increases circulation, builds strong bones, and staves off heart disease, cancer, Alzheimer's disease, and other conditions.

"I feel strongly that resistance training, cardiovascular training, flexibility, and balance are the four vital aspects of fitness for people of all ages," says Dr. Kevin Christie, a Florida-based expert on sports medicine. "But as we age, it's important to get more specific with each decade."

Dr. Gabe Mirkin, author of *The Healthy Heart Miracle*, is a prime example. The avid exercise enthusiast stands six feet tall and weighs 140 pounds—the same weight he carried in his younger days as a marathon runner. "I am eighty years old, so I no longer do impact exercises that may damage bones, muscles, and joints," he says. "Instead of running, I now cycle thirty miles three times a week at twenty miles per hour and practice interval cycling the other days to stay in shape."

Christie says that before the age of forty, any exercise that challenges the heart and builds muscle is excellent. Here's what you need to know about the benefits of exercise as you age.

Exercise in Your Forties and Fifties

For people in their forties and fifties, a key goal is strengthening the back and building a strong core. "This helps prevent disc and back pain occurrences," Christie says. "This is the age group that often hurts their back and loses function, so . . . they start to gain weight and develop cardiovascular disease."

He recommends two exercises for this purpose: "plank" and "bird dog" poses. For the plank, support your body facedown on your forearms and toes in a straight line, keeping your abdominal muscles taut and your shoulders even with your buttocks. For the bird dog, get on your hands and knees and then lift one arm in front of you and the opposite leg in back. Alternate the arms and legs. Hold each exercise for thirty seconds.

Running, swimming, cycling, and using the cardiovascular machines at the gym are also appropriate for this age group to get the heart rate up. If there are knee or hip issues, avoid impact exercises like running or jumping jacks, says Mirkin.

Balance is always a key element in aging, especially for those sixty and over, to avoid falls that can lead to life-threatening bone breaks. To improve your balance, stand on one leg and bring your opposite knee up ninety degrees to your body and hold for thirty to sixty seconds. Repeat with the other leg.

Exercise after Sixty

In your sixties, seventies, and beyond, it's harder to do strenuous resistance training exercises like lunges and squats. But you can adapt these exercises by squatting against a wall or practicing bridging to strengthen glute muscles and build hip stability.

For bridging exercises, lie on your back, bend your knees, and bring your feet close to your buttocks. Lift your hips and hold the bridge for thirty to sixty seconds. Lower slowly and repeat three times. Brisk walking and light strength training are also good ways to build cardiovascular strength and keep your muscles strong at this age.

"For flexibility, there are no age limitations on what we do to stay limber. The key is to stretch to your full range of motion and coordinate your movements with your breath," says Christie. "You may want to use machines at the gym to assist you. But it's important to include all four aspects of fitness into a daily routine to stay healthy and active longer."

Is Your Work Schedule Harming Your Health?

Setting an alarm clock might help you get up in the morning, but the growing pressure to work long days—well into the night—or be available to your boss or coworkers 24-7 might be putting your health at risk, experts say.

Scientists have long known that we all have internal biological clocks that regulate our physical and mental health over a twenty-four-hour cycle. These are called circadian rhythms, and they change as we age. This means that the work schedules we handle with aplomb in our twenties might not be as easy for us when we reach middle age and beyond.

Experts note that poor or inadequate sleep—sometimes tied to growing work-related stresses and pressures—is associated with a host of life-threatening health problems. Among them are obesity, diabetes, heart disease, depression, dementia, and even certain forms of cancer.

"One of the biggest problems people often make in today's society is create shift work through cell phones and the Internet so that they are really working close to 24-7 these days," says Dr. Matthew J. Edlund, a Sarasota-based psychiatrist who authored *The Body Clock Advantage*.

Edlund explains that this is fine if you can fit the shifts into your "morning lark or night owl" preferences, but it can wreak havoc with your health if you are constantly fighting your body's natural clock. "Countries like Scandinavia and Finland have instituted strict work-hour rules and stricter reinforcement to ensure that workers have enough time to rejuvenate and recover," he notes. "The total hours of work in America may not be going up, but they are spreading more through the twenty-four-hour day."

So what can you do about it? Experts advise trying to set aside regular non-work hours—including adequate time for sleep—and that might mean negotiating with your boss about how to handle after-hours e-mails, phone-calls, or work-related communications.

It's also a good idea to know how your biological clock might change as you age. Here are some schedules that research shows might be best for each age group.

Teens and young adults. The human brain might not grow out of adolescence until the mid- to late twenties, says Dr. Jess Shatkin, a psychiatrist at the Child Study Center at New York University Langone Medical Center. "Adolescents have this desire to go to bed later and wake up later, and that's what most people do until they are twenty-six," he says. "Adolescents start to release the sleep hormone melatonin later in the day than most adults, and that could be around ten o'clock at night. Therefore they go to bed later and wake up later."

Ideally, this group should begin work at ten in the morning and let their schedules go later.

Adults in their thirties and forties. Research shows that for most adults in this age range, the ideal work schedule should mirror personal preferences. You are either a lark, an early riser, or a night owl, says Edlund. These preferences might be linked to your genes. But whether you are a morning person or a night person, it's important to keep a regular work schedule and avoid overnight shift work.

Shift work can impair not only your body but also your brain, says Christian Benedict, a researcher at Uppsala University's department of neuroscience in Sweden. In a recent study, he found shift workers and those who worked irregular shifts for the past five years scored poorly on cognitive tests.

He also discovered that it took the irregular workers five years to improve cognitive performance when they resumed regular, steady work hours. He speculated that since shift workers often don't get enough sleep, their brains might not effectively remove cellular waste that builds up in the organ.

Adults in their fifties and older. Research recently published in the Melbourne Institute Working Paper Series suggests that a three-day workweek would be best for adults fifty and older. Working more or less than twenty-five hours a week could have negative impact on cognitive functioning, according to professor Shinya Kajitani of Meisel University in Japan, who coauthored the study.

But even though that's not practical for most full-time workers, it's important to limit your work day—as best you can—to about eight hours, experts say.

"Work can stimulate brain activity, but longer working hours are more likely to cause physical and/or mental stress," says Kajitani. "The point we are making in our study is that work can stimulate brain activity and can help maintain cognitive function for elderly workers, but at the same time, excessively long working hours can cause fatigue and physiological stress that can potentially damage cognitive functioning."

In general, studies have shown that women who work an average of sixty hours or more weekly might triple their risk of developing diabetes, cancer, heart disease, and arthritis, according to the *Journal of Occupational and Environmental Medicine*. And a 2015 study published in *The Lancet* found that working more than fifty-five hours per week might be linked to an increased risk of heart disease and stroke in men and women alike.

"Lots of people work too many hours today," noted Edlund. "If you can control the number of hours you work, that's great. But if you can't, make sure that you protect sleep time and set up a strategic naps. Lastly, learn quick rest and relaxation techniques you can use to refresh and change gears."

10

OFF-THE-GRID

HEALTH CARE

Smart Strategies That Can Boost Your Life Expectancy

Health policy reforms over the past decade have brought dramatic changes to the US health care system and Medicare that have made picking an insurance plan, keeping your doctor, and paying for drugs and services more complicated and costly than ever before. For millions of Americans, the changes have been enough to make them want to drop insurance and eschew conventional health care. If you're considering such a move yourself, here's what you need to know about how to seek out alternative medical care, find other ways to maintain your health, boost your longevity, and live off the grid.

Rising Health Insurance Undermining Preventive Medicine

Like a lot of doctors across the country, Dr. Praveen Arla is seeing a flood of previously uninsured low-income patients these days, largely thanks to expanded Medicaid coverage under Obamacare.

But Arla is also seeing a second, disturbing trend since the Affordable Care Act's (ACA) passage in 2010: many of his privately insured middle-class patients are skipping regular appointments and routine care because of skyrocketing deductibles and health insurance costs. Some are even waiting until they have serious, more costly health conditions that might have been averted through upfront routine care.

In short, he says, the calculus of Obamacare is undermining the law's primary goal of boosting insurance coverage so more Americans would seek preventive care over treatment to drive down costs and boost public health.

"We're absolutely seeing a role reversal here, in that we're seeing an increase in Medicaid patients because all their costs are paid, but patients with insurance are not coming in because they can't afford the out-of-pocket expenses," explains Arla, who runs a family practice with his father in Hillview, Kentucky. "We are definitely seeing a decrease in patients [with] high deductibles. Just today I had a patient with a $2,000 deductible tell me, 'Well, you know, I'm going to cancel my appointment; it's going to cost too much. So I'll do it later.'"

Arla, who is board-certified in pediatrics and internal medicine, worries that rising insurance costs are erecting new hurdles to health care for many Americans. He notes that his patient load used to be 45 percent commercially insured and 25 percent Medicaid, but those percentages have flip-flopped. "I agree with the idea that everyone should have health insurance—that would be great," he says. "But the issue is, if you have insurance but it doesn't cover your basic costs, you end up not seeing the doctor."

Arla's concerns are shared by many of his colleagues across the nation who have watched nervously as insurance deductibles—as well as premiums, copays, drug costs, and out-of-pocket expenses—have steadily risen in the five years since Obamacare's passage. The increases have occurred in health plans purchased through the Obamacare exchanges by nearly 16 million Americans as well as employer-sponsored policies that now cover about 150 million workers and their families.

To balance their books, under new regulatory ACA burdens, health insurers are upping premiums and deductibles—what consumers must pay themselves before insurance kicks in—and other coverage costs. That, in turn, is driving millions of Americans to put off doctor visits, postpone some procedures, and avoid filling prescriptions—all things uninsured Americans have done for years, market research shows.

According to the US Department of Health and Human Services (HHS), health insurance premiums for 2017 rose 25 percent on average in the thirty-nine states where the federal government is running Obamacare exchanges. What's more, many plans offer consumers just one insurer to choose from and narrow networks of in-network hospitals and doctors.

But some states will see much bigger jumps. In Arizona, for instance, rates rose 116 percent for a twenty-seven-year-old buying the second-lowest cost (from $196 to $422 per month). In Oklahoma, customers faced a 69 percent rate increase. In addition, the number of insurers participating in the Obamacare exchanges dropped from 232 in 2016 to 167 in 2017, a loss of 28 percent. Major national carriers—UnitedHealth Group, Humana, and Aetna—have pulled out, saying they are losing money.

You might recall that rising insurance costs and coverage limits were the primary reasons cited by ACA proponents for the need for the law's passage. Prior to 2010, many Americans couldn't get insurance because they had preexisting conditions (ACA bars insurers from rejecting such consumers today). In the decade before Obamacare, insurance premium rates rose an average of 8.7 percent each year.

In the first few years after Obamacare's passage, premium hikes ranged from 3.5 percent to 4.5 percent, according to the nonpartisan Health Care Cost Institute. But in 2015, they jumped by an average of 7.5 percent; in 2016, many insurers sought double-digit increases in many states; and in 2017, the average premium hit a near-record high of 25 percent.

Proponents note that the vast majority of the more than ten million customers who purchase insurance through HealthCare.gov and its state-run counterparts do receive generous financial assistance. But the rising rates are raising new concerns about consumers avoiding health care to save money.

Katherine Hempstead, a health care policy analyst with the Robert Wood Johnson Foundation, notes that Obamacare attempts to encourage the use of preventive care by exempting it from health plan cost sharing components, including deductibles, both in the new ACA marketplace plans and also in employer-sponsored insurance.

But the rising cost of health insurance overall is undermining that key provision.

"High insurance costs can interfere with that goal if it prevents people from getting covered," she says. "Patient share of health care expenditure is rising in health insurance—employer sponsored and on the individual market. It is an attempt to reduce utilization and maybe also put some pressure on provider prices, but it also carries the risk that some people will forgo care they need because of the cost sharing required."

A spate of market research demonstrates the real-world impact of the changes in the health care marketplace in recent years:

- The proportion of workers with annual deductibles has risen from 55 to 80 percent over the last eight years, according to the nonpartisan Kaiser Family Foundation. In real dollars, the average deductible doubled over that time—leaping from $584 to $1,217 for individual coverage.
- The biggest annual jump in "high-deductible plans"—$2,500 for an individual, $5,000 for a family—came last year, rising from 18 to 23 percent of

employees covered through workplace health plans, according to research by the benefits consultancy group Mercer. The study—representing about six hundred thousand private employers and nearly one hundred million workers—also showed that about half of the nation's large employers are pushing high-deductible plans for its workers, usually paired with a health savings account (up from 39 percent in 2013).

- A survey by the Commonwealth Fund, a nonprofit health care research organization, found that a whopping 40 percent of working-age adults skipped some kind of care because of the cost. Nearly one in three privately insured Americans with deductibles of at least 5 percent of their income had a medical problem but didn't go to the doctor or delayed recommended medical tests, treatments, or follow-ups.

- Use of hospital care among insured workers has been steadily dropping since 2010, as well as the use of outpatient care, according to insurance claim data analyzed by the Health Care Cost Institute.

Such trends are certainly likely to continue, with high deductible plans becoming even more popular. "While new plan implementations are driving up [high-deductible plan] enrollment, we are also seeing growth in enrollment in existing plans as employees become more comfortable with consumerism and employers provide them with tools to help manage the higher deductible," said Beth Umland, Mercer's research director, in a statement accompanying the report's release.

The rise in deductibles and insurance premiums has come on top of drug cost increases, climbing copays, and increases in coinsurance (the percentage of out-of-pocket costs for patient services).

Representatives for the nation's major insurance companies, who are not barred from imposing large cost increases under Obamacare, say that the increases are necessary to shoulder costs for implementing new regulations imposed by the law. Those rules require all insurance policies to meet new, higher standards of care and cover ten specific categories of federally designated "essential" health benefits—including maternity care and mental health coverage. The ACA regulations also mandate that insurers offer policies to everyone and charge all policyholders comparable rates—regardless of a person's health status, age, gender, or other factors that might influence how many health care services they might need or utilize.

Another factor that is driving up insurance costs for plans offered through the Obamacare exchanges is the fact that a high proportion of enrollees have been older, sicker individuals—and therefore more costly for insurers to cover—than expected.

Federal officials had projected about 40 percent of the exchange policies needed to be purchased by people eighteen to thirty-five years old in order to adequately cover older Americans who generally require more care and services than younger folks. But in 2014 and 2015, only 28 percent of the new enrollees were in that younger age group, federal statistics show, the net result being that insurers say they have had to raise prices on policies for nearly everyone to balance the books.

Arla is seeing the real-world impact on patients every day, particularly those with chronic conditions or multiple health problems that require regular office visits and routine blood tests to monitor the effectiveness of treatments and lifestyle changes that can prevent costly, and potentially life-threatening, complications down the road. "A lot of times, you end up needing blood tests regularly," he explains. "But when you have a high-deductible plan, where you're not covered until you reach your maximum out-of-pocket limit . . . what we're seeing is patients like that are stretching out the time [between] visits."

A poignant example of this are diabetes patients, many of whom are forgoing regular office visits and routine blood tests—generally recommended every three months—to manage the disease, which can lead to heart disease, organ damage, amputations, blindness, and other problems if left unchecked. "Studies show [that] a patient with diabetes should be coming in every three months to get a checkup [and] have their blood checked for their hemoglobin A1c," which determines how well blood sugar levels are being controlled, Arla notes. "But what's happening is patients aren't coming in every three months; instead, they're trying to stretch that out . . . because they have all these high out-of-pocket expense."

Other patients will simply call for refills of prescription drugs over and over, hoping they can "medicalize" their health problems—without the supervision of doctor. "That can be dangerous," he notes.

Ironically, perhaps, a personal physician might be in the best position to advise a patient who is struggling to pay his or her medical bills. Doctors can provide information on drug-assistance programs and lower-cost health services and even provide free drug samples and suggest other cost-saving strategies—such as pill-splitting—that can save patients money.

"We advise our patients to shop around," Arla says, noting his independent medical practice is not affiliated with a hospital network, so he is free to recommend that patients shop around for health care services. "Let's say your doctor wants you get a CT scan for pneumonia. You can call around and find one at an independent facility that will typically do it for $200–$300, but a hospital will charge $1,000 or more."

The upshot, Arla says, is that Obamacare has changed the rules of the health care game for doctors, patients, and insurance companies alike. Consequently, you have to be a savvy health care consumer. And that means not waiting until it's too late to avert disaster before booking a doctor appointment, particularly if you have a chronic health condition.

"The time when people will absolutely go to the physician is when they're acutely ill, and that's when you'll pay whatever you have to," he notes. "So when that happens, and patients do finally come in [after skipping routine appointments], it's often with added complications. . . . And that's likely to [cost] a lot more."

Money-Saving Alternatives to Conventional Health Care

In many ways, health insurance is the backbone of the nation's health care system. In fact, federal law requires all Americans to have insurance or pay a small fine to the IRS (2.5 percent of your total household adjusted gross income, or $695 per adult).

But it's not the only option. As costs have risen, a growing number of Americans are turning to alternatives that emphasize healthy lifestyles, alternative medicine (often not covered by insurance), and high-tech, low-cost options such as telemedicine and concierge practices.

The idea of going without insurance might seem like a gamble, but it makes sense financially for some Americans who are willing to take charge of their health and pay out of pocket for the health care they need.

Consider the math: A typical health insurance plan costs $8,000–$10,000 per year in premiums (twice as much for family coverage). Over a decade, that can add up to $80,000–$100,000. If you expect to require that much health care, then health insurance is a good bet for you. But if not, banking or investing that money—and paying out of pocket for the care you do need—can make a great deal of financial sense.

If you do develop a chronic health condition down the road, you can decide to sign up for insurance (federal health law requires insurers to provide health insurance to all Americans, regardless of preexisting conditions).

But in the meantime, if you are uninsured, you can pay your doctor like you would a dentist, veterinarian, chiropractor, personal trainer, dietitian, or massage therapist—with your checkbook. Many health practitioners will even offer a discount if you pay out of pocket and can direct you to low-cost drug options (such as GoodRx.com). And if you do require expensive surgery or therapy, you can explore lower-cost options abroad (in Canada, for instance) or compare prices (using an online resource such as MediBid.com).

Cost-Cutting Health Care Tips

Regardless of whether you decide to pay for insurance or not, your best defense against rising health care costs and premiums is to be a savvy consumer and look for savings wherever you can—just as you would for any other service.

Here are some smart ways to maximize your health care dollar:

RESOLVE TO STAY HEALTHY. In some ways, the best health care plan is one that minimizes your need to see a doctor or have a medical procedure. And the best way to do that is to adopt a healthy lifestyle. Eat a healthy diet, exercise, visit a doctor regularly, and account for any unique personal, familial, or lifestyle factors that can increase your health risks—such as smoking, drinking to excess, being overweight, or not getting adequate sleep.

MANAGE ANY CHRONIC CONDITIONS YOU HAVE. More than a million Americans have been diagnosed with diabetes, while another five million have it and don't know it, the US Centers for Disease Control and Prevention (CDC) estimates. Of all deaths in the United States, 1 in 9 is attributed to heart failure—causing more than 279,000 deaths each year—according to the American Heart Association (AHA). And rates of cancer expected to rise to 22.2 million people worldwide by 2030, with one person dying from cancer every minute of every day, according to the American Association for Cancer Research (AACR). But many of the nation's biggest killers are preventable. Health experts estimate that more than half of such cases are tied to obesity, smoking, poor diet, lack of exercise, and exposure to ultraviolet radiation from tanning beds or direct sunlight.

BECOME A COMPARISON HEALTH SHOPPER. You wouldn't buy a house, a car, or even a new TV without comparing costs, yet many people never think about shopping around for good deals on drugs, health care, and medical services. If you're paying out of pocket for medical expenses, you can compare prices through online resources like MediBid.com, HealthcareBluebook.com, and Medicare.gov—all of which provide average and customary costs and prices for various health care procedures and products. With such information in hand, you can try to negotiate fair fees for services with your doctor, hospital, or health care provider up front. Other consumer organizations—such as the Patient Advocate Foundation (http://www .patientadvocate.org/) also offer advice on holding down costs for care and treatment.

ITEMIZE MEDICAL DEDUCTIONS ON YOUR TAXES. Working Americans can deduct unreimbursed medical expenses on their taxes if they add up to at least 10 percent of adjusted gross income. This can save you a bundle on federal taxes. In real dollars, a worker earning $50,000 in gross income needs to have at least $5,000 in out-of-pocket health costs to file for the itemized deduction and save on federal taxes.

SAVE ON DRUG COSTS. The typical couple with average drug expenses will need about $270,000 to cover medical costs alone in retirement, according to a Bankrate .com analysis based on calculations provided by OptumHealth Financial, a United

HealthCare company. Medical costs can be much higher for people who are suffering from certain health conditions, such heart disease, cancer, or diabetes. For example, a person who smokes, has high cholesterol, and is obese might need as much as $150,000 more than a healthy nonsmoker for health care expenses in retirement, according to Bankrate.com.

If you take brand-name medicines, think about switching to generics, which are usually as effective and less costly. You can also ask your doctor to write prescriptions for over-the-counter (OTC) drugs (allowing them to be covered by insurance or paid for through tax-free health savings accounts [HSA] funds). You might also ask your doctor about pill-splitting, which can halve your prescription drug costs. And if you're income is low, ask your pharmacist about drug assistance and discount programs that pharmaceutical companies sponsor. A useful online clearinghouse for such programs is maintained by the nonprofit group NeedyMeds at http://www.needymeds.org.

EXPLORE HSAS. HSAs are tax-free savings accounts that can be used to pay for qualifying out-of-pocket medical expenses not covered by insurance. They can only be used in conjunction with HSA-eligible, high-deductible insurance plans. For 2017, the IRS set the annual limit on deductions at $3,400 for an individual and $6,750 for a family. If you're fifty-five and older, you can contribute an additional $1,000. Unlike a flexible spending account (FSA), you don't lose HSA money you don't use in a calendar year; it rolls over year to year and can be used to pay for health care as well as long-term care. HSAs are a great way to save on your taxes, particularly for people who start contributing to an HSA early and keep adding to their accounts over the years.

OTHER SAVINGS OPTIONS. In addition to looking for ways to minimize health-related costs, it might also pay to explore other financial strategies to compensate by managing other investment and spending plans for a more "holistic" approach to personal financial planning. Look for ways to lower your taxes by sheltering more of your income in retirement savings and HSAs. Create a household budget and stick to it. Clip coupons. Look for two-for-one bargains. Resolve to become a savvy comparison shopper and make an effort to negotiate prices for everything you buy.

Clinical Trials: What You Should Know about Experimental Therapies

Getting the news that you have a deadly form of cancer or Alzheimer's disease is bad enough, but it's worse if there's no effective treatment. Even in such cases, however, all might not be lost—thanks to the promise of experimental therapies undergoing clinical trials.

Clinical trials are research projects on new therapies, drugs, or vaccines that the US Food and Drug Administration (FDA) has approved for testing but have not yet been cleared for general use. In most cases, such therapies have proven to be safe and promising in early studies, usually involving laboratory experiments or animal tests. In exchange for participating, patients receive therapy at no cost.

Participants volunteer for such trials as a final step toward FDA approval, and the agency closely monitors the research. In some cases, promising experimental drugs and therapies are given "breakthrough status," which allows them to be fast-tracked so they can enter the market sooner.

Clinical trials can offer the latest and greatest in technology, medicine, and treatment methods, providing patients with cutting-edge therapies that aid healing and save lives. For instance, the new form of immunotherapy credited with saving the life of former president Jimmy Carter by putting his cancer in remission was in only experimental trials just a few years ago. But there are some caveats about clinical trials patients should know about.

Evaluating Pros and Cons

Dr. Paul Sabbatini, deputy physician-in-chief for clinical research at Memorial Sloan Kettering Cancer Center, notes that clinical trials can often provide life-saving, miracle-working treatments for many patients.

But he adds that patients need to take everything into consideration—including potential risks and benefits—before enrolling in a study. "There are many significant benefits to enrolling in a clinical trial," he says. "Participating in a clinical trial gives patients the opportunity to receive new drugs or therapies, sometimes years before they are widely available. Patients are also closely monitored for any side effects when enrolled in a clinical trial. Additionally, in most cases, there is no additional out-of-pocket cost for receiving the new treatments offered in a clinical trial.

"However, because clinical trials involve novel treatments that are not yet FDA-approved, it is important for patients to recognize that there are some possible risks involved in participating. First, a clinical trial can sometimes require more time and medical attention than normal care. This can include doctor visits, phone calls, more treatments, a hospital stay, or a more complicated treatment regimen. Next, the treatment might not work or might cause serious side effects. And even if a new approach helps some patients, it might not help every patient."

Docs Aren't Always Clued In

Because of the potential risks posed by clinical trials, they aren't always a doctor's go-to prescription for patients—even those with terminal conditions. Other factors might also keep your doctor from mentioning a potential lifesaving experimental therapy in discussing your options.

Some physicians aren't aware of the clinical studies taking place. In addition, such trials might be offered through hospitals and research facilities that are not affiliated with your doctor or only in other regions of the country. As a result, getting involved in a clinical trial is often in the hands of the patient.

The good news is that many websites and companies provide services designed to match patients with research studies that could be beneficial.

For many years, ClincialTrials.gov was the best website to use when looking for clinical trials. Sponsored by the National Institutes of Health (NIH), the web portal enables patients to find and view ongoing clinical studies and learn more about the goals and findings of such studies. The website can be intimidating, however, because of the amount of information it provides and its use of technical medical terminology that might seem to require an MD to understand.

But several online clinical trial search engines now make it easier to get involved in a study. What follows is a collection of the best options for patients.

Clinical Trials Resources

CureLauncher.com. Founded in 2012, this website offers a feature that allows patients to search for clinical trials by condition and therapy. The front page greets you with a video that explains the mission of Cure Launcher and provides a phone number for patients to be matched up with a "relationship manager." The manager sorts through the trials available to identify good options to match a patient with treatment.

MyClinicalTrialLocator.com. This free website was created to provide a window into the various clinical trials being conducted around the world. Created by West Palm Beach, Florida, doctor Bruce Moskowitz, the site also provides patients with notifications when new trials open.

CenterWatch.com. Run by a publishing and information services company, this website keeps a list of industry- and government-funded trials for cancer and other diseases. You can search by location, cancer type, drug name, and other features.

Cancer.org. This American Cancer Society (ACS) website provides a clearing-house of clinical-trial and patient-matching outfits as well as a detailed primer on what to know as a prospective study participant.

The ACS and other health advocacy organizations note that while clinical trials are vital to developing new and better treatments, patients must recognize that there are potential risks associated with becoming involved in a study.

Such trials are not primarily designed to treat health conditions, for instance, but are conducted to evaluate the safety and effectiveness of new therapies.

In many cases, trials are halted before they are completed because the researchers and FDA believe the benefits of the therapies are clear and should be offered to a wider range of patients. In some cases, they are stopped early because an unexpectedly high risk or dangerous side effect has been noted in patients receiving the treatment.

Despite the potential risks to clinical trial participants, Sloan Kettering's Dr. Sabbatini says that they are far and away the best way to evaluate lifesaving new therapies and bring breakthrough treatments from the front lines of medical research to the greatest number of patients.

"The overall benefit of clinical trials to scientific research cannot be overstated," he says. "Almost every current treatment in cancer was first tested in a clinical trial, and this research will continue to help spur future breakthroughs."

Clinical Trials: Understanding the Lingo

In general, there are four stages, or phases, of clinical trials that patients need to know about:

- **Phase I.** This stage of an experimental treatment study generally involves a small number of patients—typically twenty to eighty people—and primarily aims to evaluate safety and side effects. In essence, the participants in preliminary phase I trials are frontline evaluators in the development of a new treatment.
- **Phase II.** A step up from phase I trials, phase II studies enroll a larger group of patients—approximately one hundred to three hundred people—and are designed to evaluate the effectiveness of the treatment and to further evaluate its safety.
- **Phase III.** Such trials usually involve more than one thousand patients and are more comprehensive. The results of these studies are used to confirm preliminary trials' results that suggest the new therapy is

effective. But they also aim to track negative side effects, compare the new treatment with older standard treatments, and collect information on the optimal use of the drug or therapy. In such studies, patients are often divided into groups—one of which receives the experimental therapy, the second a placebo or older treatment. Doctors then compare the results in both groups.

- **Phase IV.** This final stage of research generally involves treatments that have been approved by the FDA. While the treatments involved in such trials might even be available to the public, follow-up research is needed to continue tracking the drug or therapy's safety, risks, benefits, and optimal usage.

Trial Patient: "I Have Made a Little Contribution to Science"

For Eduardo Angeles, a Miami truck driver, participating in a clinical trial for an experimental heart therapy not only saved his life but also made him a front-line soldier in the war on heart disease.

Angeles suffered a heart attack several years ago and underwent emergency heart surgery. During his recovery, his cardiologist, Dr. Gervasio Lamas, suggested that he enroll in a groundbreaking clinical trial of the alternative heart treatment chelation therapy.

The just-published results of that study found that heart attack survivors like Angeles who receive chelation and high-dose vitamins—a combination long used by alternative medicine practitioners—face much better survival odds than those who rely on conventional heart treatments.

Now Lamas—chief cardiologist with the Columbia University Division of Cardiology at Mount Sinai, Miami—is conducting an FDA-approved follow-up study that could lead to chelation becoming a standard treatment for cardiovascular disease alongside aspirin, statins, and other therapies.

"Dr. Lamas said I benefited from the trial 100 percent, and I started feeling a change after joining the study. Now my risk of having a second [heart attack] is very low," Angeles says. "So I feel like it helped me, but in my mind, I was also doing something for somebody else. I feel like I have made a little contribution to science."

Telemedicine Allows Doctors to Make High-Tech House Calls

You might say that Dr. Pat Basu is resurrecting the old-fashioned house call, but it's with a newfangled twist Marcus Welby could never have envisioned.

Basu is the chief medical officer of Doctor on Demand, the largest telemedicine provider in the world. The web-based operation employs one thousand medical doctors and three hundred psychologists and psychiatrists who collectively examine, diagnose, and treat thousands of American patients each day—via real-time video.

The outfit's doctors see patients—who dial in through their smartphones, tablets, or computers—in the comfort of their own homes. The doctors diagnose and treat everything from simple sinus infections to skin rashes, bacterial illnesses, and other minor conditions. The virtual consults cost patients just $40 per fifteen-minute session, and some insurance companies even cover such visits and pay doctors for such care.

"I believe telehealth is good for patients, good for doctors, and good for the health care system in general," Basu says. "I would say 95 percent of our consultations are solved at the time of the visit, and 5 percent are referred for other medical attention."

Doctor on Demand is one of a handful of companies connecting patients with physicians without patients having to wait weeks or months for an appointment or spend hours languishing in a waiting room. The approach represents a leading edge in digital medicine, offering a convenient and inexpensive alternative to time-consuming and costly office visits.

With Doctor on Demand, patients can download the company's app. To see a doctor, they just press a button and are connected to a physician licensed in their state who can see them over video. An e-consult is typically $40—far lower than a standard $125 office visit, a $300 bill for an urgent care checkup, or $1,000 or more for a trip to the emergency room.

The approach not only lowers health care costs and improves patient care and access but holds out the promise of easing doctor shortages that now face as many as one in five Americans—primarily those living in rural or remote areas far from medical centers and physician offices.

"We talk about the doctor shortage, but I call it the doctor misallocation. If you take the number of doctors and divide them by the number of patients in the country, we actually do have enough doctors," Basu says. "But the problem is, in a brick-and-mortar world, you may have some areas where there are enough doctors but also places where there [are] not enough. So you may have one doctor who is slammed with patients, but just a mile away there's another doctor who's not very busy at all. So what telemedicine allows you to do is have a patient in an [underserved area] see a doctor who isn't too busy."

Such arrangements also give doctors more flexibility to work with patients after hours, from the comfort of their own homes, Basu notes. They also leave doctors freer to spend time with those patients who require hands-on care—including those with cancer, heart, disease, and other conditions that require a doctor's close attention over time.

Despite the promise of telemedicine, however, state and federal health regulations have tied many practitioners' hands. What's more, establishment organizations like the American Medical Association (AMA) have taken a dim view of telehealth approaches, arguing that patients are best served by face-to-face meetings with their doctors.

Medicare refuses to pay doctors unless they provide hands-on care, for instance. Doctors can't be reimbursed for e-mailing elderly or disabled Medicare patients or consulting with them by phone or video.

Similar laws govern Medicaid patients in most states. At least three states—Alaska, Arkansas, and Louisiana—expressly bar doctors from writing prescriptions without physically examining a patient. And the AMA's official position is that doctors must be physically present to provide proper care.

Some states have also pressed the issue. In a widely reported case, the Texas medical board went after a firm called Teledoc—which provides telephone consultations to eleven million patients for $40 (with the doctor having access to patients' medical records)—arguing that regulators were only protecting patients.

Dr. Abraham Verghese, vice chair of Stanford's School of Medicine, has expressed the view of many doctors in applauding the efficiencies and cost-saving telemedicine will bring while saying that he's also concerned about preserving the doctor-patient relationship.

But instead of fighting telehealth approaches, regulators and medical professionals should be embracing the opportunities the technology offers, Basu argues. "The regulations have simply not caught up with the digital age," he says. "Most states have started to update their bylaws [to allow telemedicine]. The AMA has definitely gone in the direction of clearly coming out in saying we are in favor of national licensing. But it's still confusing because even though we live in the United States of America, it doesn't feel like it . . . because we have fifty states with different regulations."

Of course, telehealth isn't a solution for all medical issues, although Basu says that there have been some cases of patients with life-threatening conditions that were first identified through e-consults. Telemedicine is best suited for acute and current conditions that don't require medical imaging or a long-term relationship with a doctor but are not typically handled in routine office visits, by an urgent care facility, or ER.

The CDC estimates that there are nearly 1.3 billion patient visits each year to doctors' offices, outpatient clinics, and emergency rooms. Basu believes that telehealth consults could replace at least 400 million of them.

"We have had some cool cases where we have saved somebody. But they're not what we do generally," he explains. "The typical cases we do [are] the mother who has two kids who are sick and miserable and can't get in to see a doctor for an antibiotic, or a child with a rash, or a mother with a urinary tract infection, or a dad with a sinus infection. And literally, today we will do a thousand of these."

Other varieties of telemedicine also link larger medical centers or specialty hospitals with smaller rural clinics, urgent care centers, or other facilities.

Mayo Clinic doctors now use cameras to get detailed images of patients at smaller independent facilities in rural Minnesota. They can track vital signs, talk to patients, and direct care at those facilities—providing world-class expertise that is not available in community hospitals.

Jefferson University Hospitals in Philadelphia and Mount Sinai Health System in New York now allow primary care patients to have video consults with internists and certain medical specialists.

Mercy health system, based in St. Louis, Missouri, is opening a $54 million virtual care center to handle urgent and primary care video consultations for chronically ill and other high-risk patients.

Medical researchers at Université Laval in Quebec have found that patients who receive rehabilitation instructions via video teleconference, or "telerehabilitation," following total knee replacement surgery have comparable outcomes to patients who receive in-person physical therapy. "This study is the first to provide strong evidence for use of telerehabilitation as an alternative to conventional face-to-face care following total knee replacement surgery," said Hélène Moffet, PhD, a physical therapist and Laval professor who led the study, published in *The Journal of Bone & Joint Surgery*.

The American Telemedicine Association suggests that such telehealth applications can improve the management of chronic diseases such as diabetes, leading to fewer or shorter hospital stays. And a recent report from the research firm Towers Watson estimates that telemedicine might help employers save at least $6 billion each year in insurance costs.

Armed with such positive testimonials, telehealth experts say the HHS could—and should—expand the reach and scope of digital medicine by allowing a doctor who provides real-time video or audio consults to Medicare patients to be reimbursed for such visits.

Right now, Medicare reimburses only for a limited number of telehealth services for patients living in an officially defined "health professional shortage area" who seek care at a medical facility, not a patient's home. But expanding this policy would not only allow more elderly and disabled Americans greater access to less-expensive, high-quality care but also set a precedent for state regulators and insurance companies to follow.

Even in the absence of such federal action, insurers are getting on board, recognizing the cost savings telehealth can bring and the appeal it has for people who decide to go bare and not buy insurance.

UnitedHealthcare, Humana, Aetna, and Blue Cross/Blue Shield in several states now allow for reimbursements for video consultations offered by Doctor on Demand and similar outfits. "Other insurance companies that we don't have direct contacts with will adjudicate those claims and allow for reimbursement," Basu notes. He adds that about twenty-five states now have telehealth-reimbursement codes for doctor and patient reimbursements, and forty-seven states allow the operation's doctors to write scripts for their patients (exceptions include Arkansas, Alaska, and Louisiana).

As a result of the inroads made by Doctor on Demand, Teledoc, and other tele-health companies, the digital house-call trend is already well along—following similar digital trends in banking, retail, and music sales and distribution that have complemented or replaced brick-and-mortar operations.

Last year, nearly 20 million American patients engaged in telehealth video visits, according to the market analysis firm Tractica. By 2020, that number is projected to increase to more than 158 million, the firm estimates.

"What do I expect to happen now? It is to get more and more people who have direct contracts with us," Basu predicts. "We want to make it so you walk into our 'digital office' and it's already paid for, so the claims submission can be done on the doctor end or the patient end."

Basu—who served as White House advisor on health care and economic affairs in 2010 and 2011, shortly after passage of the ACA—believes that rising health care costs, premiums, and out-of-pocket expenses are likely to make telehealth a more attractive option for American consumers in the years ahead, as they will increasingly look for ways to lower medical bills.

"We used to define access to health care as the number of Americans who have insurance—the implication there being insurance was all you needed to have access," he says. "But true access to care—can you see a doctor in a timely factor, for instance—hasn't really increased."

He argues that Obamacare curbed some costs associated with unreimbursed hospital care, primarily provided to uninsured, underinsured, or previously uninsurable patients with preexisting conditions. But at the same time, patients are shouldering more of the costs for their own care—through higher insurance premiums, deductibles, and out-of-pocket expenses—a trend likely to drive greater consumer interest in telemedicine.

"I think the Affordable Care Act has done a lot to help curb costs in health care, but [in] access and quality, we still have a long, long way to go," he says. "The other thing it has done is it has pushed greater cost of care onto the person receiving that care . . . so quality of care and access are still gaping disasters in the America health care system.

"Nobody . . . would ever choose to go to an ER, spend three hours and $1,500, compared to spending $40 for a fifteen-minute telehealth visit. So those things are driving people to say, what am I getting for my dollar? Telemedicine is helping hold down those costs, and at the same time, by having telemedicine, you can still have a doctor available to patients from 8 a.m. to 8 p.m. So it's a win-win-win."

Desert Doc Goes off the Grid

Like a lot of doctors, Dr. Zubin Damania is disgusted with the health care changes under way in post-Obamacare America. Too much money is spent on conventional *after* care—to treat cancer, heart disease, and other conditions after they've developed—while too little is spent on prevention and wellness.

That's why Damania has gone off the grid to turn the tables on health care. As the CEO and founder of TurnTable Health, a direct-pay primary care clinic in Las Vegas, Nevada, Damania has built a facility that represents what one might describe as the "next big thing" in medicine.

A conventionally trained MD who spent ten years at Stanford University Medical Center, he is embracing alternative medicine and represents a kind of backlash to conventional fee-for-service medicine.

His practice brings together teams of holistic specialists—dietitians, personal trainers, Zumba teachers, yoga practitioners, and meditation instructors—and he even has an on-site kitchen at his clinic that teaches patients how to prepare health foods.

Members who join the clinic pay $80 a month for what Damania calls "all you can treat" access to a buffet of care, as well as on-demand access to a doctor or health coach.

The concept was developed by Iora Health, which partners with TurnTable Health, and the operation is expanding beyond Vegas and has several dozen "health coaches" at facilities across the country.

"You can't do this in a model where everything is billable and codable," Alexander Packard, chief operating officer of Iora Health, told *MedPage Today*. "You don't get paid for helping patients shop for groceries."

Oh, and one other thing: Damania has his own recording studio, where he produces PSAs on everything from Obamacare to stroke symptoms under his web-savvy alter ego, ZDoggMD.

One of his most popular music videos—called "Can't Feel My Face"—was produced in response to a recent University of California, Los Angeles (UCLA) study that showed that 73 percent of people under age forty-five wouldn't know to seek medical care immediately if they had symptoms of a stroke (http://zdoggmd.com/cant-feel-my-face/).

"Strokes aren't funny," Damania says in a blog post with the video. "They cause untold suffering, disability, and death on a massive scale each year. Having personally lost both of my grandmothers to stroke at relatively young ages, this issue is deadly serious to me. Apart from preventing a stroke in the first place (that is, controlling diabetes, hypertension, obesity, high cholesterol, stress, heart arrhythmias, etc.), recognizing the signs of stroke early is the best hope of saving brain cells—and lives."

"Can't Feel My Face" includes cameos from a variety of health care workers—nurses, stroke coordinators, and EMS students—posing as night club attendees.

It also spotlights a quick way to remember the signs of stroke: the acronym FAST, short for "face, arms, speech, time." Stroke victims often have facial drooping on one side, might be unable to lift up both arms, typically have slurred or garbled speech, and should waste no time when calling emergency services.

Other symptoms can include numbness or weakness on one side of the body, confusion, trouble seeing on one side, loss of coordination or balance, or severe headache.

PART II

Disease Directory

AGING

You might say that Dr. Alan Maisel is a modern-day Ponce de León. A cardiologist by training and an adventurer by nature, Maisel has made a name for himself by scouring the globe for medicinal remedies that have been used for centuries to boost health and longevity.

His work has taken him to the so-called Blue Zone villages in Europe, where people live inexplicably longer than most other places in the world, and to the jungles of South America, where he identified compounds in dark chocolate that improve skeletal-muscle function in heart patients.

His international travels have informed more than 150 scientific papers on heart disease and longevity, and he is widely hailed for his discovery of a cardiovascular disease biomarker now used by doctors worldwide to diagnose the condition.

But during a recent trip to Italy, Maisel stumbled on what might be the most significant finding of his career: a tiny resort village on the Mediterranean Sea that has a higher proportion of residents who have lived to age one hundred or more than anywhere else on the planet.

The town of Acciaroli, on Italy's Amalfi Coast, is home to just two thousand people—at least three hundred of whom have reached the age of one hundred or more. Even more remarkable is the fact that very few of the town's residents suffer from heart disease or Alzheimer's, even though many of its elders are significantly overweight and are quite fond of cigarettes and wine.

Intrigued by what's behind the "Acciaroli paradox," Maisel—a professor at the University of California, San Diego (UCSD)—has joined with longevity researchers from the Sapienza University of Rome to determine why so many of the townspeople are living so well for so long. "It's unclear whether this will turn out to be a kind of

Fountain of Youth find, but maybe we'll get some answers that can relate to how all of us can live better and longer, even though we don't all live in Acciaroli," he says.

The "Eureka!" Moment

The search for genuine antiaging strategies has consumed us since the time of Ponce de León and perhaps before. Why is it that some people live so well for so long, while others die prematurely or suffer terrible age-related diseases, such as cancer, heart disease, and Alzheimer's?

The answers have remained elusive to modern scientists and traditional alternative medicine practitioners alike. But the work of researchers like Maisel is offering clues to the ways that genetics, diet, lifestyle, and other factors can extend life expectancy as well as shorten it.

A primary focus of longevity researchers in recent years has been what scientists have dubbed "Blue Zones"—places like Acciaroli that have the highest concentrations of centenarians in the world. Among them are Okinawa, Japan; Sardinia, Italy; and Loma Linda, California.

Antiaging experts are attempting to determine what the people in Blue Zones have in common that might explain their longevity. While genes certainly play a role, other lifestyle factors—including diet, activity levels, stress, culture, and social issues—are also likely to figure into the equation. That means that Blue Zone elders might have important advice for the rest of us about how to improve and expand both the quality and the quantity of our lives and combat, reverse, or forestall the ravages of age-related diseases and health conditions.

"Only about 10 percent of how long the average person lives is dictated by our genes," says National Geographic explorer Dan Buettner, author of *The Blue Zones Solution: Eating and Living Like the World's Healthiest People*. "The other 90 percent is dictated by our lifestyle."

Buettner and a team of researchers scoured the world to identify three pockets of longevity and then performed exhaustive research to determine why these people lived so long. While diet and physical activity played a role, the researchers found that outlook, faith, and social connections are equally important factors.

"The best science tells us that the capacity of the human body is ninety years," Buettner told an audience during a recent TED talk. "But life expectancy in this country is only seventy-eight years. We figured the best way to get these missing years is to look at the cultures around the world where people are living to one hundred at a rate of up to ten times greater than we are."

Each Blue Zone is very different in culture, but Buettner says that these cultures share traits that people everywhere can incorporate to live a longer and healthier life. Among them are eating nutrient-rich foods, getting regular exercise, maintaining social connections with friends and family, keeping stress levels to a minimum, and having a sense of purpose in life.

The "Eureka!" Moment in Maisel's Acciaroli Study

Maisel's research on the villagers of Acciaroli mirrors what Buettner and other longevity experts have found. But he and his team are delving deeper into the interaction of genetic and lifestyle factors—nature versus nurture—with the goal of offering more detailed prescriptions for health, vitality, and aging well.

For Maisel, the eureka moment in his research came unexpectedly while vacationing on the Amalfi Coast with longtime friend and colleague Salvatore DiSomma from Sapienza, who grew up in the region.

"Salvatore has a boat, and we'd take trips to the Italian coast—to Capri, off Naples, and other places close by, and he took me a few years back to Acciaroli," he explains. "During the trip, we noticed there were a lot of older people, and they had a real joie de vivre about them—they were out and about, active, and seemed happy, and there seemed to be no stress there. It was the kind of place that made you think, 'Wow, what a great place to live!'"

Maisel also noticed something else: many of the villagers looked really old, yet they were seriously overweight, tanned a deep bronze, and smoking and drinking wine everywhere he and DiSomma went. Another curious feature of the villagers also caught his attention, a characteristic he describes as an aggressively romantic nature.

"There were two quintessential moments where we realized something interesting was happening here," he recalls. "One was walking on the beach . . . and seeing a lot of these big old fat guys smoking cigarettes, sun-tanned, and wearing speedos. And we thought, 'Geez, people don't live that long when they look like that in the United States. How can that be?'

"The second: I ran into an old lady pumping water out of a street well; she looked like she was in her nineties. And she started [hitting on] me, inviting me back to her home to have sex with her! And some of the guys we talked to, in their nineties or older, were telling me about all the sex they're still having. So I thought maybe there's something with that too, because ED [erectile dysfunction] is an aging thing too."

Maisel and DiSomma met with the town's mayor and several local doctors and discovered that birth and medical records of the townspeople indicated that a large proportion of the village was old—very old—yet remarkably healthy. In fact, 20 percent of the three hundred villagers who are over one hundred have made it to their one hundred tenth birthday—and beyond.

As a result of their preliminary legwork, the two decided to launch a formal scientific study designed to understand whether genetics, lifestyle, or diet—or all three—is the key factor in the longevity of Acciaroli. Maisel's team has enrolled several hundred residents who have agreed to undergo a series of comprehensive surveys, blood tests, and genetic analyses to determine the factors in their extraordinary vitality.

"These people have never been studied. So we've brought a lot of folks in from UCSD and University of Rome and designed what we want to do, which will include genetics and biomarkers and lots of surveys about diet, cognitive function, and health," he says.

Early Clues Point to Anchovies and Herbs

Maisel says that the research team has already gleaned some preliminary findings that might at least partly explain what's happening in the little Italian village.

Perhaps most notably, the town's residents follow a modified version of the heart-healthy Mediterranean diet. But they also eat a ton of anchovies (oily fish loaded with healthy omega-3 fatty acids) and locally grown rosemary, which contains a compound that boosts blood flow to the brain and has been shown to improve memory and cognitive function in some studies.

"They do follow the Mediterranean diet, but they seem to live a lot longer than other people who follow the Mediterranean diet," Maisel notes. "We noticed they also eat anchovies at almost every meal, and they all seem to have their own gardens, and rosemary is used in a lot of dishes too. And we know there are studies out there that show rosemary has compounds that boost cognitive function."

There is a good deal of science to back up Maisel's observations. Studies have shown that rosemary might boost mental functions by breaking down acetylcholine, a chemical found in the brain, which allows nerve cells to communicate more effectively. That, in turn, increases mental acuity and concentration and leads to a calmer disposition.

Some research has shown that simply inhaling the scent of rosemary lowers levels of cortisol, the so-called stress hormone secreted by the adrenal glands in response to stressful situations. That might be why rosemary has been used in aromatherapy and burned in incense for centuries to calm the mind.

It might also be a key factor in the longevity of Acciaroli's many residents, Maisel explains. Second, the villagers get plenty of exercise in their everyday lives.

"They don't jog or do aerobics classes, but they're pretty active people," he explains. "They're out and about a lot, walking the beach, the hills, in the garden. It's not a sedentary life."

They also have a low level of stress and a laid-back attitude, in part because the village is so removed from the hustle and bustle of modern Rome and other major cities. In many ways, the patterns of life and rural lifestyle in Acciaroli have remained unchanged for generations.

And finally, of course, there's the possibility that the *romantic* nature of the town's seniors is a contributing factor to the Acciaroli longevity paradox, and isn't just a side benefit.

The researchers hope their study will unmask Acciaroli's secrets to health and longevity—perhaps providing a prescription for living that can be adopted by the rest of us.

"I suspect it's some combination of genetics, plant genetics of the locally grown food, the diet they eat, the fact they're pretty active . . . and the laid-back lifestyle," Maisel says. "This is a place where it looks like time has kept things pretty much how they've always been. People don't seem to really move away much, and if they do, they come back—they're not really getting a lot of dilution there.

"So we have a bit of a real-world test tube there to study why these people live so long and so well; it's like a perfect little real-world laboratory for a longevity study."

Keys to Acciaroli Villagers' Longevity?

The findings of longevity researchers who are studying the villagers of Acciaroli, Italy, echo what other research has shown about the interaction of genetics, lifestyle, diet, and certain nutritional compounds as key contributors to health and long life.

The work by Maisel's team, Buettner, and others suggests that you can add years to your life by following these healthy habits embraced by the elders of Acciaroli, Sardinia, Okinawa, and Loma Linda.

Eat sensibly. The people in all these Blue Zone communities follow plant-based diets, and the animal proteins come mainly from fish along with cheese and milk from grass-fed animals.

- The Acciaroli villages follow a modified Mediterranean diet—loaded with olive oil, healthy meats, fish, nuts, vegetables, and wine—which has long been tied to health benefits and longevity. Meals emphasize whole, natural, locally produced foods and limit processed meals. But the Acciaroli diet incorporates rosemary and anchovies, two key staples that have been linked to heart health and improved cognitive function.
- The Sardinians drink a local wine that has three times more healthy polyphenols than any other wine on Earth.
- The Loma Linda group, a community of Seventh Day Adventists, shun alcohol, but the others drink moderately.
- The Okinawans have little strategies such as using smaller plates and following a three-thousand-year-old adage that suggests stopping eating when you are 80 percent full.

Stay active. Acciaroli's residents don't go to health clubs or do yoga or aerobics. But the people of the village are an active group—walking the hills and beach, spending a lot of time outdoors, and engaging in other physical activities. Making sure to get some kind of regular exercise each day can cut your risk for heart disease, stroke, diabetes, Alzheimer's disease, and certain types of cancer, studies consistently show.

Buettner's research shows that other Blue Zone residents typically don't exercise but stay fit by constantly nudging themselves into physical activity. For example, the one-hundred-year-old Okinawan women sit on the floor so they have to get up and down up to forty times a day. Many Sardinians are shepherds who walk the hilly terrain and have no conveniences to ease household work. The old folks from Loma Linda ride horses, tend gardens, and even perform manual labor like building fences.

Maintain a sense of purpose and community. The two most dangerous times in people's lives are the year they are born and the year they retire, says Buettner. So it's important to maintain a "reason to wake up every day" and stay connected with family, friends, and the community. Maisel says there is a strong sense in Acciaroli that everyone is part of an extended family, which fosters tremendous connections among the villagers.

The residents of all these places have close-knit ties to family and their "tribes," Buettner says. They also choose like-minded companions who have a positive impact on their lives. "When it comes to longevity, there is no short-term fix," says Buettner, adding that picking the right friends is "perhaps the most significant thing you can do to add years to your life and life to your years."

For the residents of Okinawa, things like teaching karate or catching fish provide a sense of purpose and connection. One 102-year-old woman finds a sense of purpose by merely holding her infant great-great-great granddaughter, which she likens to "leaping into heaven." And a 97-year-old doctor from Loma Linda still performs twenty open heart surgeries a month.

Destress your life. Daily stresses tied to work and family life can reduce the function of your immune system and increase your odds of suffering various mental and physical illnesses. Stress can be a killer because it releases hormones that can cause destructive inflammation over time.

Blue Zone residents do something for at least a few minutes every day to let go of stress—setting aside time to be introspective, taking a nature walk, sharing a glass of wine with a friend, listening to music. The Seventh Day Adventists even have "sanctuary time"—twenty-four hours every week to focus on God and family—and they go on nature walks. Faith, notes Buettner, can add anywhere from four to fourteen years to your life.

In even the most stressful urban settings, we can turn to meditation, yoga, exercise, or prayer to relax and calm the mind.

Take in the great outdoors. You might not live in a picturesque hillside village overlooking the Mediterranean or have access to a mountain path to stroll, but you should still take time daily to take in the great outdoors and breathe some fresh air. Taking a walk in a park, a local nature preserve, or even your neighborhood helps you experience nature and calm your mind.

Natural Ways to Boost Your Immunity and Stay Healthy

One aspect of the Acciaroli longevity research that Maisel's team is investigating is the role of lifestyle, diet, and other factors in boosting immunity.

A great deal of research suggests that a well-functioning immune system is your greatest ally when it comes to living a long and healthy life. Too often, however, the importance of the immune system is overlooked until something goes wrong—and by then, it's too late.

Fortunately, you can take steps to boost your immune system—through diet, exercise, supplements, and adopting healthy lifestyle habits. Taking such steps can stave off chronic diseases like heart disease, diabetes, and cancer. They can also play a role in your mood, digestive system, and healthy brain function as well.

Your Immune System

The immune system is made up of special cells, proteins, tissues, and organs that defend us against germs and microorganisms every day. The special cells, called lymphocytes and leukocytes, are located in different parts of the body, including the lymphatic system, which includes the lymph nodes, the bone marrow, the thymus, and the spleen.

In recent years, scientists have learned that a large portion of our body's immunity—at least 80 percent—is located in the gut. This makes sense because the gastrointestinal (GI) tract is the entry point for most invading organisms and toxins that come from the foods we eat.

But the vital connections among the immune system, healthy gut bacteria, and the brain are only now becoming clear. Just recently, researchers discovered a previously unknown set of blood vessels that link the immune system to the brain.

They called this the "missing link" in discovering how immunity might play a key role in protecting us from such neurological diseases as autism, multiple sclerosis, and even Alzheimer's. Some of the most important cancer treatments have come from new knowledge of the immune system as well. This new understanding of the link between and immunity and cancer has given birth to the exciting new field of cutting-edge cancer therapy known as immunology.

Why Your Immune System Needs Help

Obviously, the immune system is necessary to sustain life, but the functioning of our natural defense mechanisms declines dramatically with age.

Centuries ago, when the human lifespan was forty years, a declining immune system was not a problem. But now people are outliving their immune system's natural lifespan, sometimes by forty or even fifty years. This problem has even spawned a new medical field known as immunosenscence, which refers to the gradual deterioration of the immune system brought on by age.

Fortunately, there are natural ways to bolster your immune system. Here are some of the key ways to do it.

Antioxidant Vitamins (A, C, and E)

One of the greatest causes of damage to the immune system is simply aging. A by-product of your normal metabolism is called oxidation, and like rust on a car, this process damages the cells of your immune system as well. But antioxidants—such as vitamins A, C, and E—combat this process.

Vitamin A is the first line of defense in the immune system. Vitamin C is also essential. Along with vitamin E, both mitigate damage caused by oxidation, a study published in the journal *Toxicology* noted.

Vitamin D

Vitamin D has demonstrated its immunity-enhancement powers since before the advent of antibiotics, when it was used to treat tuberculosis. More recently, vitamin D has been shown to fight autoimmune disorders. Yet researchers find that three-quarters of Americans suffer from vitamin D deficiency.

Vitamin E

Vitamin E is known both for its antioxidant powers as well as its ability to influence the immune system, especially in the elderly. Also, a recent animal study in the *Journal of Experimental Medicine* found that adding vitamin E to food protected immune cells from such environmental stresses as UV radiation, air pollution, and tobacco smoke.

Vitamin E was discovered in 1922, when researchers doing experiments on laboratory rats discovered that the pups of pregnant females often died in the womb, but when the mothers' diets were supplemented by other foods, they didn't. They didn't know what the missing component was, so they called it "Factor X."

Eventually, this mysterious Factor X was discovered to be vitamin E, and through the years, more evidence has emerged of the role it plays in protecting the trillions of cells in our body.

Perhaps because vitamin E is such a complex vitamin—it's composed of eight different compounds; four tocopherols and four tocotrienols—researchers are finding that it is involved in preventing numerous devastating ailments.

It's often contended that we can get enough vitamin E from the foods we eat, but the National Institutes of Health (NIH) disagree. They note that most people do not eat enough of certain foods high in alpha-tocopherols (the type of vitamin E most supplements contain) and also that many conditions affect a person's ability to absorb dietary vitamin E.

In fact, a 2015 study reported in the *Journal of Clinical Nutrition* found that up to one-third of the millions of Americans with metabolic syndrome cannot absorb dietary vitamin E properly and might not be receiving its important antioxidant benefits.

Zinc

About 40 percent of Americans are deficient in zinc, which helps the immune system guard against the development of chronic disease, a study published recently in *Molecular Nutrition & Food Research* found. Also, since the body cannot store zinc, daily supplementation is needed.

Astragalus

Astragalus, an herb used in Chinese medicine for thousands of years, not only helps regulate the immune system but also functions as an antioxidant and reduces inflammation, a 2014 study in the journal *Phytotherapy Research* found.

Maitake Mushroom

The maitake mushroom is a well-known plant used in folk medicine, and its immune-boosting and antioxidant powers were also recently documented in the scientific journals *Annals of Translational Medicine* and *Molecules*.

Olive Leaf Extract

Multiple studies have demonstrated that thanks to their bioactive components, olive leaves can help optimize the immune system, protect it from environmental stress, and even reduce inflammation.

Beta-Glucan

Derived from baker's yeast, beta-glucan primes and strengthens the key immune function of neutrophils, which comprise 40 to 75 percent of white blood cells and are an essential part of the immune system. It is also considered a potential probiotic that could benefit the gut microbiome, which plays a key role in the immune system. Beta-glucan is also believed to have cholesterol-lowering and cancer-fighting properties.

Vitamin E: Aging and the Immune System

Oxidation causes aging, and this directly affects the immune system, reducing its effectiveness and leaving us more vulnerable to cardiovascular disease, cancer, and numerous other ailments as well grow older.

Most people know that antioxidants bolster the body's defenses against oxidation, the metabolic process that produces aging. But what you might not know is that vitamin E is considered "nature's master antioxidant" because of its powerful overall effect on the body.

For the past twenty-five years, evidence has built up that vitamin E is a critical factor in protecting against such ravages of aging, notes Dr. S. Moriguchi, a leading authority and author of recent research on the vitamin, published in the journal *Vitamins & Hormones*.

These include infectious diseases, cancer, and damage due to high blood pressure or radiation. "Vitamin E is an important nutrient for maintaining the immune system, especially in the aged," he says.

A number of recent scientific studies have shown just how effective vitamin E is in combatting age-related diseases tied to inflammation and oxidation:

Heart health. The excitement over vitamin E in preventing heart disease stems from the discovery that it was oxidation that fuels atherosclerosis, the disease process that results in coronary heart disease. This finding led to major large-scale separate studies in women and men, which found a 20 to 40 percent risk reduction in coronary heart disease in people taking vitamin E for at least two years, the *New England Journal of Medicine* reported. Such findings have led to vitamin E becoming a popular heart health supplement among not only people in general but cardiologists as well.

Cancer. Some studies have found that vitamin E might reduce the risk of several types of cancer. Although prostate cancer findings have been mixed, one study found that selenium supplementation reduced the risk of prostate cancer by 63 percent and that even better results were seen when selenium was combined with natural vitamin E. Similar studies have backed up this finding. For people with cancer, some supplements have been found to reduce the impact of chemotherapy, but this is not true of vitamin E, which can enhance its effectiveness and protects the body from its negative effects.

Brain health. A growing body of evidence says that vitamin E helps keep the brain sharp and wards off Alzheimer's disease, dementia, and amyotrophic lateral sclerosis (ALS), known also as Lou Gehrig's disease. Researchers who tracked fifteen thousand women found those that who had high vitamin E scored better on tests of brain function, according to a study in the *American Journal of Clinical Nutrition*. Johns Hopkins School of Medicine researchers evaluated several large studies on ALS involving more than one million people and found that the long-term use of vitamin E supplementation was associated with a 42 percent lower risk of ALS.

Lung disease. Vitamin E might protect the lungs from cellular damage due to pollution. In a 2015 study, UK researchers who looked at chemical signatures in blood samples found that those with the highest levels of vitamin E had the lowest evidence of damage from air pollution, according to research published in the *American Journal of Respiratory and Critical Care Medicine*. Previous studies had found that vitamin E could be protective against cancer, especially in smokers.

Age-related vision problems. It's estimated that by age seventy-five, 70 percent of people will have developed cataracts. One recent study that compared 175 people with cataracts to 175 without them found that those people with the highest vitamin E blood level were at a 50 percent lower risk. And a long-term study of 764 people showed that while those taking a multiple vitamin had a 30 percent lower risk, regular users of vitamin E supplements experienced a 57 percent risk reduction.

Additional research finds that vitamin E also helps prevent depression and anxiety, shingles, ataxia (loss of balance), and nerve disorders.

Younger than Your Years: How Old Are You Really?

How old would you be if you didn't know how old you were?

That's the question posed by baseball legend Satchel Paige, who seemed to defy time as he pitched professionally well into his sixties.

Paige was a prime example of how we have two different ages—chronological and biological. The first deals in time, the second in bodily function. Often they don't match up, which is why many people look and feel either younger or older than their chronological years.

"Most of us have all had the experience of being surprised to find out that someone is far younger than we had imagine," says Terry Grossman, founder and medical director of the Grossman Wellness Center in Denver. "By the same token, we will occasionally discover that someone is considerably older than we had guessed. The reason for these discrepancies is often because their biological ages are different than their chronological ages."

So which are you? Scientists can accurately measure biological age by examining a person's genes. Complicated tests in labs can also analyze the physiological function of someone's body to come up with a number. But there are also tests you can perform at home. David Kekich, CEO of the Maximum Life Foundation in Newport Beach, California, offers the following suggestions:

Lung capacity. Take three deep breaths and hold the fourth for as long as you can. A twenty-year-old can hold it upward of two minutes, but we lose about twenty seconds per decade. So if you're sixty and can hold your breath for one minute, that means you have the lung function of a fifty-year-old.

Skin elasticity. Pinch the skin on the back of your hand for five seconds and then let go. In young people, it will snap back in place instantly and take about three to five seconds for forty-five-year-olds, ten to fifteen seconds for sixty-year-olds, and thirty-five to sixty seconds for those seventy and up.

Cognitive ability. Have a pal write down a seven-digit number and tell it to you twice. Then you try to repeat it backward. Young people can typically get all the digits right, while fifty-year-olds miss one, sixty-year-olds miss two, and seventy-year-olds miss three.

Balance. Stand barefoot on a level, uncarpeted surface with your feet together and then close your eyes and raise your dominate foot about six inches off the ground. See how long you can balance that way. A twenty-year-old can do it for thirty seconds or more, but we lose about six seconds per decade. So a sixty-year-old who can do it for twelve seconds has the balance capabilities of a fifty-year-old.

Reaction time. Have a friend hold a yardstick vertically from the end. Place your thumb and forefinger about three inches apart at the eighteen-inch line. The friend lets it go without warning and you catch it between your fingers. A twenty-year-old will nab it at the twelve-inch line, but that progressively decreases to five inches at age sixty-five.

"We have a lot of control over our lifespan," says Kekich, author of the book *Smart, Strong and Sexy at 100?* "We can increase it by up to fifteen or twenty years, mostly by lifestyle—diet, exercise, meditation, stress reduction, nutritional supplements, and proper medical care.

"People can reverse their biological age dramatically. As Mohammad Ali once said: 'Suffer today and live the rest of your life as a champion.'

"These days, suffering for most people can mean skipping the donut at the office and getting some regular exercise. That's not a big price to pay to add years to your life."

Online Age Tests

Along with the home aging tests, here are three online quizzes that use blood pressure, height and weight, cholesterol level, lifestyle, diet, family history, brain function, and other data to estimate biological age:

Biological age calculator: http://www.disabled-world.com/calculators
   -charts/health-age.php
Biological age test: http://growyouthful.com/gettestinfo.php?testtype=quizb
My brain test: http://www.mybraintest.org/healthy-brain-test/

ALLERGIES AND ASTHMA

When we think of allergies, we tend to envision the sneezing and wheezing that typically comes from hay fever and seasonal pollen counts. But in fact, allergies encompass a wide range of maladies—including potentially life-threatening reactions to pollen, grass, mold, foods, drugs, and insect bites or stings.

In fact, allergies and asthma (a type of allergic disease) might be the most common afflictions in the nation, striking about fifty million people—30 percent of adults, 40 percent of children—and rising, according to the Asthma and Allergy Foundation of American.

Yet despite the high prevalence of allergies, many Americans don't know what causes them or how to treat them.

What Causes Allergies?

In simplest terms, an allergy is when your immune system has an overreaction to a foreign substance, called an allergen, that you inhale, eat, touch, or otherwise contact.

Allergies typically cause sneezing, itchy eyes, coughing, a runny nose, and a scratchy throat. But in extreme cases, they can lead to rashes, hives, low blood pressure, breathing problems, asthma attacks, and even death.

Although there is no cure for allergies, they can be managed with conventional treatments—namely, immunology shots that tamp down the immune system's response to allergens. But it's more effective to prevent them in the first place by determining what allergens provoke reactions in you and then avoiding them judiciously.

Common Indoor and Outdoor Allergies

Many people with allergies have more than one type of allergy, which can be diagnosed with simple skin-prick tests performed in a doctor's office. The most common indoor and outdoor allergy triggers include the following:

- cat, dog, and rodent dander
- cockroaches
- dust mites
- mold spores
- tree, grass, and weed pollen

Skin Allergies

Skin allergies include inflammation, hives, eczema, and contact allergies—with bugs, dust, mites, certain, foods, or latex. Poison ivy, poison oak, and poison sumac are the most common skin allergy triggers.

Food Allergies

Children have food allergies more often than adults and sometimes outgrow them. These eight foods cause most food allergy reactions:

1. eggs
2. fish
3. milk
4. peanuts
5. shellfish
6. soy
7. tree nuts
8. wheat

Drug Allergies

Allergic reactions to one or more medications affect about 10 percent of the population and up to one in five hospital patients. The following are the most common drug allergies:

- anticonvulsants
- aspirin, ibuprofen, and other nonsteroidal anti-inflammatory drugs (NSAIDs)

- chemotherapy drugs
- other antibiotics (especially those containing sulfonamides [sulfa drugs])
- penicillin (up to 10 percent of people report being allergic to this common antibiotic)

Insect Allergies

Allergies to insects affect one in twenty Americans and cause at least twenty US deaths a year, mostly due to anaphylaxis. Here are the most common causes of insect allergies:

- bee and wasp stings
- cockroaches
- dust mites
- poisonous ant bites

Diagnosing and Combatting Allergies

Identifying the cause of allergies and then avoiding those allergens is usually the first and best way to manage them. To identify an allergy, board-certified allergists use skin tests—around since the 1860s—that typically produce quick results. Here is how both types of tests are administered:

PRICK/PUNCTURE. A diluted allergen is applied with a prick or a puncture to the surface of the skin to see if it provokes a reaction, such as a raised, red, itchy bump known as a "wheal."

INTRADERMAL. Using a very thin needle, a diluted allergen is injected immediately below the skin's surface. This test is sometimes done if a prick/puncture test is inconclusive.

Allergy Shots

For people who test positive for allergies, doctors typically recommend allergy shots—a form of immunotherapy—if symptoms continue for many months of the year.

Such shots boost the immune system, allowing it to become more resistant to specific allergens and lessen symptoms. Allergy immunotherapy treatment involves receiving regular injections given in gradually increasing doses.

When allergy shots were first developed in the mid-twentieth century, they took years to be fully effective. But now, someone who begins allergy shots in January will typically experience a significant reduction, or elimination, of symptoms by April.

After a patient has built up a tolerance to allergens, allergists gradually decrease the frequency of injections. Most patients need them once every month or so in the first few years of receiving shots, but some people might eventually be able to discontinue them altogether.

Natural Alternatives

Although allergy shots are effective in combatting reactions, a wide range of natural alternatives are equally effective—and might even be preferable. Here's a list of what to do if you or a loved one has been diagnosed with a skin or nasal allergy:

KEEP YOUR HOUSE CLEAN. Pollen and allergens are often present indoors—on doormats, carpets, shoes, furniture, and curtains. Vacuum your house regularly to remove irritants that have traveled indoors. Keep the windows closed and be sure to run your air conditioning (if you have it) or whole-house ventilation system.

KEEP ALLERGENS OUTSIDE. Change clothes when you get home from work or after being outdoors so you don't bring allergens indoors. Tap your shoes outside your house to knock off any pollen. Wash your hair before getting in bed.

WATCH THE CLOCK. Levels of pollen and allergens are highest early in the morning and on dry, hot, and windy days. Limit the time you spend outdoors during peak hours so you are outside when it is cooler, less windy, and later in the day.

MAKE YOUR BEDROOM SPOTLESS. Good housekeeping habits, particularly in the bedroom, keep allergens from pets, dust mites, cockroaches, and other insects to a minimum. It's also a good idea to use pillow cases and mattress pads—to limit the growth of dust mites that feed on dead human skin—and launder all bedding in warm or hot water weekly.

KNOCK DOWN MOLD GROWTH. Check damp areas in your home—such as bathrooms, kitchens, attics, and basements—for mold growth, which can exacerbate allergies.

TRY USING A MASK. Wearing an air-filtering mask while going outdoors can help prevent allergic reactions. Some higher-end masks—equipped with a so-called high-efficiency particulate air (HEPA) filter—can be as effective as over-the-counter (OTC) remedies in heading off reactions.

AVOID CERTAIN FRUITS AND VEGETABLES. If you suffer from seasonal allergies, you might also be more likely to have allergic reactions to certain types of fruits, vegetables, and nuts. For instance, if you are allergic to birch or alder trees, you might have strong reactions to apples, cherries, or even celery. If you have grass allergies, then tomatoes, potatoes, and peaches might cause you irritation.

CHOOSE AN AIR FILTER WISELY. Cheap air filters and ionic electrostatic room cleaners can actually lead to more irritants and ions that can trigger allergies. If you're shopping for an air filter, be sure to pick one with a higher rating for removing allergens. A better option would be to use whole-house filtration systems with filters that are changed regularly.

KEEP YOUR WINDOWS CLOSED. It seems like a good idea to open windows to improve ventilation when you're feeling lousy. But doing so can allow pollen to enter your house and settle into carpet and furniture. That's why it's a good idea to keep your windows closed during allergy season.

DON'T SELF-MEDICATE. OTC remedies can ease symptoms of spring allergies but won't address the root cause. You're better off seeing an allergist, who can get to the bottom of what triggers your reactions so you can begin taking any necessary medications before the season gets under way.

TAKE ANTIHISTAMINES. Antihistamines can reduce the susceptibility to spring allergies and increase resistance. Among them are Allegra, Benadryl, Dimetane, Claritin, Alavert, Tavist, Chlor-Trimeton, and Zyrtec. Note that taking medicines for spring allergies can cause drowsiness and dry mouth.

CARRY EPINEPHRINE. If you're a risk for life-threatening anaphylaxis, it's important to carry self-injectable epinephrine, such as an EpiPen device. The condition is a severe reaction to an insect bite, food, medication, or another trigger that leads to an overrelease of chemicals that can cause shock or cardiac arrest. Such reactions can occur as long as twelve hours after the initial reaction. Symptoms include the following:

- abdominal pain
- anxiety
- diarrhea
- dizziness
- fainting
- hives or swelling
- hoarse voice
- low blood pressure
- nausea or vomiting

- rapid heartbeat
- tightness of the throat
- trouble breathing

Call 911 and get to the nearest emergency facility at the first sign of anaphylaxis, even if you have already administered epinephrine.

Allergies: By the Numbers

- About sixteen million doctor visits each year are related to allergies.
- Allergies account for more than six million lost work and school days.
- Allergic disease, including asthma, is the fifth leading chronic disease in the United States and the third most common ailment in children.
- Americans spend more than $42 billion annually on allergy-related health costs.
- Americans visit hospital emergency rooms about two hundred thousand times a year—ten thousand are admitted because of food allergies alone.
- Anaphylaxis, a life-threatening allergic reaction, is most commonly triggered by medicines, food, and insect stings.

Source: Asthma and Allergy Foundation of America

Cheaper EpiPen Alternatives

Outraged over EpiPen's $600 price tag? Get in line. Patient advocates, consumer activists, the American Medical Association (AMA), and even members of Congress have railed against the product's maker, Mylan Pharmaceuticals, for increasing the device's price 500 percent since 2007.

"We are concerned that these drastic price increases could have a serious effect on the health and well-being of everyday Americans," said US Senators Susan Collins and Claire McCaskill of the Senate Special Aging Committee in a letter to Mylan requesting an explanation for the price hike.

While the debate rages, you should know that cheaper alternatives are now available for the EpiPen—an auto-injector syringe filled with epinephrine that treats allergic reactions so severe that some people can't breathe, a condition known as anaphylaxis.

Here's a primer.

Generic Adrenaclick. *Consumer Reports* notes that the generic Adrenaclick, also referred to as an "epinephrine auto-injector," sells for as low as $140 at Walmart or $205 at Rite-Aid, with a coupon from GoodRx.com.

Pharmacists in some states—including California, Colorado, Connecticut, Florida, Vermont, and Washington—can fill an EpiPen prescription with Adrenaclick without getting a new prescription from their doctors. But in other states, you can still get the generic alternative by asking your physician to write a prescription for an "epinephrine auto-injector" or "generic Adrenaclick."

Make your own shot. EpiPen and Adrenaclick are automated epinephrine-injecting devices, but a cheaper alternative is to keep syringes and epinephrine on hand for emergencies. A three-month supply of syringes and the drug costs about $20, according to price lists.

But if you go this route, you should ask your doctor or pharmacist about how to use one and the proper dosing. You should also know that Adamis Pharmaceuticals is developing a prefilled syringe system for injecting epinephrine that delivers proper dosage through manual syringes.

Others in the works. According to the Allergy Advocacy Association, several other EpiPen alternatives—the credit card–shaped Adrenacard and a generic auto-injecting system from Teva Pharmaceuticals—are in the works and could hit the market in 2017.

The Massachusetts-based Windgap Medical is also reportedly seeking the US Food and Drug Administration's (FDA) approval for its EpiPen alternative, called Abiliject. Unlike EpiPen, which must be replaced every twelve to eighteen months, Abiliject has a shelf life of several years and might be more cost-effective for families.

Discount coupons. You should also know that in response to the outrage over its EpiPen pricing, Mylan has created a coupon savings program so that some customers can get discounts of $300 on each EpiPen two-pack.

For cash-paying customers with high deductibles, the discount cuts costs by roughly 50 percent, experts say. But the coupon doesn't apply to all customers.

Why Farmers Have Fewer Allergies: The "Hygiene Hypothesis"

You might recall this curious piece of recent health news: a landmark 2016 international study found that people who grow up on farms have dramatically lower risks of developing allergies than those who grow up in rural or urban areas.

The findings, published in the *British Medical Journal Thorax*, are based on an analysis of the medical records of people in fourteen countries, suggesting that common biological factors, rather than social or cultural ones, might have a role to play.

Experts believe that the likely culprit is something known as the "hygiene hypothesis"—a theory that suggests early childhood exposure to a variety of potential allergens and microbes might offer some protection against allergies or somehow strengthen the immune system.

Past studies have suggested that the sharp rise of asthma and allergies over the past few decades in urban and affluent areas might be partly explained by the hypothesis.

Scientific researchers who have studied the phenomenon suspect that antibacterial agents and powerful household chemical cleaners used in modern-day homes might prevent children from being exposed to bacterial, viral, and allergenic agents that would toughen up their immune systems. As a result, they are more likely to develop allergies and weaker immune systems later in life that leave them vulnerable.

Some studies have even suggested that introducing young children to peanut butter and other foods that are common allergy triggers might reduce their risk of developing allergies later on. The same has been found for kids raised in homes with dogs, cats, and other pets.

For the latest study, the researchers drew on the European Community Respiratory Health Survey II, which included more than ten thousand people aged twenty-six to fifty-four from fourteen countries in Europe, Scandinavia, and Australia between 1998 and 2002.

Participants were asked where they lived before the age of five—on a farm, in a country village, in a small town or city suburb, or the inner city. Those who had spent time as children on a farm were 54 percent less likely to have asthma or hay fever and 57 percent less likely to have allergic nasal symptoms than those living in the inner city.

Farm kids were also less likely to have had a family history of allergies than the others, were more likely to have had pets and older siblings, and were more likely to have shared a bedroom in their early childhood.

"The consistency of the findings across multicountry settings suggests that farming effects may be due to biological mechanisms rather than sociocultural effects that would differ between countries," the researchers concluded.

The upshot is that while cleanliness might be next to godliness, as the saying goes, it probably won't hurt to let the kids play in the dirt, romp around outdoors, care for a pet, and get their hands dirty from time to time.

Worst Cities for Spring Allergies

About 8 percent of Americans suffer from seasonal allergies, according to the US Centers for Disease Control and Prevention (CDC). If you are among them, it's possible that where you live is a significant factor in how miserable you feel.

The Asthma and Allergy Foundation of America (AAFA) has compiled a "Spring Allergy Capitals" report card that has identified the one hundred US cities with the right mix of factors to be considered the worst places for allergy sufferers.

Louisville ranked number one on the AAFA's most recent report, followed by Dallas, Richmond, and Birmingham. The rankings are based on the metropolitan area's pollen score, which reflects recorded pollen/mold spore levels; the duration of the peak spring season; the percentage of people in the area who are affected by those pollens; and allergy medicine use.

Even cities that rank low on the AAFA report—such as Colorado Springs, which placed last at one hundred—are considered bad for allergies. The point of the ranking, AAFA officials say, is to let allergy sufferers know that they need to take extra precautions if they live in, or are visiting, one of the nation's "spring allergy capitals."

Are Aspirin Allergies Overdiagnosed?

Aspirin is an effective, low-cost way to prevent and treat cardiovascular disease, but patients who experience side effects, such as gastrointestinal (GI) symptoms, are often told that they are allergic and must stop therapy.

But the patients are usually never tested for allergies, and according to a study presented to the American College of Allergy, Asthma, and Immunology, only 2.5 percent of patients who were told they were allergic had a true hypersensitivity to the drug.

"Our study showed none of the patients that were determined to have aspirin hypersensitivity were referred to an allergist for testing," said lead author Dr. Gabriela Orgeron. "In addition, we found that patients with GI symptoms were mislabeled as having aspirin allergy, which likely deprived them of being treated with aspirin in the future."

Probiotics Eliminate Allergy

Probiotics eliminate the cow's milk allergy in some infants, according to research conducted by the University of Chicago and Italy's University of Naples.

The immune systems of children who have milk allergies overreact to proteins in milk, making it hard to digest and putting them at risk of missing out on essential nutrients.

But infants fed a formula containing *Lactobacillus rhamnosus GG* (*LGG*), a specific type of probiotic found in many supplements, modulated the immune response and allowed some infants to develop a tolerance for milk.

In addition, the probiotic also significantly changed the makeup of the babies' gut bacteria, producing higher levels of a bacteria that helps maintain balance in the gut.

ALZHEIMER'S DISEASE AND DEMENTIA

At just fifty-nine years of age, Greg O'Brien was given the news no one ever wants to hear: you have Alzheimer's disease, and there is no cure. But instead of falling into depression or despair, O'Brien decided to turn his diagnosis into an opportunity to tell the world what it's like to have Alzheimer's and courageously chronicled its heart-rending impacts.

From the inside out.

O'Brien, an award-winning journalist, turned the story of his struggles with the memory-robbing disorder into an eye-opening 2016 memoir, *On Pluto: Inside the Mind of Alzheimer's*. The extraordinary book provides a stark yet uplifting insider's view of what it's like to live with dementia. But it also documents—in very personal terms—the astonishing genetic and med-tech advances made in recent years to diagnose the condition, the new breed of drugs used to slow its progression, and the unconventional ways O'Brien has developed to manage its symptoms.

He does not sugarcoat the hardships that he knows await him and his family. He watched his mother and grandmother die from the disease. But he says that those experiences are precisely why he wanted to share his experience, faith, and hope.

"After I started [having] the horrific symptoms, I had the brain scans . . . and clinical tests that confirmed the diagnosis," he explains, noting that he carries the so-called Alzheimer's gene—known as APOE4—and that two head injuries led to MRIs that unmasked the disease.

"Because I had a front-row seat with my family, I did go into the pity party and got angry with God. And then I . . . decided to compile about two thousand pages of notes of everything I was afraid I would forget."

O'Brien relied on his professional skills to dig into the "who, what, where, when, why, and how" of early onset Alzheimer's, which strikes before age sixty-five (about 5 percent of the five million Americans who have the condition).

In doing so, he provides a compelling glimpse into Alzheimer's and shares a handful of strategies that have helped him cope since his diagnosis nearly eight years ago. In addition, O'Brien's experiences showcase the recent progress Alzheimer's researchers have made in developing new ways to diagnose the condition early. Among them are the following:

- A handful of new drugs developed in recent decades that can slow the progression of dementia and moderate some of its symptoms.
- Brain scans that can identify biological hallmarks of the disease, including amyloid protein plaques that gum up brain functions and destroy neurons and communication between cells.
- New genetic tests that can detect the APOE4 gene linked to Alzheimer's even before symptoms surface.

Yet at the same time, O'Brien's experiences underscore the grim reality that there is no cure or effective treatment for Alzheimer's, and recent research into developing therapies to stop or reverse the disease have been disappointing at best.

"There was a dark moment when I tried to take my life, because I'd seen what happened in my family, and I didn't want to take my family and friends there," he says. "And the good Lord told me that's not my decision. So I've learned to walk in faith, hope, and humor."

O'Brien's journalistic training allowed him step outside of himself to write about the indignities and challenges of Alzheimer's, which has robbed him of about 60 percent of his short-term memory, leaving him unable to recognize familiar places and people.

"Every morning before I get out of bed, it's like putting all the files in my brain back in place because overnight, someone [has] taken the files and dumped them on the floor, and I have to go through these steps of what am I doing," he explains. "And there are times I go to the bathroom and I've brushed my teeth at times with hand soap and once gargled with rubbing alcohol. And so I write the names 'rubbing alcohol,' 'mouthwash' on some of the bottles now. You have to have strategies."

O'Brien credits his mother with providing the original spark of inspiration for his deeply personal memoir. Just days before her death, she told him, "We all have a purpose in life. Go find it!"

His hope is that *On Pluto* will expand awareness of Alzheimer's.

"Bugs Bunny once said, 'Don't take life too seriously because nobody gets out alive,'" says O'Brien, who also has prostate cancer—a condition he jokingly calls his "exit strategy" to avoid spending his final days in a nursing home. "My feeling is, as the baby boomers press forward against this tsunami, maybe we can try to do some good again. If by talking to other people I can be the canary in the coal mine, then that's given me purpose at a time when I feel I have no purpose—if that makes sense to you?"

A Growing Menace

Few ailments are as frightening as Alzheimer's, the leading cause of dementia. For most of the five million Americans diagnosed with it, Alzheimer's causes advancing memory loss, thinking problems, speaking abnormalities, and other maladies that eventually lead to death.

It is the sixth leading cause of death in the United States, and many specialists believe that figure underestimates the true impact of the disease. That's because death certificates rarely cite the condition as a primary cause of mortality but more often identify secondary ailments that result from dementia—such as pneumonia or cardiopulmonary problems—as the main reason.

And those numbers are rising. While deaths from other major causes have decreased, deaths from Alzheimer's have increased 71 percent since 2000, federal health statistics show. What's more, the number of cases is projected to more than triple by 2050 as the nation's seventy-seven million baby boomers grow older.

In addition to the physical and emotional toll it takes on patients and their families, Alzheimer's is also a costly disease from a health care standpoint. According to the Alzheimer's Association, Medicare spending for patients with dementia is three times higher than for seniors without it, and Medicaid payments are nineteen times higher.

Unfortunately, Big Pharma has logged a disappointing record of failures in attempting to develop new drugs that can reverse Alzheimer's, despite billions of research and investment dollars spent over the past three decades.

Today, doctors typically treat the disorders with drugs that merely slow, but cannot halt, its progression. The US Food and Drug Administration (FDA) has approved two types of Alzheimer's medications—known as cholinesterase inhibitors (Aricept, Exelon, Razadyne) and memantine (Namenda)—to manage the cognitive symptoms (memory loss, confusion, and problems with thinking).

And the race is on among drug companies hunting for a statin-like medication that can prevent or even cure the disease. But while Big Pharma continues to pursue what is regarded as the Holy Grail of medicine—developing what would certainly be a blockbuster Alzheimer's drug—a handful of medical, natural, and alternative approaches have proven to be promising ways to manage, slow, and combat the symptoms of dementia.

In fact, many Alzheimer's specialists believe that we are on the cusp of a new way to combat dementia that harnesses the body's own natural defenses to target and even turn back the mechanisms that lead to the disorder.

Here's a primer.

The Latest Alzheimer's Advances

In just the past two years, scientific researchers have logged more advances in the fight against Alzheimer's than in the previous four decades combined. While that progress has not yet lead to new treatments, experts expect that the research has laid the groundwork for new therapies likely to emerge in the next year or two.

Unlike past drug research, which has focused on developing medications that treat symptoms and attempt to slow Alzheimer's progression, the latest scientific discoveries have centered on compounds and substances that can change brain features and structures in ways that lead to the brain disorder.

Chief among them are amyloid plaque deposits in the brain—abnormal clusters of sticky protein fragments—and neurofibrillary tangles, which are composed of another protein called tau. As the disease progresses, the plaques and tangles build up, leading to the loss of connections between nerve cells. The cells die, causing the loss of brain tissue and, eventually, death.

Just why these tangles and deposits form is unclear (some research suggests that they might be a defense mechanism the brain uses to combat bacterial, viral, and fungal infections), but two recent studies suggest that natural substances in the brain might be used to destroy or eliminate them.

Both centered on a natural brain enzyme called neprilysin that might combat Alzheimer's by essentially digesting plaques in the brain. The first study tested a protein called IL-33—which produces neprilysin—and found that it reversed Alzheimer's-like symptoms in mice in only one week. Researchers believe that IL-33 works by activating the immune cells in the brain, called microglia, which surround amyloid plaques.

In addition to digesting plaques, IL-33 reduces inflammation in brain tissue, which previous studies have found might encourage plaque and tangle formation. Therefore, IL-33 helps clear the amyloid plaque already formed and also prevents the formation of new plaques and tangles.

Eddy Liew of the University of Glasgow, who helped conduct the study, notes that IL-33 is a protein produced by various cell types in the body and is particularly abundant in the central nervous system—the brain and spinal cord. Liew and his team found that injecting mice with the protein led to rapid improvements in their memory and cognitive functions. In the wake of the new findings, researchers have begun clinical trials of IL-33 in Alzheimer's patients to see if it is as effective in humans as in mice.

A second recent study, conducted at the Salk Institute, also involved treating Alzheimer's by increasing the amount of another natural substance found in the brain, neuregulin-1. Like, IL-33, neuregulin-1 increased levels of neprilysin to halt and reverse the buildup of plaque in the brains of mice bred to develop Alzheimer's.

The study builds on previous research that found that treating cells with neuregulin-1 lowered brain levels of a molecule that generates amyloid plaques in the hippocampus, an area of the brain responsible for learning and memory.

The Salk researchers acknowledge that they aren't sure how neuregulin-1 works or affects the brain. But lead researcher Kuo-Fen Lee says the findings offer tantalizing proof that it promotes the removal of brain plaques, can improve memory, and is a promising candidate for a new therapeutic agent.

Lee's team is now exploring whether the protein improves signaling between neurons, a function that is damaged in Alzheimer's. If ongoing studies confirm these promising early results, IL-33 and neuregulin-1 might be developed as supplements. They could then be taken to clear the brain of Alzheimer's plaques—or even prevent their formation—in much the same way that statins are now taken by millions of Americans to clear blood vessels of cholesterol and lower the risk of heart attack and stroke.

Other Promising Treatments in the Pipeline

IL-33 and neuregulin-1 are only two of a growing number of natural plaque-destroying agents recently discovered by scientific researchers.

Among the others that have shown promise are the following:

EPPS. Korean researchers have identified a compound called EPPS, which is similar to the amino acid taurine, that destroys toxic amyloid plaques that build up in the brains of Alzheimer's patients. Taurine is believed to have antioxidant properties and to improve mental and physical performance and is often added to energy drinks.

When taurine was added to the drinking water of mice that had symptoms of Alzheimer's disease, the animals' cognitive function returned to normal, and amyloid plaques were cleared from their brains.

Although EPPS hasn't yet been tried on humans, researchers believe that it has the ability to stop neurodegeneration. According to the Mayo Clinic, up to 3,000 mg of taurine a day is considered safe.

SOLANEZUMAB. The American drug company Eli Lilly has found that an experimental antibody drug called solanezumab slowed the rate of decline in Alzheimer's patients. In patients with mild dementia, solanezumab slowed the progression of the disease over the course of several years by 30 percent. Eli Lilly is now investigating whether the drug would be even more effective if given at an earlier stage of the disease. Solanezumab appears to work by deconstructing the building blocks that form the amyloid plaques and causing them to slowly disintegrate.

ADUCANUMAB. Brain scans of patients treated with another experimental antibody called aducanumab showed a reduction in amyloid plaque in patients who were in the earliest stages of Alzheimer's. The randomized, placebo-controlled trial treated patients for up to fifty-four weeks. In addition to a reduction in plaque, the study found a significant slowing of clinical impairment in patients with mild disease. The higher the dosage a patient was given, the greater the reduction in plaque and the lower the rate of clinical decline.

ULTRASOUND TECHNOLOGY. Australian researchers believe that noninvasive ultrasound can break up brain-clogging amyloid plaques and reverse memory loss. The technique has yet to be tried on humans but was effective when used on mice bred to develop Alzheimer's.

"We're extremely excited by this innovation of treating Alzheimer's without using drug therapeutics," said lead Jürgen Götz of the Queensland Brain Institute (QBI), part of Australia's University of Queensland, in a press release announcing the results. "The ultrasound waves oscillate tremendously quickly, activating microglial cells that digest and remove the amyloid plaques that destroy brain synapses. This treatment restored memory function to the same level of normal healthy mice.

"The word 'breakthrough' is often misused, but in this case, I think this really does fundamentally change our understanding of how to treat this disease, and I foresee a great future for this approach."

Are Statin-like Alzheimer's Drugs Ahead?

In September 2016, a scientist at the biotech giant Biogen shocked the world by predicting that millions of people at risk for Alzheimer's disease will one day take drugs—now in the works—that will block the condition's development in the same way that cholesterol-lowering statins are prescribed to stave off heart attacks.

Dr. Al Sandrock said healthy individuals could be treated with drugs that clear the brain of amyloid plaques, which are thought to cause the disease, decades before people experience memory loss or a decline in their thinking.

"One day you can imagine treating patients with no symptoms if they have amyloid plaques on the brain," Sandrock said. "We do that with cholesterol where people don't have cardiovascular disease."

Sandrock made the comments while discussing the publication of a new study of aducanumab, an experimental Alzheimer's drug developed by Biogen, which is being tested in large late-stage clinical trials.

The study, published in the journal *Nature*, found that the drug was able to clear significant amounts of amyloid plaque from the brain, especially at higher doses, in 166 patients who received it. Researchers reported that those who were given the highest dose of the medicine were virtually free of the sticky plaques after a year of treatment.

New Test Detects Early Alzheimer's

For years, scientists have sought a method to identify brain changes associated with Alzheimer's before memory loss and other symptoms appear so that they can stop or even reverse the changes before they severely affect people's lives.

The most significant step forward in developing such a test was reported in November 2016 by researchers at Washington University School of Medicine in St. Louis. The scientists developed a chemical compound, called Fluselenamyl, that detects amyloid protein clumps linked to Alzheimer's better than current methods.

By incorporating a radioactive atom in the compound, the location of such protein clumps in a living brain can be detected using positron emission tomography (PET) scans.

The compound, described in a paper published in *Scientific Reports*, could be used in brain scans to identify the signs of early stage Alzheimer's disease or to monitor a patient's response to treatment.

"Fluselenamyl is both more sensitive and likely more specific than current agents," explains Dr. Vijay Sharma, PhD, a professor of radiology, neurology, and biomedical engineering and the study's senior author. "Using this compound, I think we can reduce false negatives, potentially do a better job of identifying people in the earliest stages of Alzheimer's disease, and assess the effects of treatments."

Using human amyloid beta proteins, Sharma and colleagues showed that Fluselenamyl bound to such proteins two to ten times better than each of the three FDA-approved imaging agents now used for detecting amyloid beta. In other words, Fluselenamyl detected much smaller clumps of the protein, indicating that it might be able to detect the brain changes associated with Alzheimer's disease earlier.

Sharma now hopes to test the method in patients with early Alzheimer's. "Ideally, we'd like to look at patients with very mild symptoms who are negative for Alzheimer's by PET scan to see if we can identify them using Fluselenamyl," Sharma says. "One day, we may be able to use Fluselenamyl as part of a screening test to identify segments of the population that are going to be at risk for development of Alzheimer's disease. That's the long-term goal."

The Anti-Alzheimer's Diet

Grace Slick famously admonished fans to "feed your head" in Jefferson Airplane's anthemic 1967 hit "White Rabbit." But new nutritional research into the links between diet and Alzheimer's is giving the phrase a whole new meaning.

A convincing body of scientific evidence has linked sugary high-carb diets—not dietary fat—to Alzheimer's, as well as obesity, diabetes, heart disease, and certain cancers. In fact, some researchers now call Alzheimer's disease "type 3 diabetes" because chronically high blood sugar increases the odds of dementia.

In late 2015, the FDA acknowledged the dangers of sugar to the nation's collective mental and physical health, proposing new guidelines that, for the first time, aimed to limit average Americans' consumption of added sugar.

The 2015 US Dietary Guidelines call for added sugar to amount to no more than 10 percent of daily calories. The FDA has also relaxed past recommendations to limit consumption of certain fats once derided as obesity drivers.

To nutritional researchers like Dr. David Perlmutter, the changes are hardly surprising but a welcome acknowledgement of the evolution in conventional dietary thinking. The board-certified neurologist and fellow of the American College of Nutrition has long argued that sugary soft drinks and junk foods are behind millions of Americans' physical ailments as well as rising rates of Alzheimer's.

The good news, he says, is that dietary changes might be the most effective way to stave off the ravages of dementia. In fact, certain kinds of fat in the diet might actually be beneficial for brain health and keep seniors mentally sharp as they age, he notes.

"One of the key ways to help prevent [Alzheimer's] disease is through diet," says Perlmutter, author of the number one *New York Times* best seller *Grain Brain* and, most recently, the bestselling book *Brain Maker*.

Specifically, he recommends what he calls the "anti-Alzheimer's trio"—grass-fed beef, avocados, and coconut oil. All three foods are high in brain-healthy fats that boost memory and cognitive function and reduce inflammation tied to dementia. "These items are all low in carbs and high in fat, helping to reduce some of that brain-bullying inflammation—the root cause of so many ailments," he explains.

Here's why these three superfoods are critical to maintaining healthy brain function as we age:

GRASS-FED BEEF. Unlike conventionally raised livestock (fed mostly grains), cows fed grass produce meat that is much lower in inflammation-producing omega-6 fatty acids. Inflammation—from sugar, carbs, and certain types of meat common in the American diet—hikes the risk for Alzheimer's, heart disease, diabetes, and cancer.

AVOCADOS. This Mexican food staple is naturally nutrient-dense and contains some twenty vitamins and minerals. Consuming fruits and vegetables of all kinds has long been associated with health benefits, but many studies suggest that avocados are particularly helpful in combatting obesity, heart disease, cancer, diabetes, vision loss, and dementia—in part because they have anti-inflammatory properties.

Avocados contain a natural plant sterol called beta-sitosterol, which helps regulate healthy cholesterol levels. They also contain lutein and zeaxanthin—two phytochemicals that are essential to eye health—bone-strengthening vitamin K, and cancer-fighting folate, which also combats depression and other mental health disorders.

COCONUT OIL. This common oil is loaded with saturated fats, which actually raise "good" high-density lipoprotein (HDL) cholesterol and make "bad" low-density lipoprotein (LDL) cholesterol less dangerous. As a result, it can improve your cholesterol levels naturally, which lowers your risk for heart disease and Alzheimer's. Specifically, coconut oil is also a rich source of brain-healthy beta-HBA.

Other Brain Foods
A number of other foods also contain ingredients that prevent neurodegenerative disorders. Among them are the following:

BLUEBERRIES. Already known for their ability to lower the risk of heart disease and cancer, blueberries might also help fight the devastating effects of Alzheimer's, according to new research by the University of Cincinnati Academic Health Center. For the study, adults aged sixty-eight and older who had mild cognitive impairment ate freeze-dried blueberry powder equivalent to 1 cup of fresh berries or a placebo powder for sixteen weeks. Those taking the blueberry powder had a marked improvement in cognitive abilities compared to those who took the placebo powder. Functional magnetic resonance imaging (fMRI) also showed increased brain activity in those who took the blueberry powder.

BLACKBERRIES. In order to process new information, our brain cells need to "talk" to each other. Yet as we age, those cells become inflamed, making it harder for them to communicate with one another. Blackberries provide potent antioxidants called polyphenols that reduce the inflammation and encourage communication between neurons, improving our ability to process new information.

APPLES. America's favorite fruits are a leading source of quercetin, an antioxidant plant chemical that defends your brain cells from free radical attacks, which can damage the outer lining of delicate neurons and eventually lead to cognitive decline. To get the most quercetin, be sure to eat your apples with the skin on, since that is where the greatest concentration is found.

CINNAMON. Emerging research from the University of California, Santa Barbara (UCSB) reveals that two compounds in cinnamon—proanthocyanidins and cinnamaldehyde—might inactivate tau proteins in the brain, which cause cells to die in Alzheimer's patients, and help prevent age-related cognitive declines.

LEAFY GREENS. Spinach, kale, and other vibrant-green vegetables are beneficial. They have lutein, beta-carotene, folate, and vitamin K. The antioxidants in leafy green vegetables counter age-related oxidative stress, further strengthening brain cells over the years. Spinach in particular is very high in nutrients that prevent dementia. Only ½ cup of cooked spinach provides a third of the folate and five times the vitamin K of your daily needs. A landmark neurology study by the Rush Institute for Healthy Aging in Chicago revealed that eating three servings of leafy green, yellow, and cruciferous vegetables daily can delay cognitive decline by 40 percent. Of these three, leafy greens were found to be the most protective.

EXTRA VIRGIN OLIVE OIL. Amyloid B–derived diffusible ligands (ADDLs) are Alzheimer's disease–inducing proteins that are toxic to the brain. In the initial stages of the disease, they attach to brain cells, rendering them unable to communicate with one another and eventually leading to memory loss. Extra virgin olive oil is rich in oleocanthal, a compound that disables the action of dangerous ADDLs. As an added bonus, olive oil also appears to satisfy hunger pangs. One study found that restaurant goers given the option of olive oil instead of butter consume fewer calories during a meal.

SALMON. This fatty fish is a leading source of docosapentaenoic acid (DHA), the predominant omega-3 fatty acid in your brain, believed to protect against Alzheimer's disease. It is also nature's number-one source of vitamin D, a nutrient that plays an important role in the prevention of cognitive decline. Salmon protects the brain from inflammation that is thought to damage healthy neuron communication. The omega-3 fats in salmon not only fortify memory and cognition but also boost mood levels and combat depression. You'll consume 2,000 mg of omega-3 fatty acid from just 4 ounces of salmon.

TURMERIC. This unique spice is a cousin of ginger and one of the main spices used in Asian curry dishes. Turmeric is especially rich in curcumin, a compound believed to inhibit Alzheimer's disease in multiple ways. Not only does it block the formation of beta-amyloid plaques; it also fights inflammation and lowers artery-clogging cholesterol, which can reduce blood flow to your brain.

CONCORD GRAPE JUICE. Researchers are increasingly finding that what's good for your heart is also good for your brain. The same heart-healthy polyphenols in red wine and grape juice that improve your cardiovascular function can give your brain a boost. Similar to the polyphenols found in blackberries, they also improve the communication between brain cells.

ROSEMARY. England's Northumbria University found that rosemary essential oil improves the memory of people over age sixty-five. The study, which focused on prospective memory—the ability to remember when events are to take place and to remember to complete tasks at specific times—is essential for everyday functioning. Researchers diffused rosemary and lavender essential oil by placing four drops on an aroma diffuser and switching it on five minutes before the participants entered the testing room. Seniors who sniffed rosemary significantly enhanced their alertness and prospective memory compared to people who were assigned to a room with no aroma. Lavender significantly increased their feelings of calmness and contentedness compared to those who had no aroma in their testing room.

NUTS. Anything that is good for your circulatory system is also good for your brain because the blood vessels in the brain are important in terms of cognition and memory. Nuts are an excellent source of healthy fats. Research has shown that walnuts, in particular, contain compounds that promote healthy brain cell function. Perhaps that's why walnuts look like miniature brains.

YOGURT AND OTHER FERMENTED FOODS. Probiotics, prebiotics, and fermented foods help maintain a healthy balance of bacteria in your gut, which research shows can boost mental health and might even help stave off dementia.

Healthy Habits Combat Memory Loss

Dr. Kevin Passero, one of the nation's leading naturopathic physicians, agrees that dietary changes are among the wisest strategies to preventing or combating dementia. But a host of other lifestyle changes can also keep you mentally sharp as you age.

"Alzheimer's disease is a runaway train barreling down on all of us," says Passero, coauthor of *Save Your Brain from Alzheimer's and Dementia*.

In addition to cutting out sugar and choosing healthy fats—including pasture-raised meat and eggs, wild-caught fish, olive oil, and nuts—Passero notes that many studies have shown that lowering your blood pressure, cholesterol, and stress levels (via exercise, meditation, and yoga) can also reduce your risk of developing dementia.

He also believes that toxic heavy metals—such as iron, manganese, copper, zinc, and chromium—are linked to Alzheimer's. These metals are in everything, including the water we drink, the food we eat, and many household and personal care products we use. Passero's advice is to read product labels carefully to avoid household items and dietary sources of metals.

Dr. Gary Small, a professor of psychiatry and aging and the director of the University of California, Los Angeles (UCLA) Longevity Center, also believes that while it's true that brain changes are inevitable as we age, some simple yet effective steps can help us maintain our mental edge as we get older.

"Making the right lifestyle choices can have tremendous benefits for brain health," says Small, coauthor of *Two Weeks to a Younger Brain* with Gigi Vorgan and author of the *Brain Health Report* newsletter. "It's not surprising that we all have concern about age-related memory slips," he adds. "The truth is that most of these middle-aged pauses and senior moments are harmless and do not progress. But as we reach older ages, the risk that they will progress to Alzheimer's disease or some other form of dementia that interferes with daily functioning increases.

"The good news is that lifestyle changes we make every day can have a major impact on age-related brain health. Physical exercise, good nutrition, stress management, and mental stimulation can lower our risk for cognitive decline."

Here are ten other healthy habits that Passero, Small, and other experts say can keep your brain healthy:

TAKE YOUR VITAMINS. Many Americans are deficient in vitamins D and B12, which can lead to all sorts of cognitive trouble. "Both have profound effects on brain function and mood," says integrative psychiatrist Dr. James Greenblatt. "Nutritional deficiencies of these two vitamins have been found to exacerbate symptoms of depression, anxiety, and even contribute to memory loss and cognitive decline."

WATCH YOUR DRUG INTAKE. Psychoactive drugs, both natural and pharmaceutical, can impair brain function and become addictive, warn experts. "Instead, pursue a wide variety of generally accepted health measures, including rest, moderate physical exercise, mental exercise, meditation, prayer, and other practices that calm the mind and lift the spirit," says psychiatrist Dr. Peter Breggin.

GET IN TUNE. Music can soothe the wild beast—and boost brainpower. Called the "Mozart Effect," listening to classical tunes appears to improve cognitive function. "Musical activity involves nearly every region of the brain that we know about and nearly every neural subsystem," notes psychologist Daniel J. Levitin in his book *This Is Your Brain on Music*. One study showed that classical music helped with cognition and memory testing. But if you are not a classical buff, keep listening to your favorites tunes. fMRI studies indicate that listening to music sparks chemical reactions in the brain that can lift mood.

CRACK YOURSELF UP. Do something that makes you laugh. In one study, older people who watched a funny video performed better on memory tests. Humor also helps our brains stay young by lowering stress levels. Watching a half-hour television comedy has been shown to lower blood biomarkers of stress.

EMBRACE MOTHER NATURE. The great outdoors has a rejuvenating cerebral effect, according to a Stanford University study that used brain scans to compare people who walked in urban areas versus natural surroundings. "Nature experience, even of a short duration, can decrease a pattern of thinking that is associated with the onset of mental illnesses like depression," says the study's lead author, Gregory Bratman.

LEARN SOMETHING NEW. Seniors who learn new things, such as how to quilt or play a musical instrument, can improve their cognitive abilities, concludes a University of Texas at Dallas study. "It is important to get out and do something that is unfamiliar and mentally challenging," notes lead researcher Denise Park.

DITCH THE TV REMOTE. Staring at the boob tube for hours can be mind-numbing. A long-term study found that sedentary young adults who watched four or more hours of TV a day were twice as likely to suffer from cognitive decline in middle age. "This is something you can do something about," says researcher Kristin Yaffe.

BREAK THE ROUTINE. Run your normal jogging route backward, take a different way home from work, and try new restaurants in your area. Your brain gets lazy when you go to the same places and do the same things all the time, notes clinical neuropsychologist Paul Nussbaum, author of *Save Your Brain*. Give your brain a workout by shaking things up.

MAKE NEW FRIENDS. Social connections are good for brain connections. "People with rich social networks are mentally shaper and have less risk of dementia. If you take up a new activity and make friends doing it, you are doubling the brain benefits," says neurologist Dr. Marie Pasinski, author of the book *Beautiful Brain, Beautiful You*.

CHILL OUT. Stress is bad news for your gray matter because it releases the hormone cortisol, which causes brain atrophy. "You can improve your brain health by practicing stress management on a daily basis with things like deep breathing, meditation, yoga, or journaling," says chiropractor Carri Drzyzga. In one recent study, MRI tests performed on people who meditated found positive changes in the brain, including in the memory center. To get started, try the five-five-five rule: take five seconds to breathe in, five seconds to hold the breath, and five seconds to release it. Meditation not only lowers stress levels and improves mood; it strengthens neural circuits and increases mental focus.

SPELL IT OUT. If you can't seem to remember the name of someone you just met, try Small's memory technique "Look, Snap, Connect." *Look* is a reminder to focus attention. *Snap* means to create mental snapshots of what we want to remember. "For example, if the person's last name is Wolfe, picture the animal and make the connection," he explains. *Connect* is a way of linking the information to give it meaning. When something is meaningful to us personally, it becomes memorable.

SLEEP WELL. Neurologist Dr. Romie Mushtag says sleep is the key to mental health: "Sleep is sacred. When we deprive ourselves of sleep, we deprive our minds and bodies of critical rest and healing time. The end result of sleep deprivation is poor focus, declining memory and cognition, depression, imbalanced hormones, and weight gain."

Six Supplements That Boost Mental Health

A "smart pill" has long been the subject of science fiction and real-world scientific speculation. But research shows that a handful of dietary supplements might be the next best thing and can keep your brain in top form.

"Natural supplements can help our brains function better, faster, and more efficiently," says Dr. Ray Sahelian, author of *Brain Boosters*. "There is no doubt that they influence brain health and in many cases are equivalent or superior to pharmaceutical drugs."

Here are six that are worth looking into:

Ginkgo biloba. This herb has been used in traditional Chinese medicine for thousands of years. Supplements, which use the plant's leaves, boost mental functioning by increasing blood circulation to the brain. A study from the University of Miami Miller School of Medicine found that ginkgo biloba improved the brain's speed in making connections in healthy older adults by 68 percent. Researchers at UCLA examined the effects of gingko biloba in patients who complained of mild age-related memory loss and found that it improved verbal recall. Since ginkgo biloba has side effects, including insomnia and blood thinning properties, Sahelian recommends a conservative dosage of 40 mg twice a week.

Acetyl-L-carnitine (ALC or ALCAR). Several clinical trials indicate that ALC delays the onset of age-related cognitive decline and can increase cognitive function in the elderly. Sahelian believes that ALC can cross the blood-brain barrier, where it helps produce brain chemicals, keeps mitochondria (the cell's energy powerhouses) from deteriorating, and helps regenerate neurons. "You can feel mentally sharper with more mental stamina and be more focused and alert within a few hours of taking acetyl-L-carnitine," says Sahelian. He advises taking 200–300 mg in the morning on an empty stomach.

Alpha-lipoic acid. Some studies have found that this substance can enhance the body's ability to synthesize glutathione, the main antioxidant found in cells. "Alpha-lipoic acid is a powerful antioxidant that offers benefits you won't find in other antioxidants," says Sahelian. A study published in the *Journal of Neural Transmission* found that alpha-lipoic acid stabilized cognitive function in a small group of Alzheimer's disease patients. For long-term use to improve health, Sahelian recommends 10–50 mg of R-alpha-lipoic acid (the most powerful type) daily.

Omega-3 fatty acids. Researchers at Rhode Island Hospital found that the brains of older adults who took fish oil, which contains omega-3 fatty acids, suffered significantly less cognitive decline and brain shrinkage than those who didn't take fish oil. A recent study in the *FASEB Journal*—published by the Federation of American Societies for Experimental Biology—found that fish oil reduced brain inflammation and the buildup of amyloid plaque, a hallmark of

Alzheimer's. Other studies have also indicated that omega-3 fatty acids help people who have mild Alzheimer's disease. "I recommend that everyone take two capsules a day," says Sahelian. "Since current drugs used for Alzheimer's disease are not very helpful and are potentially dangerous, perhaps doctors should try omega-3 fatty acids first."

Curcumin. This active component of turmeric, a spice found in many Indian dishes, is a potent anti-inflammatory and fights free radicals that promote aging. A study at UCLA found that curcumin might treat Alzheimer's by slowing the buildup of amyloid plaques in the brain. Sahelian advises, "Take a capsule with a meal several times a week." Sahelian often suggests antioxidants in amounts smaller than recommended by other antiaging experts. "More antioxidant supplements may not lead to more benefits," he says. "There comes a point where a supplement, no matter how benign, can become unhealthy if the doses are too high."

Pycnogenol. An extract of French maritime pine bark, this supplement can significantly improve memory, attention span, decision making, and the ability to manage everyday tasks, according to the latest research. A recently published yearlong study compared the effects of a healthy lifestyle, with and without Pycnogenol supplements, on seventy-seven people between the ages of fifty-five and seventy. Everyone in the study ate a healthy diet with reduced caffeine, salt, and sugar; exercised regularly; and slept at least eight hours per night. Although this type of lifestyle program is good for overall health, by itself, it did not produce significant cognitive improvement in attention span and mood. But by the end of the study period, thirty-nine people who did not take the supplement experienced slight declines in memory and the ability to deal with people and manage money. By contrast, thirty-eight people who took 50 mg of Pycnogenol twice daily experienced improvements in attention span, memory, ability to manage finances, interpersonal skills, and judgment.

"It's a super antioxidant, and it works on the collagen and elastin in the body," explains Dr. Fred Pescatore, an integrative physician in New York City and author of *The Hamptons Diet* and other health books. "If you keep the collagen and elastin healthy in the blood vessels, it keeps them open. And if you keep blood vessels open, you allow more blood flow to get to all of your organs, and when you allow more blood flow, you allow more oxygen, and everything stays healthier." More than three hundred studies have tested the supplement and found many benefits, from reduced blood pressure, cholesterol, diabetes, wrinkles, and jet lag to improvements in allergies, asthma, premenstrual syndrome (PMS), menopause symptoms, osteoarthritis, endometriosis, attention deficit hyperactivity disorder (ADHD), and circulatory problems.

In addition to these six supplements, Sahelian says that a healthy diet, especially one that includes a wide variety of vegetables, is essential for a healthy brain. "People who eat their vegetables daily keep their minds sharp into old age," he says. "Vary the fruits and vegetables you eat because each vegetable and fruit has a unique combination of carotenoids and flavonoids."

He recommends consuming juices daily made from vegetables as well as fruits, especially carrots, beets, celery, cucumbers, oranges, apples, green leafy vegetables, and berries. "These juices add hundreds of types of antioxidants and other natural anti-inflammatories that can't be found in capsules or tablets," says Sahelian. "A diet dense in nutrients should be your first step to a healthy brain. Then add brain-boosting supplements."

Is It Memory Loss or Signs of Dementia?
Five Signs That Could Spell Trouble

Nearly all of us have done it—misplaced the car keys, forgotten why we've walked into a room, or been unable to come up with the name of an acquaintance. But when are simple memory lapses a sign of a deeper problem or early dementia?

Here are five examples of normal age-related memory changes versus symptoms that might indicate that you or a loved one is be suffering early signs of dementia and should consult a health care professional:

Daily tasks. Normal: You are able to function independently, despite occasional memory lapses. Caution: You have difficulty with simple tasks such as paying bills, dressing, or practicing good personal hygiene.

Forgetfulness. Normal: You are able to recall and describe periods of forgetfulness. Caution: You can't recall the times when memory loss caused problems.

Sense of direction. Normal: You sometimes need to ask for directions but don't get lost in familiar places. Caution: You get lost in familiar surroundings or can't follow directions.

Speech patterns. Normal: You occasionally have difficulty finding the right word but can carry on a conversation. Caution: Words are frequently misused, forgotten, or garbled. Phrases and stories are repeated during a conversation.

Judgment. Normal: Judgment and decision-making ability are the same. Caution: You have trouble making choices, exhibit poor judgment, or have inappropriate social behavior.

Not Your Average Joe: Namath Working to End Injury-Related Dementia

Joe Namath has been known for many things. His dazzling performance on the gridiron earned him a spot in the Pro Football Hall of Fame. His larger-than-life persona off the field garnered him the nickname "Broadway Joe." And he even had a minor acting career, starring in several 1970s movies and TV series.

But now Namath is working to make his name synonymous with something else entirely—namely, finding a cure for NFL players suffering from traumatic brain injuries sustained on the field that can lead to or accelerate Alzheimer's disease.

The legendary New York Jets quarterback has lent his name and considerable celebrity to a small medical start-up in South Florida—the Joe Namath Neurological Research Center—that is using hyperbaric oxygen therapy to treat traumatic brain injuries.

Since the center's founding in 2015, the center's medical director—Dr. Lee Fox, an old friend and golfing buddy of Namath's—has been bringing new hope to NFL players and others suffering from brain injuries. Among them, Namath himself.

"After seeing some of my teammates, a couple of [them] literally deteriorate and pass on . . . I began to analyze and monitor myself, so to speak," Namath says, explaining what motivated him to become the center's first patient for the treatment of mild symptoms that he attributes to repeated head injuries he sustained during his NFL career.

He recalls thinking, "How is my mind working these days?" or occasionally walking from one room of his home into another and wondering, "Why did I come in here?" So Namath approached Fox to see if hyperbaric therapy could improve his condition. He went through a battery of tests—for memory and cognition—as well as single-photon emission computerized tomography (SPECT) brain scans. Then he underwent dozens of treatments over nearly seven months.

After even the first few treatments, Namath says he could feel his mind becoming sharper—his thinking more focused, his memory getting better. And today, he says he's never felt better.

"My thinking is much clearer," says Namath, seventy-four. "Finding the right words has become easier, and I remember events with more clarity. One of the really great results is that my sleep has improved; I sleep more soundly and have vivid dreams."

What's more, Fox notes, is that SPECT scans of Joe's brain showed notable improvements in blood flow and activity in key areas tied to memory and higher-level thinking. Regions that had appeared dark in scans—suggesting brain cell death—began to light up after his therapy, showing new neurological activity that indicates the neurons were "coming back to life," he explains.

"He went through 120 treatments over 200-plus days . . . and he continued to improve the whole time," says Fox, chief of radiology at Jupiter Medical and codirector of the center with Dr. Barry Miskin.

Namath could also see for himself the improvements in the brain scans as he continued to receive therapy. "I was able to literally see the change take place in my brain," he recalls. "Each one showed a marked improvement to where my most recent one is wonderful."

Follow-up tests conducted a year after he completed his therapy showed that the benefits of the therapy were lasting and permanent. "We put him through the testing again—the cognitive testing, the SPECT scan—and all the improvements he had over the previous year were all maintained," Fox explains. "His SPECT scan remained normal; his cognitive exam remained normal. And to this day, he continues to feel great."

Questions about the long-term effects of repeated blows to the head have become a major focus of the NFL and neurological researchers in recent years. League officers have changed the rules of the game, outlawing certain helmet-to-helmet tackling techniques that were once common and put players at risk. The NFL recently reported that as many as one-third of players—who sustain hundreds or even thousands of head blows over a career—can be expected to show brain injury.

At the same time, a growing number of studies have tied head injuries to an increased risk for suicide and a variety of mental health problems—including depression, dementia (including Alzheimer's), Parkinson's, and Lou Gehrig's disease. Research out of the University of Pennsylvania and Boston University has also found that football players and others who suffer head injuries often have certain types of brain damage that has been linked to aggressive behavior and violence.

And crime statistics tell us that domestic violence arrests are three to four times higher among NFL players than in the general population.

Several high-profile cases have brought the issue to national attention in recent years—including the recent Ray Rice domestic violence affair and the suicides of Kansas City Chiefs linebacker Jovan Belcher, Philadelphia Eagles star safety Belcher Andre Waters, Chicago Bears safety Dave Duerson, and Atlanta Falcons safety Ray Easterling.

Hyperbaric therapy is an alternative medical practice, and its effectiveness in treating brain injuries tied to Alzheimer's has only recently been studied. Such injuries occur when brain cells can't get enough oxygen to produce new cells. Doctors feed high volumes of oxygen into the brain to awaken dormant brain cells, reduce the extent of brain damage, and speed recovery and rehabilitation.

Namath's interest in oxygen therapy as a potential treatment for head injuries was sparked by the tragic suicide of former NFL linebacker Junior Seau in 2012. An autopsy revealed the forty-three-year-old suffered from chronic traumatic encephalopathy (CET)—a progressive degenerative brain disease found in athletes and others with a history of repetitive brain trauma.

At the time, Namath wasn't certain if he himself had any personal neurological issues, but Seau's death prompted him to wonder if he unknowingly suffered any lasting effects as a result of at least five concussions he sustained during his thirteen seasons in the NFL.

"Although he clearly had a history of head trauma by playing in the NFL, Joe wasn't suffering from chronic brain injury, but he had some very mild symptoms," Fox says. "He started to notice some of the very earlier signs of [mild] cognitive impairment—certainly nothing severe, [but] enough to kind of say, 'Maybe I should kind of check this out?' And when we evaluated him, we thought we could actually help him, even with his mild symptoms. And so he was our first patient to go through our trial."

The scans performed on Namath's brain showed that he did have signs of injury, particularly on the left side of his brain—where he would have received the most impact during sacks as a right-handed quarterback—and the back of his head from falls he likely suffered while trying to hold onto the ball while being tackled.

According to Fox, "after his first group of treatments, he noticed a remarkable result. His SPECT scans . . . had turned completely normal . . . His cognitive examination improved. And subjectively, he felt much better. His sleep is better, his memory is better, his word finding is better."

As his treatments continued, so did the improvements in Namath's scans and cognitive functions. Today, he says is grateful for the benefits he has seen and hopeful that they will translate into improvements for potentially millions of other Americans with traumatic brain injuries.

Fox hopes the center's clinical trial will build on Namath's success so such treatments might become standard care.

"The ultimate goal is to generate enough data so that this could be covered treatment for insurance companies," he says.

He also credits Namath for allowing the center to take its research to the next level, noting that it was not an easy decision to go public with his own mental health struggles.

"It speaks volumes of his character," says Fox, sounding as much like a long-time friend as Namath's personal physician. "The fact that he is willing to put himself out there an example to raise awareness . . . shows the kind of man he is.

"He's concerned about himself, but even more concerned about people suffering with chronic brain injury. And we're fortunate to have him in our community and to be in support of our hospital. But I think the county is lucky to have him as a spokesperson for such an important disease."

For more information, visit the Joe Namath Neurological Research Center's website at http://www.namathneurocenter.com.

Music Rejuvenates Alzheimer's Patients

"Where words fail, music speaks." That famous quote, attributed to Hans Christian Andersen, is being given new meaning by a growing body of research showing that music has extraordinary healing powers for dementia sufferers.

A spate of new studies has found that music can not only improve the mood of Alzheimer's disease patients, but listening to favorite songs also boosts their memories, thinking, and cognitive skills in ways scientists are just beginning to understand.

Mental health specialists say new studies provide compelling evidence that music is making significant gains in the treatment of Alzheimer's—an incurable disease with no effective therapy.

"There is relatively strong evidence with respect with music's ability to affect behavior, such as reducing anxiety and agitation," says Sarah Lock, senior vice president of policy, research, and international affairs at AARP, which recently spotlighted the latest in the emerging field of music therapy for dementia patients in the organization's *AARP Bulletin*.

Lock notes the most exciting scientific findings show people with dementia who listen to their favorite style of music score better on tests of cognitive skills, including memory and learning. "A study out of Boston University found people can learn things better if they're listening to . . . their favorite songs," she explains. "So if we could understand more about that and apply to it to people in treatment, it would really help."

Scientists believe that music might affect the brain in ways that are beyond the normal channels of intellectual processes that are damaged by dementia. That might explain why some Alzheimer's patients can remember songs they learned as children, even when they can't remember the names of their own kids.

For this reason, music might be as important—or more so—than medication to dementia patients, says neurologist Oliver Sacks in his book *Musicophilia*, adding that music "can have a power beyond anything else to restore them to themselves."

Lock, who lost both of her parents to Alzheimer's, says she has seen the benefits of music therapy in dementia care facilities and in her personal life. "We don't know exactly why, but people talk about the ability of music to affect the natural rhythms [of the brain]," she says. "My father, who was not musically inclined, could sing the 'Battle Hymn of the Republic' until the very last."

Among the many research projects involving music therapy and Alzheimer's, a handful of studies stand out:

- Neurologists at the Boston University Alzheimer's Disease Center have found dementia patients have a much easier time recalling words that are sung to them rather than spoken. This approach might help them learn tasks, such as when to take their medication (with instructions encapsulated in songs).
- George Mason University researchers have found that dementia patients who regularly sang songs like "Somewhere over the Rainbow" and "Isn't It Romantic?" scored better on cognitive and memory tests over a four-month period.
- Music therapist Connie Tomaino, who founded the Institute for Music and Neurologic Function, has conducted numerous studies showing people with dementia respond to songs that are meaningful to them, triggering and strengthening memory.
- Other researchers have found that pairing music with everyday activities helps dementia patients better recall how to do them, singing songs from a person's youth can spark other memories, and up-tempo tunes stimulate both mental and physical activity.

Some states, including Wisconsin and Utah, are incorporating music therapy into their Alzheimer's care facilities and home health care programs. Documentary filmmaker Michael Rossato-Bennett also chronicled the rise of music therapy in his recent film *Alive Inside*, which profiles Music & Memory—a program that is now used in one thousand nursing homes worldwide.

With no effective treatments for Alzheimer's—available drugs merely slow its progression—Lock predicts that music therapy will gain popularity in the decades ahead, as the number of Americans with Alzheimer's grows as the baby boomers grow older.

"[There are a lot] of good reasons for that," she says. "It's cheap, it's effective, it involves the caregiver in terms of interaction with the patient, and . . . although there is no cure for people with dementia, music can greatly enhance their quality of life."

She adds that AARP is developing an app to help caregivers find individualized music for patients. But even burning a CD or creating an iPod playlist of favorite songs for a friend or relative with dementia can have a positive effect on that person's quality of life.

"The whole idea of individualized music is that you can connect with people with that kind of music," Lock says. "It's absolutely critical from a policy perspective that you can actually positively affect people's lives."

Glen Campbell's Farewell Song Hits Home

Glen Campbell has become the most visible face of Alzheimer's since Ronald Reagan. The country music legend's swan song and video, "I'm Not Gonna Miss You," is a heartrending musical reflection on his battle with dementia—one that has hit home with relatives and advocates of Alzheimer's sufferers across the country.

The song, which went viral shortly after its 2015 release, was just one in a series of courageous efforts by Campbell; his wife, Kim; and their three children to publicize the singer-guitarist's struggles with the memory-robbing disease.

Jimmy Webb—the legendary songwriter who wrote the rhinestone cowboy's biggest hits, including "Wichita Lineman" and "By the Time I get to Phoenix"—says the Campbells' decision to go public with his story is both difficult and brave: "Believe me, if there were a way for me to change this lyric, I would. Glen is one of my dearest friends."

Campbell first revealed he had Alzheimer's several years ago, when the condition forced him to curtail his touring and recording. He then went on to do a farewell tour that was filmed for a 2014 documentary, *Glen Campbell . . . I'll Be Me*, which followed him on the road and chronicled the progression of his disease.

Webb says the early indications of Campbell's advancing dementia were subtle. He'd occasionally forget the words to some of his favorite songs while the two were performing together several years ago, Webb recalls. But only those who knew him well would notice the memory lapses.

"It just started out with him like maybe forgetting a couple of lines in a song, and I'd kind of look at him and I'd think, you know, time to cut back on the red wine or something like that," says Webb.

But before long, it became clear that those little episodes were more than just minor bouts of forgetfulness. Webb and his wife, Laura Savini, have been in close contact with the Campbell family through the various phases of the disease.

"There's certain stages of the disease where—I don't know how to put this, but—it's almost like cute. There's an endearing quality to it, almost like having a child, having a very precocious child," Webb says. "But then it goes from there very quickly to a place where it's no longer that; it's something else. And it really requires constant attention."

Webb hails Campbell as "a true musical genius" who was an important inspiration in his youth. He first heard Campbell on the radio as a teen growing up on a farm in Elk City, Oklahoma, and decided he wanted to write music.

He calls "Wichita Lineman," which won a Grammy in 1968, "a perfect record." In light of Campbell's advancing dementia, the song has taken on a poignant new meaning—particularly in the fading walk-off line: "He's still on the line."

Although Webb's songs have been performed by many artists over the years—including Frank Sinatra ("Didn't We"), Art Garfunkel ("All I Know"), Kris Kristofferson, Johnny Cash, Willie Nelson, Waylon Jennings ("The Highwayman"), the Fifth Dimension ("Up, Up and Away"), Joe Cocker ("The Moon's a Harsh Mistress"), Donna Summer, Richard Harris ("MacArthur Park"), and Brad Paisley ("Galveston")—Campbell has been the most public voice for his music.

"We were counting up the other day that he's recorded about seventy or eighty different songs of mine," Webb says. "So basically, he would record everything that I wrote, and out of those songs came some hits. But certainly not all of them were hits, and some of them are just absolutely gorgeous and nobody ever heard them.

"He recorded 'The Highwayman' first—before Johnny Cash and Willie and Kris and those guys. And he recorded so many other things of mine. He was the first to record them, and they actually went on to become hits for somebody else."

Campbell's final release, "I'm Not Gonna Miss You," was recorded in 2013.

"I'm still here, but yet I'm gone; I don't play guitar or sing my songs," Campbell begins, and then pays tribute to his wife, Kim, singing, "You're the last person I will love, you're the last face I will recall."

In the accompanying video, Campbell's moving lyrics are punctuated by personal videos and clips of performances marking his five-decade musical career.

Among the film's most striking images is footage of a doctor showing Campbell X-rays of his brain and explaining how the disease will steal his memory.

Is Alzheimer's Caused by Infections?

Alzheimer's disease might be linked to the brain's attempt to battle past infections, according to a new study suggesting that debris left over from the fight leads to the condition.

The study, published in the journal *Science Translational Medicine*, suggests that in an effort to fight off infections, the brain's defense system creates a sticky cage made of beta-amyloid proteins to trap invading microbes. The remains of those cages over time become the plaque commonly associated with Alzheimer's.

"Our findings raise the intriguing possibility that [amyloid proteins] may play a protective role in innate immunity and infectious or sterile inflammatory stimuli may drive amyloidosis," said the researchers, led by Dr. Michael W. Weiner, a radiology professor at the University of California, San Francisco.

The idea that infections might be a cause of Alzheimer's isn't new—a contemporary of Alois Alzheimer proposed the idea in 1910, but it's been mainly ignored by modern scientists.

But that might be changing as new research confirms this century-old idea. If it proves true, antibiotics, antivirals, and antifungal medicines might prove to be promising new ways to treat Alzheimer's.

Magazine: ADHD Epidemic and the Massive Overprescribing of Stimulants

An epidemic of ADHD is spreading across America, and vast numbers of American children and adults are being diagnosed and treated with amphetamines.

Doctors have diagnosed ADHD in about 15 percent of American children, and they routinely prescribe stimulants such as Adderall and Ritalin to help kids focus and concentrate. But the diagnosis is correct only about a third of the time, says Alan Schwarz, author of *ADHD Nation: Children, Doctors, Big Pharma, and the Making of an American Epidemic*. He argues that doctors are prescribing ADHD drugs for millions of children who don't need and shouldn't be taking them.

Schwarz began investigating the overuse of stimulants after he learned that kids in high school were abusing the medications.

"Kids were abusing and snorting Adderall before taking their ACTs," says the Pulitzer Prize–nominated investigative reporter for *The New York Times*. "I saw it as an academic pressure thing," he says. "That in itself was horrifying, but when

I started researching, I found out how the kids got the medication. They were either faking ADHD to their doctors or buying the pills from someone who had been diagnosed."

Further research revealed that the American Psychiatric Association's Diagnostic and Statistical Manual of Mental Disorders claims that ADHD affects 5 percent of American children—far fewer than the actual number who are being diagnosed and treated for the disorder.

"That's millions of children being told there is something wrong with their brain when there probably isn't," Schwarz says. "It was abundantly clear that the system by which the kids got diagnosed with ADHD and got the prescriptions was completely out of whack."

ADHD: A Real but Overdiagnosed Condition

Schwarz doesn't deny that ADHD is a real condition or that millions of children and their families have been helped by treatment with Adderall and other stimulants.

"I've never questioned the legitimacy of the ADHD diagnosis itself," he said. "It's not for me to say. Some kids really struggle with it. The problem is we're diagnosing 15 percent of children, not 5 percent."

ADHD is a complex disorder that can affect a child's success in school and also their relationships with family and friends. It can be difficult to diagnose, and symptoms vary but include the following characteristics:

- constant motion
- daydreaming
- distractibility
- excessive talking
- fidgeting
- impatience
- inappropriate outbursts of anger
- not finishing tasks, whether chores or homework
- not paying attention when spoken to

"If the kid fits the constructs of ADHD, intervening at that point with medications is not a bad thing to do," Schwarz says. "Parents may be at their wit's end. They have tried everything to help their child and are desperate. But we're doing a rotten job of distinguishing the kids that actually have ADHD from others who are having problems but don't have ADHD. Adderall might not be the treatment they need."

Why Are Drugs Overprescribed for ADHD?

Children are overprescribed ADHD medications for several reasons. First, the condition is difficult and time-consuming to diagnose properly. Many physicians just take note of symptoms and bow to the parents' demands that their children be diagnosed with the condition and medicated.

Second, drugs are often the first-line treatment option, even though nondrug alternatives—such as cognitive behavior therapy (CBT)—are viable options that have been proven to be very effective in many cases.

"CBT is expensive, and it's difficult to find a provider who is qualified, so it's much easier to give [the child] the drug, which is inexpensive, and see if it helps," Schwarz says. "The medical establishment tells parents that studies have shown that medication works best, which is actually not true. Parents have been getting all of these signals saying 'Give them the drugs, it'll be OK' from doctors, friends, experience, and ads from the pharmaceutical companies."

Third, pharmaceutical companies have undertaken long-term, successful marketing campaigns that have expanded the perception of ADHD to include relatively normal behavior such as impatience and carelessness, says Schwarz. Big Pharma has also exaggerated ADHD medications' benefits.

It's also true that some parents think that a prescription of Adderall or Ritalin is the passport to good grades, so they push doctors to prescribe the drugs, Schwarz notes.

But a recent study at Florida International University in Miami, which was published in the *Journal of Consulting and Clinical Psychology*, found that stimulants might not help improve grades and that behavioral therapy was more effective than stimulants.

Drug Prescriptions Continue to Rise

Schwarz argues that the current situation is intolerable, noting that if prescription trends continue, five hundred thousand more children will be diagnosed with ADHD in 2017.

"While we need to find the kids that would benefit from stimulant medication, we don't need to give the medication to those who wouldn't benefit," he says. "It's not appropriate therapy for them. You wouldn't give chemotherapy to a kid with pneumonia, so why are we giving amphetamines to kids who are struggling but don't have ADHD?"

These misdiagnosed children suffer the consequences. "Giving millions of kids medicine they don't need doesn't make any sense," says Schwarz. "I don't know of any other medical condition that allows for that high rate of misdiagnosis. It's indefensible, and yet the powers that be argue that everything's hunky-dory. I don't see how anyone could make that case."

Natural Help for ADHD

For children who truly have ADHD, many natural treatments have shown promise.

Test for food allergies. Pediatric neurologist Dr. Joseph Edgar has found that 90 percent of children with ADHD have allergies or intolerances. In most cases, removing the offending food from the child's diet can solve the problem.

Clean up the diet. Removing all foods containing dyes and additives (monosodium glutamate, aspartame, and hydrolyzed vegetable protein) from a child's diet can also help.

Eliminate sugar and high-glycemic foods. Many children with ADHD suffer from hyperglycemia, and taking them off sugar and high-glycemic foods can make a difference.

Use nutritional supplements. Giving kids a multivitamin/mineral tablet daily can boost brain development.

Try bacopa. Bacopa is a traditional Indian medicinal plant that is found throughout the world in tropical and subtropical regions. It has been used in Ayurvedic medicine for at least 1,500 years to improve neurological and cognitive functioning. A twelve-week double-blind clinical trial of children with ADHD found that those who took 50 mg of bacopa twice a day showed significant improvement in ADHD symptoms, improving concentration and focus, calming the mind, and boosting academic performance. The children's response was evaluated four weeks after stopping the herb and still showed improvement, suggesting that the effects were long-lasting.

Include DHA in diets. DHA is an omega-fatty acid found in cold-water fatty fish, such as salmon, and in fish oil supplements. Studies show that sufferers of both ADHD and autism have significantly lower levels of omega-3 fats in their diets.

Six Treatable Conditions That Mimic Dementia

Memory loss. Confusion. Disorientation. Depression. These are among the most common symptoms of Alzheimer's disease. But in some cases, they might actually be caused by an unrelated problem whose symptoms copycat dementia, experts say.

"Certain medical conditions and situations can mimic the symptoms and confuse the diagnosis," notes Dr. Gary Small, a noted expert on Alzheimer's disease and coauthor with Gigi Vorgan of the best-selling book *The Alzheimer's Prevention Program*.

He explains that "a long list of medical conditions" can cause dementia syndrome. "That is why it's important, if you are concerned about your memory, to consult with your doctor because one of these treatable conditions can be the real culprit. Also, if the cause turns out to be nonreversible like Alzheimer's disease, early detection and treatment leads to better patient outcomes."

According to Harvard University research, more than fifty conditions can cause or mimic the symptoms of dementia. Here are six of the most common examples:

Normal pressure hydrocephalus (NPH). This condition causes a gradual buildup of spinal fluid in the brain that leads to swelling, pressure, and brain damage. The symptoms of NPH include problems with memory and thinking, lack of concentration, and urinary incontinence. Sufferers also tend shuffle when they walk and hold their legs wide apart for balance. A neurologist can identify the problem with a combination of medical history, CT scan, MRI, or spinal tap. A shunt surgically inserted into the brain drains the fluid and usually corrects the problem.

Medication. People who take certain prescription drugs might suffer from memory glitches caused by long-term buildup of the medication. Tell your doctor about all drugs you are taking, including supplements, and ask for options. Don't stop taking any prescription medications without checking with your health care provider.

Urinary tract infections (UTIs). UTIs in older people are hard to diagnose because they don't have the typical symptoms of a high fever and pain. Instead, they might suffer from memory loss, delirium, dizziness, agitation, and even hallucinations. Since older folks have a tougher time emptying their bladders, bacteria builds up internally, interfering with the brain's ability to send and receive signals.

Diabetes. According to the American Diabetes Association, 25 percent of Americans over the age of sixty have diabetes. Too much or too little blood glucose damages blood vessels in the brain, causing memory problems, confusion, irritability, and lack of attention.

Thyroid disorders. According to the American Thyroid Association (ATA), approximately thirty million people over the age of fifty have thyroid disease and might feel sluggish, depressed, forgetful, and anxious. Since thyroid disorders develop slowly, the symptoms are often mistaken for normal aging, say experts. Your primary care physician or endocrinologist can perform a simple blood test to measure thyroid levels. Thyroid disorders can usually be treated with medication but sometimes require surgery to correct.

Vitamin B12 deficiencies. Another common dementia impersonator is caused by a vitamin B12 deficiency that leads to pernicious anemia over time. As we age, our bodies cannot absorb this crucial vitamin as well, and the deficiency leads to nerve damage, confusion, personality changes, irritability, and forgetfulness. Blood work can easily measure B12 levels. If levels are low, supplementation taken orally or by injections most often corrects the dementia-like symptoms of pernicious anemia.

ARTHRITIS

It's the nation's leading cause of disability. It strikes more than one in six Americans. It includes more than one hundred different diseases and conditions. As the US population ages, the number of adults with it is expected to increase sharply.

It's arthritis, and drugs to treat some forms of it can cost as much as $30,000 a year, with many carrying serious potential negative side effects.

If you suffer from arthritis pain, the good news is that scientific research is increasingly finding that natural, drug-free alternatives can help you cope with the pain without emptying your wallet.

By 2020, sixty million Americans, or 18 percent of the population, will be suffering from some form of arthritis, by some estimates. It is already the leading cause of disability in the United States, resulting in more than five million hospitalizations per year.

But a handful of alternative nondrug treatments can ease the pain, stiffness, and disability tied to arthritis. Among them are glucosamine and *Boswellia serrata*.

What Is Arthritis?

The word *arthritis* comes from the Greek words *arthron* ("joint") and *itis* ("inflammation"). It is a broad category that includes more than one hundred different rheumatic diseases and conditions, including rheumatoid arthritis, fibromyalgia, osteoarthritis, gout, lupus, and Lyme disease.

Symptoms include pain, aching, stiffness, and swelling in or around the joints. An estimated 27 million adults have osteoarthritis (also called degenerative joint disease), and 1.3 million are estimated to have rheumatoid arthritis (chronic inflammation of the body's synovial joints).

Although it is more common among adults aged sixty-five years or older, people of all ages (including children) can be affected. In fact, nearly two-thirds of people with arthritis are younger than sixty-five. Arthritis is more common among women (26 percent) than men (19 percent) and more prevalent among obese individuals.

How Do Glucosamine and Boswellia Work?

Glucosamine is a natural chemical compound found in the body. It is available in supplement form and is most often used to ease the joint pain caused by arthritis. Glucosamine helps keep the cartilage in joints healthy, but levels of it drop as people age, which can lead to gradual deterioration of the joint.

Many studies have shown that glucosamine supplements can counteract this effect, easing the pain of mild to moderate osteoarthritis of the knee. It has also been used to treat rheumatoid arthritis and other conditions, such as inflammatory bowel disease, asthma, allergies, chronic venous insufficiency, sports injuries, temporomandibular joint problems (TMJ), and chronic low back pain.

Although glucosamine supplements are often manufactured from the outer shells of shellfish, there aren't any natural food sources of glucosamine.

Some people experience mild side effects including upset stomach, heartburn, drowsiness, and headache. Although health experts say it is a fairly safe supplement, people taking heart medicines, insulin, and blood thinners should check with their doctors before taking glucosamine.

Boswellia is a potent anti-inflammatory agent. It has been used in traditional Ayurvedic medicine for centuries. *Boswellia serrata* is a branching tree that grows in dry mountainous regions of India, Northern Africa, and the Middle East. It contains a variety of compounds that—like aspirin—block enzymes responsible for inflammation in the body.

Problems with Conventional Treatments

Natural alternatives to conventional medicine offer a significant advantage over drugs and painkillers used to treat arthritis.

For the past fifty years, nonsteroidal anti-inflammatory drugs (NSAIDs) have been the primary treatment for arthritic disorders. But if this medication fails, more powerful steroids or other drugs, such as chemotherapeutic agents, are employed.

In many, if not most, cases, such drugs alleviate the symptoms of arthritic disorders—often temporarily—but they do little to halt or reverse the progression of the illness.

In addition, NSAIDs and the newer drug therapies are toxic to the body and can actually inhibit healing and weaken the immune system.

Research suggests that more than 16,500 patients with rheumatoid arthritis or osteoarthritis die annually from the toxic effects of NSAIDs.

Studies have also shown that the prolonged use of NSAIDs inhibits cartilage formation in arthritic patients and actually worsens arthritic conditions. NSAIDs are also known to decrease blood flow to the kidneys.

A newer category of arthritis medications, called disease-modifying antirheumatic drugs (DMARDs)—such as methotrexate, Humira, Imuran, and Enbrel—have been touted by some doctors as preferable to NSAIDs. But DMARDs also have clear immune-suppressing properties and have been associated with serious side effects.

Healthy Habits Help

In addition to taking glucosamine and *Boswellia serrata* supplements, alternative medicine practitioners say a handful of healthy habits and strategies can help manage and reduce the symptoms of arthritis.

Marcy O'Koon, senior director for consumer health at the Arthritis Foundation, notes that something as simple as adding more anti-inflammatory foods to your diet can have a big impact on pain.

"An anti-inflammatory diet is good for overall health," she notes. "The Mediterranean diet is considered a good model for eating a diet that reduces or at least doesn't promote inflammation. Go for cold-water fish that are high in omega-3 fatty acids, such as herring, mackerel, trout, salmon, and tuna; high-fiber foods, such as whole grains and vegetables; and extra virgin olive oil [in moderation] too."

Here are ten simple ways to lessen arthritis pain without drugs:

GET MOVING. Staying—or getting—physically active can ease pain naturally. Jogging, running, weight lifting, cross training, swimming, hiking, bicycling, and even low-impact activities (such as gardening and housework) can all alleviate inflammation and pain and improve mobility, studies show. If you're just starting an exercise program, talk to your doctor first and start slow. Go for a quick warm-up instead of an hour-long session and work your way up to a more intense workout over time.

MAINTAIN A HEALTHY WEIGHT. People can reduce their risk of developing arthritis—and ease the pain associated with it—by controlling their weight and avoiding injuries.

AVOID UNHEALTHY FOODS. Steer clear of foods that boost inflammation in the body—including those with refined sugar, salt, oil, and flour, which are chief components of fast food, processed meals, and junk snacks. Eat a whole-food diet including unrefined sugar, salt, oil, and flour and as much organic produce as possible. Many arthritic patients need to avoid nightshade plants such as tomatoes, potatoes, peppers, and eggplant. People with arthritis should also limit foods that are high in purines, such as red meats and shellfish. Better alternatives include thin-sliced bologna, turkey, and chicken. Alcoholic beverages also contain high levels of purines. Those with gout need to be mindful of purines, since higher amounts lead to greater levels of uric acid.

TAKE SUPPLEMENTS. Most arthritic patients have multiple nutritional deficiencies, including low levels of vitamins A, B6, B12, and C and should consider taking supplements along with glucosamine and Boswellia. Magnesium and selenium are also important.

STAY HYDRATED. Drinking adequate amounts of water can help arthritic patients significantly improve their condition. It's a good idea to cut out sugary soda, which can boost weight gain, weaken bones, and increase inflammation in the body.

DRINK CONSERVATIVELY. Research shows that women who drink as little as three cocktails per week are likely to reduce symptoms of rheumatoid arthritis. But there are caveats: drinking too much beer might increase knee and hip osteoarthritis pain and might also increase your weight, which puts added pressure on joints.

CHERRIES. These antioxidant-loaded fruits provide a remedy for your arthritis. The bright-red color of cherries comes from antioxidants known as anthocyanins. Research suggests that these compounds can reduce inflammation and cholesterol levels and can ease pain caused by arthritis or gout. Cherries can be eaten alone or added to meals, salads, cereals, and other dishes. Experts say it takes just a couple days for the benefits of consuming as few as a dozen cherries per day to take effect.

CURRY WITH FOOD. Turmeric—the main spice in curry that gives Indian dishes their yellowish coloring—has been proven to have potent anti-inflammatory properties that can help battle arthritis-related symptoms.

GO WITH OLIVE OIL. Although canola and vegetable oils are popular for cooking, olive oil is the preferred choice when reducing arthritis pain, experts say. A compound in olive oil called oleocanthal prevents the production of proinflammatory COX-1 and COX-2 enzymes—easing pain in the same way that ibuprofen works. AARP suggests adding olive oil to salad, tossing it with pasta, or using it to flavor vegetables.

RELAX YOUR BODY. Acupuncture, massage, Tai Chi, and yoga are alternative means of healing arthritis that aim to relax the body and mind to ease pain. Acupuncture and Tai Chi have been shown to be effective treatments for pain caused by rheumatoid arthritis and osteoarthritis, according to a study at the University of Aberdeen in Scotland.

Eagles Founder Glenn Frey's Death
Spotlights Arthritis Drug Dangers

The death of Eagles founder Glenn Frey in January 2016—tied in part to rheumatoid arthritis (RA) medications he was taking that likely compromised his immune system—spotlights the dangers of powerful drugs used to treat the condition.

Frey died from complications of RA, ulcerative colitis, and pneumonia. His manager, Irving Azoff, said that the RA drugs the legendary musician had taken for years left his body vulnerable to infection.

Frey's death is a cautionary tale about the risks of such prescription medications that should push arthritis patients—and the doctors who treat them—to seek out safer available alternatives.

For many of the 1.5 million Americans with RA, doctors prescribe corticosteroids, biologics, and DMARDs—such as methotrexate, Humira, Imuran, and Enbrel—all of which suppress the immune system and leave patients vulnerable to bacterial and viral infections like pneumonia.

But natural remedies and healthy lifestyle changes can offer relief to patients and are far less risky than RA drugs.

Holistic health specialists say that the four following strategies can help manage RA and other forms of arthritis that strike tens of millions of Americans. They recommend discussing the options with your doctor when weighing the pros and cons of taking more powerful medications.

Boost your nutrition. Many studies show that diet plays a key role in arthritic symptoms. The first step in any holistic plan is to clean up the diet. Eat a whole-food diet including unrefined sugar, salt, oil, and flour and as much organic produce as possible. Cut processed foods loaded with carbs, refined salt, flour, and sugar—the staples of most packaged and fast foods—proinflammatory items that increase the redness, warmth, swelling, and joint destruction associated with arthritis. Drinking adequate amounts of water can also alleviate arthritic symptoms. To determine how much water you should drink, divide your weight (in pounds) by two. The resulting number is the amount of water, in ounces, you should drink daily.

Hit the gym. Numerous studies have shown that exercise and physical therapy strengthen the muscles around joints, which can alleviate arthritis pain. Low-impact activities—such as swimming, water aerobics, Tai Chi, and yoga—are good bets and can also stave off heart disease, cancer, osteoporosis, and Alzheimer's disease.

Apply heat and cold compresses. Applying heat or cold compresses to painful, inflamed joints can alleviate pain by naturally increasing blood flow (heat) or dulling the sensation (cold) in those areas.

Ask your doctor about antibiotics. Research has found that antibiotics might help some people with arthritis because the condition might be tied to bacterial infections. Mycoplasma, a bacterium, was first suggested as a cause of RA in the 1930s, and later research has confirmed the connection. Thus low-dose antibiotics might help.

The big picture here is that boosting the body's natural defenses—not weakening them—should be the goal of treating RA and other chronic conditions.

CANCER

In August 2015, former president Jimmy Carter joined the ranks of the 1.7 million Americans who are diagnosed with cancer every year. At age ninety, Carter developed an advanced case of deadly melanoma skin cancer that spread to his liver and brain. With no standard treatment that could stop it from killing him, Carter said at the time that he believed he had only weeks to live and put his fate "in the hands of God."

But within six months, in February 2016, Carter's doctors revealed that tests had found that he was "cancer-free." The good news came as a welcome shock to relatives, friends, and well-wishers. But some doctors on the front lines of the war on cancer, who have been logging steady progress against the nation's number-two killer, were not entirely surprised by Carter's recovery.

Why? The former president was treated with what some are hailing as a genuine breakthrough in cancer treatment: a newly approved immunotherapy drug called Keytruda, which works by enlisting the body's natural defenses to fight cancer. While the drug is not a cancer "cure" exactly, it might be the next best thing—representing the greatest medical advance in decades.

"Some people may be surprised by how well Jimmy Carter is doing, but to be honest with you, I'm not terribly surprised," says neurosurgeon Dr. Lee M. Tessler, executive director of the Long Island Brain Tumor Center in Lake Success, New York. "Usually when I see sick patients as old as this, the thought is to use palliative care [which only alleviates pain] or to call hospice. But we now have to rethink this because Jimmy Carter's case shows us that there are obviously patients who can tolerate the treatment and survive."

Tessler adds that Carter's case spotlights the promise of the latest immunotherapy drugs like Keytruda. Such treatments combat cancer in an entirely new way—by boosting the body's immune system to combat tumors—and represent a safer and more effective alternative to conventional surgery, chemotherapy, and radiation.

"This is very good news for Jimmy Carter. It shows that the cancer treatment is working and that any disease he has, whether in his brain or elsewhere in his body, is now under control," Tessler says. "I think this is the new horizon for cancer treatment, absolutely. There is no question about it."

A Holy Grail of Medicine

The idea of harnessing the natural power of the body's immune system to combat cancer and other illnesses has been a kind of Holy Grail for medical researchers for nearly a century. With the advent of Keytruda, it has become a reality. And it's just one of many drugs now entering the market or in the pipeline.

The US Food and Drug Administration (FDA) approved the new drug (also known as pembrolizumab) in October 2015 for patients with advanced non-small-cell lung cancer whose tumors have a specific genetic mutation. It was given a "breakthrough therapy designation" and a fast-tracked approval because it was deemed to be a significant improvement over available treatments based on the results of clinical trials.

Other studies have found it to be effective against advanced melanoma, and it also holds promise in the treatment of lymphoma, leukemia, and breast, bladder, and colorectal cancer, among others—on its own or in combination with other therapies.

Dr. Richard Pazdur, director of the office of hematology and oncology products in the FDA's Center for Drug Evaluation and Research, says that Keytruda is just one in new generation of treatments designed to work with the body's immune defenses to combat cancer.

"Our growing understanding of underlying molecular pathways and how our immune system interacts with cancer is leading to important advances in medicine," Pazdur notes. "[The] approval of Keytruda gives physicians the ability to target specific patients who may be most likely to benefit from this drug."

Among them, Jimmy Carter.

Better than Chemo, Radiation, and Surgery

For decades, the gold standard of conventional cancer treatments involved surgery to cut out tumors, chemotherapy to poison them, and radiation to burn them away. But all those approaches destroy healthy tissues as well as tumor cells, knock down the body's natural immune defenses against cancer, and can cause serious side effects—including the potential to spread the disease.

That's why many alternative medicine practitioners have argued that conventional cancer treatment is barbaric and, for some patients, does as much harm as good. A better option, they say, is to use herbs, nutrients, healthy habits, botanical treatments, supplements, mind-body medicine, and natural healing practices to boost the body's natural defenses to combat cancer and other diseases.

In some ways, immunotherapy represents a *coming together* of both sides—combining the best of both worlds, so to speak. Unlike chemo, surgery, and radiation, Keytruda and other forms of immunotherapy target cancer indirectly by arming and enhancing the tremendous power of the body's immune system to identify and destroy tumors. This leaves healthy tissues unharmed and does not carry the risk of debilitating side effects that conventional treatments can pose.

Specifically, Keytruda blocks a cellular pathway found in the body's immune cells and some tumors, helping the immune system target and fight cancer cells. The drug works in patients with a cancer-linked genetic mutation, which the FDA requires patients be tested for in order to be eligible for the treatment.

Although the drug has only recently entered the market, early studies involving small numbers of cancer patients—as well as Carter's experiences—suggest that the drug holds tremendous promise. As a result, many oncologists predict that drugs like Keytruda will become standard first-line cancer treatments likely to replace chemo, as well as some surgical and radiological treatments, in the years ahead.

Immunotherapy drugs, which the FDA began fast-tracking just two years ago, are now used to treat melanoma, Hodgkin lymphoma, and cancers of the bladder, kidney, head, and neck. But the FDA's approval of Keytruda represents, by far, the biggest nod for this type of therapy.

The FDA approved the drug after it was tested on 550 advanced lung cancer patients, sixty-one of whom had already been treated (unsuccessfully) with chemotherapy. In 41 percent of patients, tumors shrank after treatment with the drug, and their cancers remained in check for more than nine months.

A follow-up study, published in December 2015 by the University of California, Los Angeles (UCLA), found the drug to be more effective against lung cancer than chemotherapy in a head-to-head comparison. The study, published in *The Lancet*, involved 1,034 patients who were randomly given Keytruda or the chemotherapy drug docetaxel. Those treated with Keytruda fared substantially better than those taking the conventional therapy drug, the UCLA researchers found.

"This treatment provides real hope of long-lasting responses while avoiding the toxicities of typical chemotherapy," says Dr. Edward Garon, a UCLA researcher who helped conduct the study. "We are excited that these results have identified a larger group of patients for whom in general, immunotherapy is a superior treatment option than traditional approaches."

Since then, follow-up studies have only confirmed Keytruda's benefits in targeting cancer. In October 2016, the FDA cleared the way for Keytruda to be offered as the main drug treatment of lung cancer, making it the first time an immunotherapy has been approved as the first-line drug treatment for nonsmall metastatic lung cancer (NSCLC)—the nation's number-one killer when it comes to cancers.

The regulators approved the drug based on two new studies, including one that hailed the drug's effectiveness as a breakthrough at a meeting in Copenhagen of the European Society of Medical Oncology.

While Keytruda is not for everyone, it is perhaps the most compelling example that immunotherapy is coming of age and is already helping people with cancer—including those well into their nineties—who would have died just a few years ago.

Tessler adds that medical scientists still have much to learn about how immunotherapies work to treat cancer and other diseases. As Carter himself demonstrates, individual factors—such as an active, healthy lifestyle—might be keys to the success of new treatments like Keytruda in ways researchers are just beginning to understand.

"I would rather treat a patient who is ninety and gets sick for the first time than someone who gets sick in their sixties," Tessler notes. "You always think that the person of ninety is going to do worse, but they've got something in them, whether it's genetics or a certain type of strength, that has enabled them to reach that age."

Although immunotherapy has yet to move fully into the mainstream, there is no question that we have entered a new era in medicine—one that future medical historians might view as a turning point in using the body's own natural defenses to target disease, boost overall health, and increase human longevity to its fullest potential.

Carter: Beneficiary of Two New Therapies

Doctors who are treating former president Jimmy Carter have used not only the breakthrough new drug Keytruda but also a leading-edge form of radiation that holds great promise for other patients who are fighting the malignant disease.

Carter had a small tumor removed from his liver in August 2015, which subsequent testing revealed had originated as a form of melanoma and had also spread to four spots in his brain.

To treat the former president, doctors at Emory University's Winship Cancer Center in Atlanta used Keytruda (pembrolizumab) and an advanced form of radiation called stereotactic radiosurgery, sometimes referred to as "Gamma Knife" treatment.

Like conventional chemotherapy, traditional radiation does not distinguish between tumors and healthy cells—it destroys both. But stereotactic radiosurgery focuses the beams better on the tumor, so it can kill the cancer cells more effectively while sparing the healthy ones.

Follow-up tests in January and February 2016 showed that the former president has no signs of the cancer. By March, his doctors declared that the treatments had been so effective that he no longer needed to receive therapy.

Carter made the announcement at the Sunday school class he teaches in Plains, Georgia. Carter Center spokeswoman Deanna Congileo said the former president will "continue scans and resume treatment if necessary."

Immunotherapies in the Pipeline

Keytruda, the landmark immunotherapy drug used to treat Jimmy Carter, has become the poster child for this new form of cancer treatment. But many other therapies, designed to combat cancer by boosting the body's immune defenses, have shown promise or are in the pipeline.

Here's a look at the most exciting prospects and treatments:

"Checkpoint inhibitors." Keytruda is one of a new class of drugs known as "immune checkpoint inhibitors" that target immune system "checkpoint proteins" (such as PD-1 and CTLA-4) that cancer cells sometimes enlist to avoid being attacked by the immune system. Three others have also been approved: (1) Yervoy (ipilimumab), which targets CTLA-4; (2) Opdivo (nivolumab), which targets PD-1 (made by Bristol-Myers Squibb); and (3) Tecentriq (atezolizumab), by Genentech.

Monoclonal antibodies. More effective forms of monoclonal antibodies—which attach to drugs or other substances to make them more powerful and/or boost immune defenses and are used to treat many kinds of cancer—are being designed. One new approach combines parts of two antibodies such that one part attaches to a cancer cell and the other to an immune cell, bringing the two together to kill tumors.

Cancer vaccines. Researchers are working to develop new vaccines delivered with other substances that arm the body's immune system and "infect" tumors. Some are made with actual cancer cells that have been removed and then "killed" and injected back into the patient to provoke the body's natural defenses against other similar tumors still in the body. Others enlist "dendritic cells"—special cells that help the immune system recognize cancer cells—and reengineered viruses, bacteria, or yeast cells that have been altered so they no longer cause disease but still provoke a strong natural defense against tumors.

Others. Some other forms of immunotherapy are being studied to try to boost specific agents of the immune system, including T-cells and tumor-infiltrating lymphocytes.

Radical Remission: Why Some Terminal Cancer Patients Beat the Odds

Every year, countless terminal cancer patients—some given only months to live—somehow survive to beat the odds, even after doctors have told them conventional treatments are not working. So how do they do it? Is it just a matter of luck or are there common characteristics of such remarkable, long-term cancer survivors?

Dr. Kelly Turner, a Harvard-educated cancer researcher who spent a year examining cases of "spontaneous remission," says there is much more to these recoveries than random chance and that scientists are only beginning to understand the physiological mechanisms at work.

In her best-selling book *Radical Remission: 9 Key Factors That Can Make a Real Difference*, she details her findings from interviews with more than one hundred cancer patients in ten countries who have experienced such recoveries. She also analyzed one thousand other similar cases to identify commonalities in against-all-odds survivors.

"I was looking for the most common thing or the top common things among all of these radical remission survivors, and I found over seventy-five different things that they were doing to try to get well," she says. "Not everyone did all seventy-five, but almost everyone that I've studied did nine of these things."

According to Turner's findings, the following seven factors were common to all of the "radical remission" cases she examined:

Taking control of your health. The most dramatic recovery Turner recounts involved a Japanese kidney cancer patient who underwent unsuccessful surgery, radiation, and chemotherapy. But once he started taking control of his health—drinking filtered water, eating healthy food, and watching the sunrise every day—he went into remission. "He did all the nine factors in my research, and twenty-five years later and counting, he is completely cancer-free and has grandchildren," she says.

Radically changing your diet. Not surprisingly, all the long-term survivors had taken aggressive steps to boost the nutritional value of their diets—a factor Turner calls "the big one" among the patients she studied. "And that was a shift really into fruits and vegetables and away from things like meat, wheat, sweets, and dairy," she explains.

Using herbs and supplements. No single anticancer natural remedy was uncovered by Turner's research. But she says that most survivors used three types of herbs and supplements—those that aid digestion and increase the body's absorption of nutrients, those that help detoxify the body of bacteria and viruses, and those that boost the immune system (such as probiotics, prebiotics, aloe vera, turmeric, and vitamin C). "I wish that I could say there was one magic bullet, that everyone was taking this one herb from Indonesia and—*poof!*—their cancer was gone," she notes. "[But] what I found . . . is there were three categories of herbs that almost everyone I studied was taking."

Embracing social support. A wide variety of research has found that close connections with family and friends can boost cancer survival—something Turner's research confirmed in the individuals she studied. "They would say to me, 'You know, I don't know how to explain it, Dr. Turner, but I know that the love that just came pouring in helped me heal,'" she notes. "Well, scientifically, we know that that's actually possible, because when you feel loved, oxytocin is released in huge amounts form the master glands of your brain, and that increases [the immune system's] natural killer cells and white blood cells."

Increasing positive emotions, releasing negative feelings, and having strong reasons for living. Three other characteristics of long-term survivors were interrelated: embracing positive emotions, letting go of negative feelings, and developing stronger reasons for living. Turner found that the patients she studied made time every day to do these things, just as they made time to eat, sleep, and exercise. "Even if it was just for five minutes a day—so [they're] not trying to be happy positive all the time, because that's just not possible— but making sure [to] get five minutes of joy every day," she says. "They [also] released suppressed emotions that they were holding onto from the past, such as stress or regret or sadness."

Following your intuition. Learning to trust your gut instincts was also a key factor Turner observed in the patients she studied. "They used their intuition to help make decisions," she says. "And intuition is interesting because it actually can sense danger and paths to safety long before the front of your brain—which is the thinking part of your brain—even knows what's going on."

Deepening your spiritual connection. Turner found that faith itself was not necessarily a key factor in helping cancer patients live longer, but the practice of some form of spirituality—praying, meditating, or interacting with the natural world—has measurable impacts on the immune system.

"Faith, according to my research, actually doesn't help them survive. What helps them survive, according to the people I studied, is not what they believe but how they practice their spirituality," she explains.

"So there are certain spiritual practices—such as prayer or meditation or even walking in nature—that will change . . . the physiology of your body and put you into the parasympathetic nervous system, and that's when your immune system really lights up. So it actually becomes scientific—if you do these spiritual practices that calm your body down and sort of connect you to [what] some people would say [is] a divine energy . . . really you're just turning on your parasympathetic nervous system. If you do that every day, you're really going to help your immune system."

She adds that this aspect of research challenges the notion that people with strong personalities who embody a "fighting spirit" in taking on their cancer have an advantage. In fact, such an approach might be counterproductive, she suggests.

"Research has shown that having a fighting spirit and fighting against your cancer actually doesn't lengthen survival time. And that's exactly what I found among my radical remission survivors as well," she says. "Many of them weren't fighting their cancer; many of them were just simply focused on enjoying life for as long as they had it. And so, again, that's moving them out of fear and out of . . . this fight-or-flight mode and into the rest-and-repair mode, where you're enjoying life, you're relaxing, you're taking happiness when you can get it. And that is actually better for your immune system than being in a fight with something."

Functional Foods That Destroy Cancer Cells

It's no secret that certain foods contain powerful compounds that can fight many dreaded diseases. But research shows that specific foods might prevent and even control the growth of cancer cells in the body.

"The main mechanism behind these foods is their anti-inflammatory properties," Dr. Dimitri Alden, a renowned New York City–based cancer surgeon, says. "Inflammation causes cancer cells to grow and spread, so by eating these foods, you can prevent this process."

Here are ten of the most recognized functional foods that destroy cancer cells:

GRAPES AND RED WINE. Resveratrol, the powerful ingredient found in grapes and wine, is an extremely powerful antioxidant. It also inhibits cyclooxygenase-2 (COX-2) production, which is related to cancers and other types of inflammation. COX-2 inhibitors such as resveratrol have been shown to decrease the incidence of cancer and precancerous growths.

SEA VEGETABLES. These delicious treats from the sea include nori, arame, kombu, and wakame. They contain a variety of antioxidant and anti-inflammatory compounds that will prevent and reverse the damage done by foods and other factors that cause inflammation and oxidative stress—two known contributing factors to many types of cancers.

TURMERIC. The miracle ingredient in the spice turmeric, found in most Indian dishes, is curcumin. Curcumin is an extremely powerful antioxidant and anti-inflammatory that reduces the metastases of tumors and might destroy or prevent their growth in the first place. Alden says the spice inhibits the formation of new blood vessels in cancer cells—a crucial step in delaying development.

GREEN TEA. Green tea owes its cancer-destroying abilities to a group of plant flavonoids known as catechins. One of these catechins—epigallocatechin gallate (EGCG)—is the most powerful anti-inflammatory and also disrupts the development of cancer cells.

CRUCIFEROUS VEGETABLES. We all know that veggies are healthy, but cruciferous vegetables like broccoli, arugula, cabbage, cauliflower, and kale contain chemicals called glucosinolates, which create compounds that fight cancer. According to the Linus Pauling Institute, they work by eliminating carcinogens before they can damage DNA.

GARLIC. According to researcher Dr. Carmia Borek, PhD, many populations have used garlic as a remedy for cancer for thousands of years. The National Cancer Institute says that garlic might reduce the risk of stomach, colon, esophageal, and breast cancer. The Iowa Women's Study revealed that women who consumed the most garlic had a 50 percent lower risk of cancer of the colon. Borek recommends taking aged garlic extract (AGE) for the most consistent cancer fighting benefits.

HEMP OIL. Hemp oil is known to speed up the healing process throughout the body and also raise melatonin levels. Melatonin has been shown to reduce or even completely stop the growth of certain types of cancers, so the extra production of it thanks to hemp oil is a great asset in your body's fight against cancer. Hemp oil can be consumed through gelcaps or even directly out of the bottle.

MUSHROOMS. These tasty fungi have antiviral and anticancer effects that have been proven through numerous in-vitro and animal research studies. Mushrooms have been used for more than five thousand years in ancient and traditional medicines due to their powerful effects on a number of diseases and conditions—including cancer.

GINGER. Certain compounds found in ginger make it a powerful anti-inflammatory and antioxidant to reduce oxidative stress that your body has to fight daily. Studies have shown that ginger can reduce cancerous tumors by as much as 56 percent and have also shown it to be a more effective remedy than traditional medical treatments like chemotherapy in the case of certain types of cancers.

TOMATOES. These red fruits and products made from them contain lycopene, a compound known for its ability to destroy cancer cells. Scientific studies show that lycopene helps prevent prostate, lung, and stomach cancers. This powerful antioxidant offers a double whammy, as it also reduces your risk of heart disease by lowering "bad" low-density lipoprotein (LDL) cholesterol and blood pressure.

Four Natural Supplements That Fight Cancer
In addition to cancer-fighting foods, a handful of dietary supplements have shown promise in combatting the development, growth, and spread of tumors:

CURCUMIN. This powerful anti-inflammatory stops cancer cells from forming, kills existing cancer cells, and prevents them from spreading.

POMEGRANATE SEED OIL. Pomegranate seeds have powerful anticancer properties and chemicals. In one cellular study, punicic acid from pomegranate seed oil showed dramatic antitumor effects and inhibited cancer cell proliferation.

GRAPE SEED EXTRACT. Grape seed extract is high in oligomeric proanthocyanidins complexes (OPCs), which have excellent antioxidant activity and are known cancer fighters. Cellular studies indicate that grape seed extract has powerful aromatase inhibitors that stop enzymes from converting androgens into estrogens, which might fuel certain forms of cancer.

VITAMIN D3. Clinical research has shown that more than 75 percent of breast cancer victims were vitamin D deficient. Other studies conclude that high levels of vitamin D might reduce the risk of developing breast cancer by a whopping 50 percent and might also combat other forms of the disease.

Viruses and Cancer: What's the Link?

Cancer is not contagious and can't be spread like the common cold or flu. But the truth is that some viruses, which are contagious, are tied to tens of thousands of certain cancers each year. For instance, human papillomavirus (HPV) causes

- 91 percent of cervical cancers,
- 95 percent of anal cancers, and
- 70 percent of oropharyngeal cancers.

In addition, the hepatitis B and C viruses are responsible for approximately 80–95 percent of all liver cancers.

The good news is that most of these cancers can be prevented or eradicated with available vaccines and screening, says Carolyn Aldige, founder of the Prevent Cancer Foundation, which is dedicated to preventing the dreaded disease.

The bad news, however, is that most Americans aren't aware of the link and haven't taken advantage of the medicine and technology available.

"I realized that after my own father died from cancer . . . I wanted to do everything in my power to educate people about cancer prevention," says Aldige. "We want to raise awareness of the connection between certain viruses and cancer. The campaign is focused on three of these viruses directly linked to cancer: HPV, hepatitis B, and hepatitis C."

Three HPV vaccines are available that protect against related cancers, and they have been approved as safe and effective. HPV vaccines are given as a series of three shots over six months. All three have been approved by the FDA for women, while two of the vaccines are approved for men.

The US Centers for Disease Control and Prevention (CDC) recommend the HPV vaccine for boys and girls ages eleven and twelve, and all vaccines are available for women through the age of twenty-six.

"These are the ages when the vaccines are most effective," Aldige explains. "Unfortunately, many parents believe that having their children vaccinated will lead to promiscuity. So only one-third of adolescents have received the protocol."

Even with vaccination, experts recommend that women still have regular Pap smears for cervical cancer screening.

But cervical cancer isn't the only link to the HPV virus, which is the most common sexually transmitted infection. The virus can also cause vulvar, vaginal, penile, and anal cancers, as well as cancer of the head, neck, and back of the throat, including the base of the tongue and tonsils, called oropharyngeal cancer. Actor Michael Douglas suspected that his throat cancer was caused by the HPV virus.

Hepatitis B and C are viruses that have also been linked to several forms of cancer. But the most common is the link to potentially deadly liver cancer. Hepatitis B is a liver infection transmitted through bodily fluid from an infected person. Hepatitis C is a blood-borne virus most commonly transmitted by sharing needles or other equipment used for injecting recreational drugs.

The best way to prevent hepatitis B is to get vaccinated. The CDC recommends that all children receive their first dose of hepatitis B vaccine at birth and complete a three- to four-dose series between six and eighteen months of age.

While there is no vaccine for hepatitis C, it is recommended that people reduce their risk by avoiding activities that spread the virus, especially using injectable drugs. It's also important to have blood tests that screen for the virus, as there are treatments available that reduce the chance of developing cirrhosis or liver cancer.

"Tens of thousands of Americans are suffering each year from cancers caused by viruses—all the more heartbreaking when you consider that infection with these viruses is mostly preventable," says Dr. Erich M. Sturgis, professor of the department of head and neck surgery at the University of Texas MD Anderson Cancer Center.

"As a physician who treats cancer patients daily, I'm disheartened to learn that research shows most people are unaware of the link between viruses and cancer. We need to educate the public and health care providers on the steps they can take to prevent viral infections and ultimately cancer."

Coping with Cancer: A Doctor's Perspective

Dr. Herman Kattlove, a medical hematologist/oncologist and former spokesperson for the American Cancer Society (ACS), notes that just about every family in the nation is affected directly or indirectly by cancer. He offers the following perspective on diagnosing, treating, and coping with the disease.

Q: How are most cancers diagnosed?

A: Only a handful of cancers are diagnosed early by specific exams. These are breast cancers, diagnosed by mammograms or physical exam or by a patient's self-exam; colon cancers diagnosed by colonoscopy; cervical cancers by Pap smears; and prostate cancers by blood tests.

Most of the others are picked up because of symptoms. Although lung cancers are sometimes found by chest X-rays looking for other problems, most patients diagnosed with lung cancer come to the doctor because of chest pain, constant cough—perhaps with blood in the sputum—shortness of breath, or lung infection because of the cancer.

Women with ovarian cancer often have abdominal discomfort and loss of appetite. The same is true for people with pancreatic cancer. People with colon or rectal cancer may see blood in their bowel movements or just have abdominal pain and appetite loss.

Q: What is the usual reaction of patients and their family?

A: Most patients who are diagnosed with cancer, even when it is advanced, react with optimism and hope. I think this is because they are feeling well in spite of their symptoms and can't picture getting worse. But if they have had experience with friends or family dying of cancer, they may be less optimistic. When it is more advanced and causing major symptoms like fatigue or pain, then the reaction is also more guarded, and there is less optimism. Patients with strong faith will often accept their diagnosis as the will of God and put trust in their religious faith to see them through the cancer.

Q: What advice do you have for people who have been recently diagnosed?

A: The first step for anyone diagnosed with cancer is to see a qualified specialist, which is most often a medical oncologist. The patient should bring along a close family member or friend. This is important because many studies have shown that with the stress of a cancer diagnosis, patients forget what they are told. They are also reluctant to ask questions. Having another person in the room can overcome this problem.

A second opinion with a major cancer institution is also helpful both for reassurance and to help plan therapy. In these situations, treatment can still be given by a local oncologist, especially if the cancer center is located far from the patient's home. Let close friends and coworkers know because it is important to have support during potentially difficult treatment.

Q: What tools have been shown to help enhance the outcome of cancer treatment and survival?

A: The most important factor in having the best outcome is sticking to the program. Cancer therapy can be difficult, with many side effects. Anything that helps a patient such as meditation, support groups, and helpful friends and family can contribute to a patient's success in undergoing treatment. Also, it has been shown that maintaining a healthy lifestyle such as exercise and proper eating habits can reduce the chances of a cancer recurrence.

Could Aspirin Be Our Best Defense against Cancer?

It's cheap, safe, and has been effectively used for millennia—in various forms—to treat pain, fever, and minor illnesses. Now that old standby headache pill, aspirin, is poised to become the latest weapon in the war on cancer.

Federal health experts say that aspirin, long taken to prevent heart disease, also appears to reduce the risk of developing cancer and should be used as a primary means to prevent the disease. In new guidelines issued in April 2016, the US Preventive Services Task Force (USPSTF)—charged with crafting national health recommendations—indicated that a daily low-dose aspirin (81 mg) is best used as a preventive measure against heart disease for people in their fifties. The panel also said that aspirin helps people in their sixties cut their risk for heart attack and stroke to a lesser extent.

But the biggest surprise in the new guidelines was that the inexpensive painkiller cuts the risk of colon cancer, the third leading cause of cancer-related death in the United States. Previously, the task force had suggested only that low-dose aspirin could help men forty-five to seventy-nine and women fifty-five to seventy-nine prevent heart disease.

Age-Old Medicine

Aspirin is one of the oldest known medicines, first used by the ancient Greeks, who used a naturally occurring form of it—derived from tree bark—to treat pain and fever. Today, millions of Americans take a low-dose aspirin daily for heart-healthy benefits, and a growing number of studies have suggested that the medicine might prevent a variety of cancers as well.

Health experts note that traditional cancer-prevention strategies—colonoscopies, maintaining a healthy weight, and eating a diet high in fiber—should not be abandoned in favor of aspirin alone to stave off colorectal cancer, which kills fifty thousand Americans a year.

But USPSTF recommendations say that adults in their fifties who have a 10 percent or greater risk of heart disease over the next ten years should consider taking a low-dose aspirin daily to prevent heart disease and colon cancer.

As with any drug, patients and their doctors must balance the benefits and risks of aspirin, a nonsteroidal anti-inflammatory drug (NSAID) that can reduce blood clotting and lower inflammation. Even low doses of aspirin can cause sometimes deadly internal bleeding in the stomach, intestines, and brain of some people.

But under the careful supervision of a doctor, millions of Americans who don't face bleeding risks can benefit from aspirin. The USPSTF, whose recommendations form the basis for medical policy, is also very specific about who benefits most from aspirin.

"Persons who are not at increased risk for bleeding, have a life expectancy of at least ten years, and are willing to take low-dose aspirin daily for at least ten years are more likely to benefit," the task force says in its recommendations.

"The USPSTF found adequate evidence that aspirin use reduces the incidence of colorectal cancer in adults after ten years of use."

What Research Shows

USPSTF guidelines follow a spate of new studies that have spotlighted aspirin's anticancer properties. A landmark 2012 analysis of fifty-one studies involving more than seventy-seven thousand patients found, for instance, that aspirin not only reduces a person's risk of developing colorectal cancer and other forms of the disease but can also stop tumors from spreading to other parts of the body.

The research, published in the journal *The Lancet*, found that cancer death rates were significantly lower among people taking aspirin.

"Aspirin has a big effect on the spread of the cancer, which is important, as it's the commonest reason that cancer kills people," said Oxford University researcher Peter Rothwell in a statement issued with the findings. "We found that after five years of taking aspirin, there was a 30–40 percent reduction in deaths from cancer."

More recently, Yale University researchers found that taking a low-dose aspirin for more than ten years might lower the risk of developing pancreatic cancer by up to 60 percent. In addition, the 2014 Yale study indicated that taking a daily aspirin for just three years lowered the chances of developing the deadly cancer by nearly 50 percent.

Other aspirin-cancer studies are also moving forward in the wake of the USPSTF guidelines. Boston-based researchers, for instance, have launched a new $10 million study to determine if aspirin is an effective way to treat breast cancer. The federally funded clinical trial—by the Dana-Farber Cancer Institute and Brigham & Women's Hospital—will test whether aspirin helps breast cancer survivors avoid recurrences and live longer.

"Although chemo and hormonal therapies have helped women with breast cancer live longer, they are expensive and have many side effects," said researcher Wendy Chen, MD. "The results of this trial, if positive, could have a huge impact."

Seven Proven Ways to Beat Melanoma

Melanoma is the deadliest form of skin cancer—the most common of all cancers—killing one person every fifty minutes. According to the CDC, the incidence of new melanoma cases has doubled over the last three decades and continues to climb, despite the hype about using sunscreen.

But according to the new book *Win the Fight*, written by noted fitness expert Lisa Lynn and Yale University–based surgical oncologist Dr. Deepak Narayan, sunscreen is *not* a magic bullet that protects us from the sun's potentially deadly rays and prevents cancer.

"People think that putting on sunscreen makes them invincible," says Narayan. "They misjudge how long they've been exposed to the sun and think they're protected for the whole day."

While Lynn and Narayan acknowledge the advance of immune-boosting drugs to fight melanoma over the past five years, they say that prevention is still the key. Here are their top tips to "win the fight" against this dreaded disease.

Limit sunburn. There's no such thing as safe tanning. Avoid tanning beds and sunbathing, especially if you have light-colored eyes and fair skin. Every five sunburns you've suffered in the past increase your risk of melanoma by 74 percent.

Cold, cloudy days are not safe. You're not safe from the sun on cold or cloudy days. The sun's rays can be just as intense on cloudy days and during winter months. They can even penetrate through windows. The top states for melanoma are actually "cold" states, but because of their higher altitude, people are closer to the sun's rays.

Sunscreen is not armor. All it does is provide us with some protection when we're out in the sun. Look for a broad-spectrum sunscreen with at least a sun protection factor (SPF) of thirty-five. Apply a liberal amount—the size of a golf ball—every hour or two. Spray sunscreens do *not* give you enough protection. Check expiration dates for maximum effectiveness. Wear protective hats, sunglasses, and clothing.

Boost your nutrition. Eat lots of foods with cancer-fighting compounds. Numerous studies have shown that a diet rich in colorful fruits and vegetables helps fight cancer.

Sleep for immunity. Use the healing power of sleep to boost immunity. Our bodies produce melatonin, a powerful compound that helps us sleep and heal. If you're having trouble sleeping, consider taking 3 mg of melatonin in supplement form before going to bed.

Exercise the right way. Aim for thirty minutes of exercise daily, but don't overdo it. Even light exercise lowers blood sugar levels and releases hormones that reduce stress and depression while also boosting your body's natural defenses.

Reduce stress. Research shows that stress plays a role in lowering the body's immune system, making it more susceptible to cancer. Apply stress management techniques and increase your intake of omega-3 fatty acids, AGE, and curcumin.

Changing Guidelines on Mammograms Raise More Questions than Answers

In a major shift in policy, the ACS now recommends that most women get annual mammograms starting at age forty-five rather than at age forty, and that those who are fifty-five and older scale back screening to every other year.

The new guidelines, issued in late 2015 in the *Journal of the American Medical Association*, are nearly in line with guidelines from the USPSTF, the government-backed expert panel that recommends biennial breast cancer screening starting at age fifty for most women.

Both sets of guidelines were based on studies suggesting the benefits of detecting cancers earlier did not outweigh the risk of false-positive results, which needlessly expose women to additional testing, including a possible biopsy.

When the USPSTF first recommended pushing back mammogram screening from forty to age fifty, many advocacy groups, including the ACS, decried the change, claiming it would lead to more women dying from breast cancer.

New guidelines from the USPSTF note that some women in their forties might benefit from screening and that decisions should be made on an individual basis and discussions between a woman and her doctor.

But the changing guidelines have left many women confused, health experts say. What's more, some women's health specialists believe the new ACS recommendations could cost some women their lives.

"Since the 1990s, annual breast cancer screening is the only thing that has been proven to decrease breast cancer rates," says Dr. Kathleen A. Ward, a medical director of breast imaging at the Loyola University School of Medicine. "I think it is likely that this decision is economically motivated and comes from a desire to cut health care costs, but there are other places that we could be doing that."

Shifting Health Stances

The change in the ACS guidelines signaled a major shift in the organization's stance in the continuing controversy over mammography. The world's leading cancer advocacy organization is recommending that women who do not face higher-than-normal risks of breast cancer get annual mammograms starting at age forty-five rather than at age forty and that women aged fifty-five and older scale back screening to every other year.

Previously, the society had been in the forefront of recommending an aggressive annual screening program for women beginning at the age of forty. By comparison, the USPSTF recommends mammograms every other year for women ages fifty to seventy-four and advises against routine annual mammograms for women ages forty to forty-nine.

Women's health advocates say that the screening guidelines are important because breast cancer is one of the four most common cancers. This year, 231,840 new cases of breast cancer will be diagnosed, and 40,290 deaths due to the disease are expected in the United States.

In issuing its new guidelines, the ACS stressed that they apply only to women with no history of breast cancer or known risk factors based on genetic mutations, family history, or other medical problems that would make them more likely to develop the disease. Women at greater risk for breast cancer should consult their doctors about the benefits of mammograms as early as young adulthood.

Even so, Ward was "very surprised and disappointed" to hear about the change. "This is the wrong thing to do," she says. "Annual mammography is the best tool we have to find breast cancer early so it can be treated without the need for disfiguring surgery or toxic chemotherapy."

Best Bet: Talk to Your Doctor

Many experts say that while the differences among the various sets of guidelines might lead to confusion, they indicate that there is no single or correct answer for when and how often women should be screened for breast cancer.

In announcing the new guidelines, the ACS was careful to stress that women should make final decisions in conjunction with their doctors.

Although the organization no longer recommends mammograms for women ages forty to forty-four, it said those women should still "have the opportunity" to have the test if they choose to, and that women aged fifty-five and older should be able to keep having mammograms once a year.

Are New Federal PSA Guidelines Putting Men at Risk?

One in seven. That's how many men develop prostate cancer. But only about one in every thirty-eight men with prostate cancer will actually die from the disease.

The reason being, prostate cancer is often a slow-growing disease, and early detection of aggressive tumors through prostate-specific antigen (PSA) testing can lead to early treatment—surgery, chemo, or radiation—that increases a man's odds of survival. Or at least that was the operating assumption doctors have made since the FDA approved the PSA test in 1986.

But in 2012, the USPSTF—which sets medical policies for the nation—recommended against routine PSA screenings after concluding that the blood test is not foolproof and that harms from overtreatment outweigh the benefits.

Many men's health experts criticized the change in the guidelines at the time. Some even predicted that the change would leave men vulnerable by discouraging the tests.

Sadly, those dire predictions have come true.

A recent study led by Vanderbilt University Medical Center investigators has found that new diagnoses of prostate cancer have plummeted since the USPSTF recommended against routine PSA screening.

Just twelve months after the new guidelines were issued, diagnoses of new cancers had fallen by 38 percent, while colon cancer cases remained stable. New prostate cancer diagnoses also dropped by up to 29.3 percent among men over age seventy.

"These findings suggest that reduced screening may result in missed opportunities to spare these men from progressive disease and cancer death," said lead researcher Dr. Daniel Barocas, an assistant professor of urological surgery and medicine. "The results raise concern that if this trend continues, more men may be diagnosed at a point when their disease is advanced."

Trend Worsening

A second study, published in late 2015 in the *Journal of the American Medical Association*, indicates that this trend has only worsened over time. That study tracked 446,000 men since 2005 and found that for every 100,000 men—age fifty and older—the number of new cases of prostate cancer diagnoses has fallen from 535 to 416. In addition, the percentage of men who reported PSA screening fell from 41 percent in 2008 to 31 percent in 2013.

Dr. David Samadi, an expert in robotic prostate surgery at Lenox Hill Hospital in New York, says the new numbers are troubling and that the new PSA guidelines do not take into account many studies that provide a strong endorsement of PSA testing. That's particularly true for men in their forties who have an increased cancer risk because of their family history, genetics, race, and other factors.

One 2014 study, published in the *British Medical Journal* (*BMJ*), found that men with high PSA test results as early as age forty-five are three times more likely than those with lower levels to develop a life-threatening form of prostate cancer that spreads to other parts of the body within fifteen years. "We know the PSA test has reduced the mortality of cancer by 40 percent, so it has been an effective test," says Samadi.

PSA Testing Not Perfect

Even backers of PSA testing acknowledge its shortcomings. An elevated PSA can flag other noncancerous conditions, such as prostatitis, inflammation, and benign prostatic hyperplasia (BPH). Harmful side effects of aggressive cancer treatment include incontinence, erectile dysfunction (ED), and radiation cystitis.

But Samadi notes that PSA screening is the best test available and can be an effective tool in the hands of a doctor who specializes in its use. "There's an art to managing the PSA test, and it should be handled by doctors who use the PSA all the time," he says. "I don't just look at the value alone, but I look at the trend over time."

His recommendations are as follows:

- Men should start PSA screening at forty-five as a baseline.
- Every year afterward, men should have a PSA test to track for changes. Doctors consider PSA levels of 4.0 ng/mL of blood and lower to be normal. Those with PSAs of 4.0 or higher are often sent for a prostate biopsy to check for cancer.
- Men at increased risk for cancer should start PSA screening at forty—including African Americans, those with a family history of the disease, and men with variations in the genes BRCA1 and BRCA2 (tied to both prostate and breast cancer).

"Medicine is really like detective work," Samadi explains. "You have to use the art to decide who should have the PSA test and who should not. You have to look at the [results of] a physical exam, the race, family history, then the genetic package . . . and then decide who should be screened."

Cancer Prevention Beats Treatment

If you could take a pill that could cut your risk of developing cancer in half, would you take it? Of course you would. Unfortunately, no such pill exists today. But you can slash your risk of developing or dying from cancer by 50 percent by simply making a few lifestyle changes, experts say.

"If people did everything we know about preventing cancer, ideally, we could eliminate half of cancer incidence and prevent half of deaths," says Carolyn Aldige, president and founder of the Virginia-based Prevent Cancer Foundation.

Here are experts' top cancer-prevention tips:

Quit smoking. Using tobacco has been linked to various types of cancer, including cancer of the mouth, lungs, throat, larynx, pancreas, bladder, cervix, and kidneys. Even exposure to second-hand smoke increases your risk, says Dr. T. J. Patel, chief of hematology and oncology at Kelsey-Seybold Clinic in Texas.

Limit sun exposure. "Skin cancer is the most common of all cancers," Patel adds. "Reduce your risk by seeking shade in the middle of the day, covering exposed skin with sunscreen, protective clothing, hats, [and] sunglasses and reapplying sunscreen as needed."

Manage stress. Dr. Lauren Richter, DO, with the Center for Integrative Medicine at the University of Maryland School of Medicine, says that finding ways to manage stress is critical to boosting your immune system to combat cancer.

Hit the gym. Health experts endorse federal guidelines recommending exercise for at least thirty minutes daily to head off a range of obesity-related cancers.

Limit toxin exposures. Avoid hormone-disrupting toxins such as household chemicals, pesticides, parabens, and other pollutants that contribute to about 6 percent of cancer deaths, according to the ACS.

Lose weight. Dr. Gabe Mirkin, a leading health expert from Orlando, Florida, and the author of *The Healthy Heart Miracle*, says it's critical to lose excess weight and watch your blood sugar levels. "Obesity is a significant cancer risk," he says. "Everything that raises your blood sugar levels also increases that risk—being overweight, eating sugar-laden foods and drinks, lack of vitamin D, not exercising, and so forth."

Eat a healthy diet. Include a lot of fruits and vegetables in your diet, increase your fiber intake, and limit consumption of red meat, simple sugars, and alcohol. It's also a good idea to include as many of the following foods—loaded with cancer-fighting nutrients—as you can in your diet:

- **Leafy greens.** Kale, spinach, romaine lettuce, collard greens, Swiss chard, and other dark leafy greens contain compounds called carotenoids. Some studies show that they might reduce your risk of mouth, pharynx, and larynx cancer and slow the proliferation of the cells that cause breast, skin, lung, and stomach cancer. Carotenoids might work by soaking up potentially cancer-causing free radicals.
- **Cruciferous vegetables.** Broccoli, brussels sprouts, cabbage, and cauliflower are just a few members of this extended veggie family that might help you keep diseases like lung, prostate, and colorectal cancer at bay. The culprit here might be a group of cancer-fighting compounds in cruciferous veggies called isothiocyanates (ITCs). Studies reveal that ITCs might halt the growth of cancer cells and kill them as well as reduce inflammation. These superfilling, low-cal veggies can help you maintain your weight or shed a few pounds. Cutting and chewing cruciferous veggies helps release the anticancer compounds, so slice them up and eat them raw with your favorite dip or oven roast them with sea salt and olive oil.
- **Allium vegetables.** This smaller family of veggies—including garlic, leeks, onions, scallions, and chives—packs a powerful punch in terms of taste and cancer protection. Research reveals that allium veggies might have an impact on stomach cancer, and lab studies credit compounds in garlic—like quercetin, allixin, and organosulfur compounds—with slowing the development of prostate, bladder, colon, and stomach tumors. According to the American Institute for Cancer Research, "Recently, [one garlic component, called diallyl disulfide] proved able to kill leukemia cells in the laboratory."
- **Legumes.** Lentils, garbanzo beans, peas, kidney beans, black beans, split peas, and peanuts are some of the more well-known legumes. Not only are they loaded with fiber, iron, folate, potassium, magnesium, and B vitamins, but they're rich in protein so they're ideal for vegans and vegetarians. They also contain potential anticancer substances called lignans, which are plant chemicals, as well as resistant starch and an array of antioxidants. Some evidence links diets loaded with legumes to a decreased risk of stomach, colorectum, and kidney cancers.
- **Fish, milk, cereals, and other vitamin D-fortified foods.** You know that vitamin D can help keep your bones and teeth in tip-top shape. But some studies suggest that people who had higher levels of this nutrient in their bodies had lower rates of breast, ovarian, renal, colon, pancreatic, and prostate cancers. "Laboratory studies provide some strong

biological evidence to support a role for vitamin D in cancer prevention," according to the ACS. This vitamin might work by regulating various genes that cause cancer cells to proliferate and by reducing inflammation. Foods rich in vitamin D include cod, shrimp, salmon, eggs, fortified milk, and cereals.

Cancer: By the Numbers

- Each year, an estimated 1,685,210 new cases of cancer are diagnosed in the United States; 595,690 people will die from the disease.
- The most common cancers are breast cancer, lung and bronchus cancer, prostate cancer, colon and rectum cancer, bladder cancer, melanoma of the skin, non-Hodgkin lymphoma, thyroid cancer, kidney and renal pelvis cancer, leukemia, endometrial cancer, and pancreatic cancer.
- Cancer mortality is higher among men than women (208 per 100,000 men and 145 per 100,000 women). It is highest in African American men (262 per 100,000) and lowest in Asian/Pacific Islander women (91 per 100,000).
- The number of people living beyond a cancer diagnosis reached nearly 14.5 million in 2014 and is expected to rise to almost 19 million by 2024.
- Nearly 40 percent of men and women will be diagnosed with cancer at some point during their lifetimes.
- In 2014, an estimated 15,780 children and adolescents under age nineteen were diagnosed with cancer and 1,960 died of the disease.
- National expenditures for cancer care in the United States totaled nearly $125 billion in 2010 and could reach $156 billion in 2020.
- The overall US cancer death rate has declined since the early 1990s. Since 2003, cancer death rates decreased by 1.8 percent per year among men, 1.4 percent per year among women, and 2 percent per year among children.
- Cancer is among the leading causes of death worldwide. In 2012, there were 14 million new cases and 8.2 million cancer-related deaths worldwide.

Source: National Cancer Institute

Do X-Rays Raise Cancer Risks?

Radiation is a double-edged sword. Thanks to its use in diagnostic testing, the need for exploratory surgery to seek out cancer has dropped dramatically. On the other hand, many of these tests use radiation, which raises the fear that they might be causing exactly the disease they are designed to find.

The use of such radiation has historically been viewed in terms of the benefits outweighing any risks, but the use of medical imaging has skyrocketed in recent years, which suggests more people are being exposed to higher levels than ever before.

About sixty-two million CT scans, which use X-rays to create images, were performed in 2006 in the United States, compared with just three million in 1980. And in 1990, fewer than three million nuclear studies were performed in the United States, but this number has more than tripled since then, statistics show.

This proliferation prompted the White House advisory group known as the President's Cancer Panel Report to recommend recently that doctors make sure that "radiation doses are as low as reasonably achievable without sacrificing quality."

Among those concerned is top cardiologist Dr. Chauncey Crandall, chief of the cardiac transplant program at the world-renowned Palm Beach Cardiovascular Clinic in Palm Beach Gardens, Florida.

"These tests emit ionizing radiation, which is the type that can damage DNA, and that is linked to the development of cancer over time, and so I am concerned about the amount that patients are getting," Crandall says.

It's well known that children who are exposed to large amounts of radiation to treat certain cancers are more likely to develop a second cancer later in life. But little data exist on the dangerous effects of radiation from diagnostic testing on healthy adults, or whether such radiation poses a problem to cancer patients.

Most of what is known about the effects of ionizing radiation comes from long-term studies of people who survived the World War II atomic bomb blasts, which have shown a slight but significantly increased cancer risk.

"There is so much fear of radiation today, but this comes from people at Nagasaki and Hiroshima who were exposed to it during World War II. These were extremely high doses, and this experience is irrelevant to the type of radiation in use today," says Dr. James Welsh, a radiation oncologist at Loyola University Medical Center in Maywood, Illinois.

He's concerned that people will either pass on needed tests or insist too little radiation be used. "Simply put, you need a minimum [of] X-ray photons striking it, and if you don't have that, you don't get an adequate image, and then the study needs to be redone, exposing the patient to more radiation," he says.

But Welsh agrees that patients should not be exposed to radiation unnecessarily, so he suggests asking the following questions when such tests are ordered:

- What information will this test provide?
- Are you ordering this test in accordance with the recommendations established by the leading clinical guidelines?

- Are there any tests that don't use radiation that can provide you with the information you need? Many diagnostic tests emit little or no radiation, including EKGs, echocardiograms, and MRIs.

If the answer to any of these questions is yes, here are follow-up questions to ask the radiation medical physicist, the person at the facility who deals with the use of radiation during such testing:

- Will the machine being used emit the lowest amount of radiation needed to get the information my doctor is seeking?
- Can you customize the amount of radiation to suit my physiology? As Welsh notes, "More radiation is needed to provide images of a 400-pound man than a 120-pound woman, so you should if the amount of radiation you will get has been recalibrated from the person whose test was done before you."

CHRONIC FATIGUE SYNDROME

Yuppie flu. Shirker syndrome. For nearly three decades, people with chronic fatigue syndrome (CFS) faced such derisive nicknames for the condition that left them feeling tired all the time. Doctors, bosses, coworkers, and close friends and relatives sometimes accused them of imagining their symptoms or suggested they had mental health problems.

Even the Centers for Disease Control and Prevention (CDC) acknowledged in 1999 that millions of dollars allocated by Congress to study CFS had been diverted to other research programs because scientists just didn't believe it was a real health condition. But in the last decade, the CDC recognized that studies have proven CFS is linked to genetic mutations and abnormalities in gene expression involved in key physiological processes.

In other words, CFS sufferers aren't malingerers or imagining things; CFS is a bona fide health disorder that now garners $6 million a year in public awareness campaigns sponsored by the CDC. What's more, the agency has released studies suggesting that it is far more common than previously believed—striking at least one million Americans who might suffer symptoms as debilitating as AIDS, cancer, or other chronic conditions.

What Is CFS?

Chronic fatigue syndrome, also known as myalgic encephalomyelitis (ME), was first identified in the 1980s. For reasons scientists don't fully understand, it afflicts more women than men, causing extreme fatigue, sleep disorders, cognitive problems, malaise, and other symptoms.

Typical symptoms of CFS, and its painful cousin fibromyalgia, include

- pain
- tingling
- headaches
- irritability
- sleep disturbances
- numbness in hands and feet

Because it is not easily diagnosed—there are no specific lab or blood tests for it—doctors typically identify sufferers on the basis of characteristic symptoms and history of illness. There are no effective conventional treatments, so doctors typically prescribe medications to manage symptoms, with widely varying degrees of effectiveness.

Studies suggest CFS is likely tied to problems in the nervous system, the immune system, cognitive functions, the stress response pathways, and perhaps other biological processes.

It's also possible that it might have multiple causes, as yet undetermined—including genetic factors, exposure to microbial agents and toxins, and other physical and emotional traumas. Some studies have also suggested it might be caused or triggered by infectious diseases, such as Lyme disease, Q fever, Ross River virus, parvovirus, and mononucleosis.

According to the CDC, only 20 percent of those with CFS are diagnosed with the illness. Even so, health care costs associated with the disease are estimated to be $18–$51 billion annually in the United States.

Managing and Treating CFS

Dr. Jacob Teitelbaum, a CFS specialist and author of *The Fatigue and Fibromyalgia Solution*, refers to CFS as a "human energy crisis." The pain comes from having too little energy, which causes muscles to lock in a shortened position, making you hurt all over.

"What's going on is an energy crisis, so anything that causes you to spend more energy than you're able to make—whether it happens to be hormonal problems, nutritional deficiencies, infections, chronic stress, autoimmune diseases like lupus, basically anything that drains your energy account, can cause you to blow that circuit breaker," he says. "And then once that happens you can't sleep and you're on that slippery slope going downhill."

Unfortunately, mainstream medicine has not taken fibromyalgia and CFS seriously, which historically has been a typical reaction to diseases affecting mainly women, he notes. "We've seen this over and over in illnesses that affect women, and especially if there's no good blood test for it," he says. "And we saw the same thing with rheumatoid arthritis, lupus—women used to be considered neurotic—multiple sclerosis, which was called hysterical paralysis. All these are illnesses of the immune system that affect women. And until they had a test for it the doctor said: 'I don't know what's wrong with you so you're crazy.' It's really a nasty thing to do to people. But we're seeing it now with fibromyalgia and chronic fatigue syndrome."

The good news is that fibromyalgia and chronic fatigue syndrome are highly treatable conditions, he says. With thirty years of experience treating hundreds of patients a year, Teitelbaum has developed a five-step treatment approach known as the "SHINE" protocol—short for sleep, hormones, immunity, nutrition, and exercise. The regimen includes the following:

SLEEP. Aggravated by pain and body stiffness, insomnia is common in people with CFS and fibromyalgia. Nevertheless, sleep is a critical component for a condition that depletes energy and you should look to get between eight and nine hours of sleep per night.

HORMONES. Most sufferers also have hormone deficiencies. So checking hormone levels and possibly getting on thyroid medication can improve symptoms for some.

INFECTIONS. Underlying viral, bacterial, bowel, sinus, and yeast infections are common and can be a chronic feature. Get treatment as soon as symptoms of infections occur.

NUTRITION. Make sure to get optimal nutrition because the entire nervous system is depleted and under duress in people with CFS and fibromyalgia. Teitelbaum recommends using vitamin powder to ensure the body gets the right amount of vitamins and minerals and to avoid having to swallow handfuls of pills.

EXERCISE. Even walking for just thirty minutes a day can help ease symptoms and strengthen the body and mind.

"I know what people live through with this," Teitelbaum says. "I had chronic fatigue syndrome and fibromyalgia back in 1975. It knocked me out of med school for a year. That's how I learned about it. We've treated thousands of people. This is a very, very treatable disease."

He is also critical of doctors who continue to dismiss patient's symptoms as imaginary or linked to mental illness. "It is no more appropriate for a doctor to say 'I don't know what's wrong with you so you're crazy', then it was when multiple sclerosis was rudely called hysterical paralysis," Teitelbaum says. "If a doctor is so hopelessly out of date that they still do this to you, walk up to them, give him a big hug, and tell them 'Thank you for letting me know quickly what an utter and completely out of date idiot you are so I don't waste my time with you.' And walk out the door."

Gut Bacteria: Key to Treating CFS?

Heart disease. Diabetes. Cancer. Depression. Autism. Alzheimer's disease. Autoimmune disorders. A growing body of scientific research has linked these conditions to imbalances in gut bacteria—the makeup of "good" and "bad" microbes that live in our digestive tracts.

Now, a new study suggests chronic fatigue syndrome—a hard-to-diagnose condition—might be influenced by a person's gut bacteria. The findings, say Cornell University researchers, are the first to seriously refute the idea that the syndrome is a psychological disorder, often dismissed by doctors as not real.

Maureen Hanson, a professor of molecular biology and genetics who led the study, found that people with CFS have a different profile of bacterial species in their gut microbiome than healthy individuals.

Specifically, sufferers have less diversity or different types of bacteria, the researchers found. They also tend to have more types of microbes that promote inflammation.

Up to four million Americans have CFS, also known as myalgic encephalomyelitis, according to the CDC. But only one in five with the condition know it or have been diagnosed. Symptoms include severe fatigue, malaise, joint and muscle pain, headaches and gastrointestinal problems such as irritable bowel syndrome.

For the Cornell study, researchers evaluated forty-eight people diagnosed with the syndrome and thirty-nine healthy individuals. All provided stool samples, which were tested for bacterial DNA—tests that pointed out the differences.

The researchers noted the lower level of microbial diversity seen in the chronic fatigue patients is similar to those seen in people with two Crohn's disease and ulcerative colitis.

Hanson notes that many species of gut bacteria are beneficial to healthy bodily functions, including the immune system. She adds that the findings might be used to develop a new diagnostic test to determine if someone has CFS.

The study adds to the expanding list of research on various health conditions that has identified what experts call the gut-brain axis. Such findings suggest adjusting the diet might be one way to ease symptoms by altering and improving the gut environment in ways that are beneficial to health.

Probiotics and foods that contain "good" bacteria—such as yogurt, aged cheeses, and kimchi—have been shown to help many people with digestive disorders.

The Cornell study was published in the journal *Microbiome*.

Medications That Can Cause Fatigue

While CFS is a distinct physical disorder, millions of Americans experience less debilitating feelings of low energy and listlessness that can make life difficult. Research shows that one surprising factor can contribute to fatigue: common medications used to treat everything from allergies to hypertension to heartburn.

Among the prime culprits are the following:

Beta-blockers. Prescribed as the first-line treatment for high blood pressure, these drugs reduce stress on your heart by slowing your heart rate. It is this same mechanism that leaves many patients feeling fatigued and lethargic. In 2014, the Joint National Committee on Detection, Evaluation and Treatment of High Blood Pressure (JNC) released an update on managing blood pressure relegating beta-blockers to second-line treatment.

Alternate treatment with drugs called thiazide-diuretics, calcium-channel blockers, and angiotensin-converting-enzyme (ACE) inhibitors might have fewer side effects. If you are on a beta-blocker and feeling extremely tired, ask if you can switch to another type of blood pressure medication. An omega-3 fish oil supplement might also help lower blood pressure naturally, but always check with your health care provider before making any changes in your medication.

Proton pump inhibitors (PPIs). These ubiquitous drugs used to treat gastro-esophageal reflux disease (GERD) and other similar disorders are prescribed to a whopping twenty million Americans. Long-term use of PPI medications can reduce the absorption of important nutrients such as magnesium, iron, and vitamin B12.

Imbalances in these levels can lead to everything from osteoporosis to anemia, which is a significant source of fatigue. The majority of patients with heartburn and reflex should only take a finite course of these drugs, experts say, and then focus on lifestyle modification, weight loss, exercise and avoiding trigger foods.

Antihistamines. These drugs used to relieve the symptoms of allergies or the common cold are central nervous system (CNS) depressants. First-generation antihistamines like diphenhydramine (Benadryl) are the worst offenders. Second-generation drugs like cetirizine (Zyrtec), loratadine (Claritin), and fexofenadine (Allegra) are better options. But natural approaches to easing congestion—such as nasal irrigation using a neti pot—often work as well but carry no side effects.

Sleep aids. You'd think that using sleep aids would relieve fatigue, but in fact, experts note that common drugs like benzodiazepine (Valium, Xanax) and zolpidem (Ambien) prescribed to treat insomnia can actually leave you feeling exhausted during the day.

They work by dampening the "awake" centers in the brain. But some of these drugs stick around in your system for extended periods of time, making you tired the next day. They can also cause memory problems, dependence, and rebound insomnia.

For long term-management of insomnia, you're better off using nonmedication alternatives such as practicing good sleep hygiene. That means going to bed and waking at the same time every day, keeping your bedroom as dark as possible, and not watching TV or using a cell phone, tablet, or computer right before bedtime—all emit "blue light," which disrupts the release of the natural sleep hormone melatonin.

Seven Surprising Energy Thieves

If you're chronically tired and lack energy, you might also want to take a closer look at the consumer products you use and foods you eat. Certain chemicals and compounds in many foods, consumer products, and even upholstery can disrupt thyroid function and leave you feeling fatigued and less energetic.

It all has to do with the function of the thyroid gland. The butterfly-shaped gland located just below the Adam's apple in your neck uses iodine to manufacture hormones that regulate metabolism throughout the body. But chemicals and compounds in many foods, consumer products, and even upholstery can disrupt thyroid function and leave you feeling fatigued and less energetic.

"The thyroid hormones are crucial for energy," says Dr. Ajay Rao, an endocrinologist at the Lewis Katz School of Medicine at Temple University in

Philadelphia. "Classic symptoms of an underactive thyroid are fatigue, weight gain, cold intolerance, constipation—basically, the whole body slows down."

The most common cause of an underactive thyroid, called hypothyroidism, is the autoimmune disease Hashimoto's thyroiditis. "Other causes include surgery to remove the thyroid, certain medications, long-term steroid use, and iodine deficiency," Rao says. "There are also some chemicals that disrupt thyroid function, but they are hard to nail down, as there is still active research in this field."

Here are seven surprising things that might disrupt thyroid function:

Toothpaste. If your toothpaste contains fluoride, you might want to consider switching brands. While fluoride is good for teeth, it's not so good for the endocrine system. In fact, fluoride was once used to treat an overactive thyroid. And a British study in 2015 strongly liked fluoridated water to hypothyroidism. The problem? Your thyroid will typically absorb fluoride over iodine, which inhibits its ability to produce its key hormones.

New cars. Love that new-car smell? Well, it doesn't love you. The chemicals used to create it also emit fumes that you typically inhale in a confined space. One of them, the fire retardant bromine, is another compound that the thyroid will sop up instead of iodine. Eventually, the effects of the chemicals fade away, which is why old cars might not tickle your olfactory nerves but are healthier for your thyroid.

Swimming pools. Swimming is great exercise, but if you're doing it in a chlorinated pool, you could be handicapping your thyroid. Like fluoride and bromine, chorine also hogs your thyroid's attention at the expense of iodine. Even if you don't swim, you ingest chlorine in your drinking water and even absorb it through your skin during showers.

Selenium deficiency. The thyroid produces hydrogen peroxide to help it metabolize iodine, but that process also creates free radicals that can damage the gland. That, in turn, can trigger autoimmune diseases including Hashimoto's. But the trace mineral selenium protects the thyroid by neutralizing the free radicals. Brazil nuts are the best source of selenium, but it can also be found in sardines, yellowfin tuna, grass-fed beef, poultry, eggs, and spinach.

Super greens. Leafy greens and cruciferous vegetables such as kale, arugula, bok choy, cabbage, watercress, mustard greens, broccoli, and cauliflower are packed with nutrients, but they are also goitrogenic foods. That means they have compounds that can disrupt the thyroid's absorption of iodine. Taken in normal amounts, the greens won't hurt thyroid function. But eating massive quantities of these veggies raw, especially through juicing, might be too much of a good thing, warn experts.

Smoking. Here's one more reason to quit tobacco. As if heart disease and cancer aren't bad enough on their own, cigarette smoke wreaks havoc on the thyroid gland. One problem is that the cyanide in the smoke boosts excretion of iodine, limiting its availability to the thyroid.

Caffeine. Drinking too much coffee or caffeinated soft drinks stimulates the release of the stress hormones cortisol and adrenaline, which can interfere with the way the thyroid hormones T3 and T4 interact, making them less effective. So if you need a morning pick-me-up, you might want to try a cold shower instead of hot cup of java.

UK Study CFS Therapy That Cures Two-Thirds of Patients

British scientists have launched a clinical trial of a new chronic fatigue syndrome therapy that has been found to cure two-thirds of children with the condition in early studies.

The trial, on 734 children, will use intensive online therapy sessions to modify sleeping habits and activity levels. It also uses a form of behavioral therapy to help children with the disease adapt the way they live.

Esther Crawley, a children's doctor from the University of Bristol, is leading the study, supported by the British National Health Service, to see if online consultations work and are cost-effective.

Studies of the technique in the Netherlands showed that 63 percent of the patients given therapy had no symptoms after six months.

The technique aims to change the way children think of the disease and reduce the time spent sleeping and sometimes cut activity levels.

COLD AND FLU

The average American catches two to four colds each year, while the flu infects millions—sending about 200,000 people to US hospitals annually, according to the Centers for Disease Control and Prevention (CDC). In addition, influenza kills about 36,000 Americans in a typical flu season, with the annual death toll ranging from 3,300 to 49,000 over the past three decades.

To combat influenza, the CDC recommends everyone older than six months get a flu shot annually. In addition, US consumers are spending billions of dollars on cold remedies to prevent and treat respiratory infections, coughs, sore throats, and stuffy noses.

But what really works and what doesn't when it comes to combating the common cold and flu? Here's a primer.

Flu Shot Myths, Facts

Few public health campaigns are as visible and aggressive as the CDC's annual pitch for Americans to get a flu shot. Many mainstream medical studies show that the vaccine is the best way to prevent influenza, which strikes about 20 percent of Americans each year, yet only about four in ten actually get a flu shot each year.

Why?

First of all, many myths surround the shot—including the falsehood that it can actually cause influenza (it can't) or that it might cause serious allergic reactions or complications (which are possible but extremely rare in individuals allergic to eggs, which are used to make some vaccines).

Others opt not to get the shot because of widely circulated social media claims that it isn't effective—claims that are largely false but do contain of kernel of truth.

In fact, the flu shot is not 100 percent effective. Studies show the vaccine is only 63 percent effective in a good year and far less so during several recent seasons. But that still means more than six in ten individuals exposed to the flu virus won't catch it if they've been vaccinated.

Some years, however, the flu shot is even less effective. The severe 2014–15 flu season's flu shot was disappointingly ineffective, for instance. The CDC reported that people who got the shot were just 19 percent less likely to get the flu than people who did not get vaccinated. That's about a third less protection than previous seasons' shots. During the 2012–13 flu season, for instance, the flu shot reduced the risk of contracting the flu by 56 percent.

The reason being, the 2014–15 flu shot was a mismatch between the flu strains included in that vaccine and the viral strains that were circulating. Most flu illnesses were caused by a viral strain known as H3N2. But about 80 percent of the H3N2 viruses in circulation were different from the H3N2 strain included in the flu shot, because the virus's genetic material changed slightly over time.

As a result, that year's flu season was particularly severe for older adults, who had the highest rate of flu hospitalizations in a decade, according to the CDC. Between October 2014 and April 2015, there were about 322 hospitalizations per 100,000 people among US adults ages sixty-five and over. Previously, the highest rate of hospitalizations for this age group was 183 flu hospitalizations per 100,000 people, which occurred during the 2012–13 flu season.

Even so, federal health officials and nearly all mainstream medical doctors argue that vaccination is the best way to reduce the odds of getting seasonal flu and spreading it to others.

Here are some common questions and answers about the flu vaccine.

When Is Flu Most Active?

In the United States, flu season generally runs from late fall into spring, but sometimes starts earlier and runs later. Flu activity typically peaks in January or later.

Who's Most at Risk?

Young children, people over age sixty-five, pregnant women, and individuals with certain medical conditions—such as asthma, diabetes, or heart disease—face a higher risk of flu-related complications, including pneumonia, ear and sinus infections, and bronchitis.

Why Do You Need an Annual Vaccine?

Flu strains mutate every year, which means vaccines need to be revised annually to combat the strains that CDC specialists and others believe will be circulating in a particular season.

Flu vaccine manufacturers devise and distribute shots based on the viral mutations the flu has undergone as it travels eastward through Europe and Asia before arriving in the United States.

Flu vaccines work by boosting the body's ability to develop antibodies to fight future exposure. The vaccines are "inactivated," which means that the flu virus used to produce them is killed and the inactivated components stimulate the antibody production that protects against the virus.

What Options Are Available?
Until 2016, the FluMist nasal spray was available as an alternative to needles. But the CDC determined the FluMist's effectiveness was just 3 percent during the 2015–16 flu season; the injected vaccine had a 63 percent effectiveness rate.

The CDC recommends everyone six months and older receive an annual flu vaccination, but some forms of the shot are only recommended for certain demographics.

- The regular-dose shot (which usually offers protection against several strains of the virus) is the most common form of the vaccine and is recommended for most people, including pregnant women.
- Children ages six months to eight years old should get two doses, one month apart, for their first shot. For every subsequent season, they will only need one dose.
- A high dose shot is recommended for people sixty-five years of age or older.
- An alternative form of vaccination—Flublok—is recommended for people over age eighteen with severe egg allergies.

Late September or early October is the ideal time to get your flu shot, but if you have concerns about possible local outbreaks, contact your health care provider. Keep in mind that it takes up to two weeks for the vaccine to offer full protection against the flu. As a result, it's not uncommon for people to develop the flu after receiving a shot, but it is only because they were exposed to the virus before the vaccine became effective—*not* because the vaccine caused the infection.

What Are the Most Effective Ways to Avoid the Flu?
Experts recommend frequent hand washing, using hand sanitizers, covering your mouth when you cough, not touching your hands to you face and eyes, and wiping down surfaces with disinfectant to reduce the risk of contracting the flu.

What Are the Symptoms of Flu?
Here are the typical signs and symptoms of the flu:

- cough
- high fever
- body aches or headache
- extreme fatigue
- sore throat
- nasal congestion
- runny nose

Can Anything Treat the Flu?

The Food and Drug Administration (FDA) has approved three influenza antiviral drugs to treat the virus: Tamiflu (generic name oseltamivir), Relenza (generic name zanamivir), and Rapivab (generic name peramivir).

These meds can lessen the severity and duration of influenza, although research has shown the effects might not be significant in many people. But they are most effective when taken within a forty-eight-hour window from the onset of symptoms.

Preventing and Treating the Common Cold

Over-the-counter (OTC) cold remedies typically fill more drugstore aisles than the cereal shelves in supermarkets. But the latest research suggests a large number of those medications do little to stop or treat viral and bacterial infections that strike during winter months.

However, a recent analysis of sixty-seven cold-remedy studies—by Dr. Michael Allan, director of medicine at the University of Alberta—found strong evidence that certain OTC remedies are reliable and effective. Among them are zinc, which can help prevent a cold, and pain relievers and decongestants, which are reliable treatment options.

The review, published in the *Canadian Medical Association Journal*, found that probiotics—"good bacteria" in yogurt and other food products—can also block cold infections.

But Allan's findings were inconclusive on the benefits of homeopathic remedies and certain vitamins. Allan added, however, that despite the lack of scientific evidence for many cold and flu remedies, many of his patients still swear by some—in part because they believe the treatments are working.

"People have individual reactions to medicines that are not predictable," he said. "There is also, of course, the placebo effect—you think it's going to work [and you feel better]."

Here's what you need to know about the latest word on common cold prevention and treatment strategies based on Allan's analysis and other studies.

ZINC. Lozenges and OTC tablets that contain zinc (such as Zicam and Cold-Eeze) have been shown to ease symptoms and shorten the duration of the common cold. They also might help prevent infections from taking hold. Two studies indicated that children who took 10–15 mg of zinc sulphate daily had fewer colds and absences from school. Although the studies were carried out on children the researchers concluded, "There is no . . . reason why zinc could work only in children and not adults." But not all zinc products are safe. In 2009, the FDA warned consumers not to use some zinc-based nasal products, which have been linked to a loss of taste and smell in some people.

DECONGESTANTS. OTC decongestants relieve stuffy sinuses by shrinking blood vessels that cause congestion. The most effective ones contain pseudoephedrine (the active ingredient in Sudafed). But FDA restrictions implemented in 2005 limit how much an individual can purchase because the drug can be used to make methamphetamine. That said, it is safe and among the most effective cold remedies. Spray-based decongestants are also effective, but they should only be used short term.

EXPECTORANTS, ANTIHISTAMINES. Products designed to help you cough up mucus (such as Mucinex) can ease coughs, but drinking more water or using a humidifier can have the same effect. Combining expectorants with antihistamines, however, can also alleviate cold symptoms but should not be used in children under five years of age, health officials warn. In addition, antihistamines and allergy medicines—such as Claritin, Zyrtec, and Benadryl—can help treat a runny nose or sore throat.

PAINKILLERS. For fever, acetaminophen (Tylenol) and ibuprofen (Advil) can be helpful, as well as anti-inflammatories like naproxen (Aleve). But some individuals with heart disease, asthma, or stomach problems should consult a doctor first about which medication is the safest and most effective to take, Allan notes. Theraflu contains acetaminophen and other anticold ingredients but can pose a risk of liver damage at high doses or if taken with alcohol or other acetaminophen-containing products.

PROBIOTICS. Allan said scientific research has shown that probiotics might help prevent colds, perhaps by boosting the body's immune system. But the types and combinations of organisms varied in the studies, as did the formulations, making comparisons difficult. Because many foods with probiotics contain other healthy ingredients, there are few downsides to adding them to your diet during cold and flu season.

VITAMIN C. Taking megadoses of vitamin C became popular in the 1970s after Nobel laureate Linus Pauling claimed it could prevent and treat the common cold.

But studies of the antioxidant have been disappointing. A review by the Cochrane Collaborative—a scientific organization that analyzes multiple studies to reach consensus conclusions—found vitamin C supplements had no effect in preventing the common cold but might shorten an infection's duration. But be aware, high doses can cause nausea, diarrhea, and stomach cramps. A healthier option is to eat foods loaded with vitamin C, such as citrus fruits, to stay healthy.

HOMEOPATHIC REMEDIES. Products such as Defend and Sambucol promise to fight multiple symptoms of a cold, but the National Institutes of Health (NIH) has concluded that there is little to no evidence that such homeopathic remedies are effective preventive measures. In addition, they are not as stringently regulated as drugs.

OTHER STRATEGIES. The benefits of frequently used remedies such as ginseng (found in ColdFX), gargling with salt water, or using honey are unclear, Allan concluded. His team also noted that most colds are caused by viruses, with only about 5 percent due to bacterial infections, so antibiotics won't help, even though they are often prescribed inappropriately for viral infections.

In addition to these findings, health experts say the following strategies can ward off a cold or ease symptoms:

- **Fastidiously wash your hands** and use alcohol-based hand sanitizers and disinfectants to keep cold and flu bugs at bay.
- **Avoid close contact** with people who have a cold, especially during the first few days, when they are most likely to spread the infection.
- **Drink lots of fluids**—including water, fruit juices, and even warm lemon water with honey—to loosen congestion and prevent dehydration. Avoid soda, coffee, and alcohol, which can make dehydration worse.
- **Use saline nasal drops and sprays** to ease stuffiness and congestion. Such products carry few risks, even for children, and don't lead to the rebound effect—a worsening of symptoms when the medication is discontinued—seen in other types of nasal products.
- **Eat chicken soup**, or even clear broth, which might actually relieve cold and flu symptoms by acting as an anti-inflammatory and speeding up the movement of mucus.

Echinacea: Nature's Cold and Flu Fighter

Echinacea has been the Rocky Balboa of natural cold and flu remedies since the 1990s—called a champion for your health one year, only to be knocked down by health experts the next.

In the late 1990s, it was the king of the ring, racking up impressive annual sales of $206 million after research suggested that it can effectively combat winter viruses. By 2010, it was practically washed up after some studies showed that it had little or no benefit, with annual sales plummeting to a paltry $115 million.

But the most recent research suggests that Echinacea is ready to reclaim its crown. "There seems to be some benefit from taking it throughout the cold season," says Dr. Tod Cooperman, president of ConsumerLab.com, which recently published an extensive product review of Echinacea.

How a big a benefit? A 25–50 percent reduced risk of catching a cold, Cooperman says. That's on par with other prevention strategies designed to boost the immune system—such as getting regular exercise, eating a healthy diet, and managing stress levels.

If you're one of miserable millions who catch cold after cold through the winter, that's huge. Here's a primer.

WHAT IS ECHINACEA? A flowering plant that is native to the United States and Canada, echinacea includes nine different species—three of which have been used medicinally: *Echinacea purpurea*, *Echinacea angustifolia*, and *Echinacea pallida*. Of these, *E. purpurea* seems to be the most effective.

HOW DOES IT WORK? Researchers believe that Echinacea prevents colds and flus because it stimulates the immune system. In laboratories, the herb has been shown to increase production of infection-fighting white blood cells.

HOW IS IT USED? "Echinacea is typically used as a preventive product," explains Cooperman. "That's how it's most effective." He advises taking about 900 mg of Echinacea extract per day divided into two or three doses.

ARE ALL PRODUCTS THE SAME? In a word, no. Not any product will do. "Make sure it has the right species and part of the plant," Cooperman cautions. It's best to choose extracts or tinctures that contain either *E. purpurea* or *E. angustifolia*, which are the two best-studied species. It's also important to choose extracts made from the above-ground (aerial) part of the plant, such as its flowers, leaves, and stems. Such information should be listed on the label. Beware of products that list Echinacea as part of part of a "blend" or "proprietary formula" without specifying the type or amount. Based on the ConsumerLab.com report, the top three picks are

1. Swanson Superior Herbs Elderberry Echinacea Goldenseal Immune Complex
2. Gaia Herbs Echinacea Supreme Liquid
3. A. Vogel Echinaforce

WHAT DOES THE RESEARCH SHOW? A. Vogel Echinaforce is a Swiss-made product that was used in a large-scale study published in 2012. During the study, 755 participants took either A. Vogel Echinaforce or a placebo for four months. The Echinacea group caught fewer colds than the placebo group (149 versus 188), which wasn't statistically significant. But the Echinacea group experienced 26 percent fewer cold "events," which was statistically significant.

Such an "event" was defined as a combination of a cold and its duration. In addition, the Echinacea group was significantly less likely to catch more than one cold. When they did come down with a cold, they took less pain medication. The researchers noted that Echinacea was particularly effective at preventing colds in people who smoked, had high levels of stress, or had trouble sleeping.

DOES IT TREAT VIRUSES? Although most research supports the use of Echinacea to prevent colds and flus, some studies suggest that it also might be a valuable treatment. A 2015 study showed that a hot drink blend of Echinacea and elderberry is just as effective as the prescription drug Tamiflu at treating symptoms of influenza.

The preparation is available in Europe and Canada and is expected to hit the US market sometime in 2016. At the first sign of a cold, Cooperman recommends starting a 900 mg daily course of Echinacea extract divided into two or three doses per day. If you take this amount for one to two weeks, you might be able to decrease the severity of your illness and shorten its duration.

IS IT SAFE? For most people, Echinacea is a relatively safe herb. If side effects occur, they're usually mild ones, such as stomach upsets. Because Echinacea stimulates the immune system, however, it should not be used by people who have autoimmune conditions such as rheumatoid arthritis or Crohn's disease or those who take immune-suppressant drugs such as steroids.

Echinacea also should be avoided by people with allergies to related plants such as daisies, sunflowers, marigolds, chrysanthemums, and ragweed.

Flu-Fighting Strategies for Holiday Travelers

About thirty-eight million Americans typically take flights to visit family and friends for Christmas and New Year's celebrations. While it's a great time to spread cheer, it's also high time for the spread of influenza and winter colds.

Health experts note that your chances of catching a nasty virus increase dramatically if you're traveling during the holidays, with airplanes and airports teaming with pathogens—not to mention holiday parties and get-togethers.

"We've seen an increase in influenza in December, January, and February in the past few years, and holiday travel is probably a reason," notes Dr. Stephanie Haridopolos, a board-certified family practitioner in Melbourne, Florida, and president of the Brevard County Medical Society. "With travel, you're more vulnerable to colds and flu."

But you can take steps to reduce your risks and make sure your holidays are happy and healthy. If you're traveling by air, be aware that certain surfaces on plans and in airports are loaded with disease-causing germs. A recent analysis by Travelmath.com, which helps people calculate the driving and flying time between cities, found that airports and planes tend to be dirtier than the average American home, in terms of germs.

The study also found that bathrooms have fewer germs than other areas you might not consider hotbeds of infectious pathogens. Tests showed that the dirtiest place on most planes is the tray table—the surface most travelers touch as they eat and drink in-flight foods and beverages. Other hotbeds for bacteria, fungi, and viruses include overhead air vents and seat belt buckles, which harbor as many microbes as dirty lavatory flush buttons, the analysis showed.

In airports, the findings were comparable, with tests showing that drinking fountain buttons were far more contaminated with germs than bathroom stall locks. "Bathrooms were some of the cleaner surfaces tested, which may be contrary to conventional thought," the researchers reported. "Regular cleaning schedules mean these surfaces are sanitized more frequently. This is a good thing."

To reduce your risk of catching a cold, the flu, or something worse while on the road this holiday season, health experts recommend the following precautions:

- Ask to move your seat if someone near you is coughing or bring a mask you can wear if someone next to you appears sick.
- Boost your immune system by staying active, eating well, and getting plenty of rest in the days leading up to your travel.
- Don't use courtesy airline pillows and blankets, which might be loaded with germs from previous fliers.
- Drink water or use a saline spray to keep nasal passages moist and hydrated. The air on planes can be dry, which hikes your risk of contracting a respiratory infection.
- If the plane's circulation is shut down during a ground delay, complain to the crew.

- Open the air vent "gaspers" overhead, which improve circulation, and point the vents over your head so the air flows in front of your face to deflect any airborne viruses or bacteria.
- Pack and use sanitizer wipes to clean plane trays, bathroom surfaces, and anything else you touch. Keep your hands away from your face and eyes to avoid spreading germs. Try not to touch the seat-back pocket in front of you or the armrests.
- Try to sit near the front of the plane, where ventilation is best, and avoid aisle seats, which will put you in greater contact with potentially sick passengers.
- Wash your hands frequently or use an alcohol-based hand sanitizer. Avoid shaking hands with fellow passengers.

Haridopolos also advises limiting close contact with family and friends as much as possible over the holidays because this increases your risk of catching a cold or the flu. Limit hugs and kisses if you're feeling under the weather and wash your hands frequently.

In addition, be on the lookout for signs of cold or flu—fever, body aches, chills, fatigue, sneezing, sinus congestion, sore throat, coughing, headache, nausea, or diarrhea—and seek care and treatment. People who come down with the flu are infectious during the first seven days of the onset of symptoms; for children, it can even be longer—up to twenty-one days.

Finally, if you're feeling sick, don't travel at all—for your own good and the sake of fellow travelers, Haridopolos recommends. Some airlines will even waive the cost if you cancel your flight because you're sick.

Germ Hotspots on Airplanes

The tourism website Travelmath.com recently ranked the dirtiest places in airports and airplanes, based on samples gathered by a microbiologist who was dispatched to examine five US airports and four flights.

The website found that airports and planes tend to be dirtier than the average American home. And the places that harbor the most disease-causing germs might surprise you. For instance, the samples gathered show that bathrooms in airplanes and airports have fewer microbial pathogens than other areas that you might not consider hotbeds of infectious agents.

Bathrooms Cleaner than Trays

"Bathrooms were some of the cleaner surfaces tested, which may be contrary to conventional thought," the researchers reported. "Regular cleaning schedules mean these surfaces are sanitized more frequently. This is a good thing."

By contrast, the tests showed that the dirtiest place on most planes is the tray table—the surface most travelers will touch as they eat and drink in-flight foods and beverages. Researchers found that the tray table had 2,155 colony-forming units (CFU)—a measure of the number of bacteria or fungal cells that are able to multiply—per square inch. That compares to just 265 CFU on the lavatory flush button, 285 CFU on the overhead air vent, and 230 CFU on the seat belt buckle.

In airports, the findings were comparable, with tests showing that drinking fountain buttons had 1,240 CFU per square inch, compared to only 70 CFU on bathroom stall locks.

Here is Travelmath.com's ranking of the dirtiest places on airplanes and in airports that you should try to avoid:

1. **Tray table:** 2,155 CFU
2. **Drinking fountain buttons:** 1,240 CFU
3. **Overhead air vent:** 285 CFU
4. **Lavatory flush button:** 265 CFU
5. **Seatbelt buckle:** 230 CFU
6. **Bathroom stall locks:** 70 CFU

The only good news here is that all the samples were negative for fecal coliforms like *E. coli*, which can make people fatally ill. But the presence of the microbes suggests that other infectious pathogens are also likely present on planes and in airports, experts say.

The Travelmath.com researchers noted that while it might seem counterintuitive that bathrooms are cleaner than tray tables and countertops, the tests suggest that airlines and airports are sanitizing restrooms, which can easily spread disease if not cleaned properly.

"The bad news is that airlines and airports don't appear to be doing a good enough job of cleaning other things," the researchers noted. "Travelmath points out that the pressure on airlines to board a plane quickly has increased in recent decades, meaning tray tables often don't get cleaned until the end of the day."

According to research by the National Sanitation Foundation, some of these airplane and airport surfaces have higher concentrations of microbes than household toilet seats, cell phones, and even money. Still, some surfaces in the home—including pet bowls (306,000 CFU), pet toys (19,000 CFU), and kitchen countertops (361 CFU)—can pose a greater risk.

To reduce your risk of picking up a nasty bug while traveling this summer, experts advise you to do the following:

- Avoid eating anything that comes into contact with your tray table.
- Carry portable hand sanitizers and use them often.
- Wash your hands frequently while traveling.

Don't Just Do Something, Stand There, Doc Advises

When you're feeling sick, the temptation is that you push your doctor for an antibiotic or try an OTC remedy. But health experts note that those might not be the most effective ways to combat a cold or the flu—and might even do more harm than good.

Antibiotics only treat bacterial infections and do nothing to combat viruses that cause influenza and the common cold. But taking them can kill "healthy" bacteria in your gut, which are important to a functioning immune system and help fuel the risk of drug-resistant superbugs.

In addition, some OTC cold and flu remedies might put your health at risk, notes Dr. Janet Sluggett, an internationally respected researcher at Monash University in Melbourne, Australia. "Cough mixtures can interfere with other medicines," she says. "The cough suppressant known as dextromethorphan, for instance, is not suitable for people taking some antidepressants because it can increase risk of side effects."

Dr. Susan Smith, a professor of primary care medicine at the Dublin-based Royal College of Surgeons in Ireland, is also skeptical of OTC cough and cold remedies. She's has exhaustively researched whether such treatments are worth buying and found they often aren't.

A review published by the Cochrane Library—an esteemed international medical group—recently reported the findings of an analysis of studies involving nearly five thousand people treated with OTC old remedies led by Smith.

The striking conclusion: "We found no good evidence for or against effectiveness of OTC medications in acute cough." In addition, nineteen studies reported adverse effects, "such as nausea, vomiting, headaches, and drowsiness" in people taking such products.

This is particularly true for cold remedies designed for young children, for whom "potential for harm" from OTC preparations exists, Smith says.

For most people, she prescribes what might be a hard pill to swallow but also might be the most effective remedy for the common cold: simply let it run its course naturally. Most will go away on their own within a few days.

DEPRESSION, ANXIETY, ADHD, PTSD, AND OTHER MENTAL ILLNESSES

Antidepressants are among the drug industry's biggest sellers, with more than one in ten Americans taking such medications as Prozac, Paxil, Zoloft, and Celexa to combat depression.

Millions more take psychoactive drugs for other mental health conditions, such as anxiety, post-traumatic stress disorder (PTSD), phobias, and sleep disorders.

All told, one in six US adults takes a psychiatric medication, according to a 2016 analysis by the nonprofit Institute for Safe Medication Practices in Alexandria, Virginia. Among the specific findings, published in the journal *JAMA Internal Medicine*, are the following statistics:

- About 17 percent of adults filled one or more prescriptions for antidepressants such as Zoloft; sedatives and sleep drugs, including Xanax and Ambien; or antipsychotics, used to treat schizophrenia and bipolar disorder.

- Among the one in six who reported use of these drugs, 12 percent said they had taken an antidepressant, and 8 percent reported filling a prescription for anxiety medicine, sedatives, or sleep aids.
- Nearly 2 percent had taken antipsychotic drugs.
- Whites were about twice as likely to use these medications (21 percent) as African American and Hispanic adults.
- Eight of ten taking such drugs reported long-term use and increased usage with age, with one-quarter of those aged sixty to eighty-five reportedly taking them compared to 9 percent of eighteen- to thirty-nine-year-olds. Women also were more likely to report using psychiatric drugs than men.
- Among the ten leading psychiatric medications were six antidepressants: Zoloft (sertraline), Celexa (citalopram), Prozac (fluoxetine), Desyrel (trazodone), Lexapro (escitalopram), and Cymbalta (duloxetine).
- Also in the top ten were three anxiety drugs, Xanax (alprazolam), Klonopin (clonazepam), and Ativan (lorazepam) and the sleep aid Ambien (zolpidem).

Downsides of Drugs Are Significant

What is most troubling about these statistics is that many of these are expensive, don't work for all patients, and can have serious negative side effects.

But what if a natural supplement was just as effective as powerful prescription drugs without the cost and adverse effects? That's exactly what Dr. Ajay Goel and his colleagues at Baylor University found in a recent groundbreaking study of curcumin, a compound in turmeric, the spice used in popular Indian curry dishes.

Goel, director of epigenetics and cancer prevention at Baylor University Medical Center, says his research is the first clinical trial to show that curcumin is nearly as powerful as Prozac when it comes to easing depression symptoms. "It was a surprise to us to see that curcumin actually worked as good as the antidepressant," he says. "So this is amazing news."

Past research, primarily involving laboratory animals, suggested that curcumin has antidepressant properties. So Goel and his team sought to examine its effects on people with depression. They enlisted three groups of twenty volunteers for the study: one group took 500 mg of curcumin twice a day, the second was given Prozac, and the third received a combination of the two.

After six weeks, the team evaluated the symptoms of the patients using a standardized test of depression that tracks mood, suicidal thoughts, insomnia, agitation, anxiety, weight loss, and other factors. The results showed the spice compound had roughly the same beneficial impact as Prozac on the patients.

"Yes, we still need to validate, we need to do further studies," says Goel, who reported his findings in the journal *Phytotherapy Research*. "But this initial evidence is very encouraging, considering that curcumin is safe, it is nontoxic, and it has many more beneficial effects . . . besides its ability to control depression."

He adds that medication is an appropriate treatment for depression but can pose long-term risks. "These antidepressants . . . are fine if you're taking them for a short time, but as you know, depression is a chronic disease, so the problem happens when you take these antidepressants for a long time," he says. "And when you do that, you put yourself at risk for developing side effects and toxicity."

By contrast, the turmeric spice is a natural, nontoxic compound, even at high doses. "The exciting aspect is that curcumin is extremely safe, there is no virtual toxicity, there have been multiple human studies that have [shown] even when you take curcumin up to 12 grams a day for six months, virtually there is no toxicity," he explains. "So this is very encouraging."

Although you can derive the benefits of curcumin by eating foods that contain turmeric, such as Indian curry dishes, most people in the United States don't eat enough of it to make a difference. Consequently, taking a curcumin supplement—Goel recommends a formulation known as BCM-95, which is ten times more potent than standard curcumin—makes more sense for most Americans.

"In order to get the benefits of curcumin, you'll need to eat enough turmeric probably multiple times a day—two to three meals loaded with turmeric," he explains. "For people in the Western world . . . I think it would be best to consume curcumin as a health supplement."

Other Promising Natural Remedies for Depression

While curcumin might be the most promising natural treatment for depression and anxiety, a number of other nondrug alternatives have been shown to combat these mental health problems. Among them are the following:

ST. JOHN'S WORT. Extracts of this plant contain high levels of a chemical called hypercium, which studies have found to be as beneficial as prescription antidepressants and antianxiety medications. In Germany, it is the most commonly prescribed antidepressant.

OMEGA-3 FATTY ACIDS. A great deal of research has shown that low levels of omega-3 fats—in fish and fish oil—significantly increase one's risk of developing depression and anxiety. The most effective component is docosapentaenoic acid (DHA), which is used almost exclusively by the brain. Eicosapentaenoic acid (EPA) has also been shown to reduce depression.

COCONUT OIL. While not an omega-3 oil, coconut oil has been shown to reduce brain inflammation and combat depression and anxiety.

PHYTOCHEMICALS. Several plant phytochemicals have antidepressant and antianxiety properties, research shows. These include hesperidin, quercetin, ginkgo biloba, resveratrol, berberine, and luteolin.

METHLYCOBALAMIN AND FOLATE. These natural forms of vitamin B12 have been shown to reduce depression by combatting inflammation.

ZINC. Several studies have shown that low zinc levels are associated with depression and that supplementation can improve symptoms.

Is Your Diet Making You Depressed or Anxious?

You are what you eat, as the saying goes. And nowhere is that idea more true than when it comes to diet and mental health. In fact, the latest research shows an undeniable connection between junk foods that boost inflammation and depression.

"We've gone light years beyond the notion that certain foods like carbohydrates create a good mood," says Dr. James M. Greenblatt, a Boston-based psychiatrist and author of *Breakthrough Depression Solution: Mastering Your Mood with Nutrition, Diet, and Supplementation.* "We know from many research studies that a poor diet causes a variety of mental disorders, including depression."

Greenblatt says that a recent US Centers for Disease Control and Prevention (CDC) study that found suicide rates have jumped by 24 percent over the past fifteen years are partially a reflection of our junk-food society.

"Particularly at risk, in my personal experience, [are] adolescents with eating disorders," he says. "The most dramatic increase in suicide rates was seen among girls between the ages of ten to fourteen. Since 1999, the suicide rate for this group has exploded by an incredible 200 percent. Part of this is due to social media, but a large part is due to malnutrition. The adolescent diet is characterized by increased intake of refined grains and processed sugars and devoid of essential nutrients."

Greenblatt explains that your brain consumes a whopping 25 percent of our metabolic energy and therefore needs the correct food sources of protein, vitamins, and minerals, along with omega-3 fatty acids to ensure optimum functioning. "Research has shown that low levels of vitamins D and B12, magnesium, and particularly omega-3 essential fatty acids have been linked to depression and increased risk of suicide," he says.

Dr. Adrian Lopresti, PhD, a clinical psychologist and senior researcher at Murdoch University in Western Australia, has more than eighteen years of experience working with people suffering from a range of mental health conditions, including depression and anxiety-related disorders. He explains how important a nutrient-dense diet is to prevent depression and other mental disorders: "Our diet can affect mood in a number of ways. Brain chemicals often associated with mood are known as neurotransmitters. These neurotransmitters are reliant on several nutrients derived from food. For example, to produce the mood-lifting neurotransmitter serotonin, we must eat protein. This protein then gets broken down into an amino acid called tryptophan, which in turn gets converted to serotonin."

Lopresti adds that we also need enzymes to facilitate this process. For those enzymes to work properly, they require adequate levels of vitamins and minerals. The B vitamins from the fruits and vegetables we eat are especially important for the conversion.

"Foods that we eat can also have an impact on inflammation of the body," he says. "Too much inflammation has a negative impact on several hormones and neurotransmitters. So eating inflammatory foods such as fast foods and soft drinks can lower the levels of mood-lifting neurotransmitters.

"Excess inflammation is damaging to the brain. On the other hand, eating a healthy diet composed of lots of fruit and vegetables, spices and lean protein has a protective, anti-inflammatory effect on the brain." Spices like turmeric and saffron are particularly beneficial, says Lopresti.

One of the best nutrients to protect the brain and stave off depression is omega-3 fatty acid, say the experts. "Eating fatty fish at least three times a week or taking a supplement is highly recommended," says Greenblatt. "As we age, it becomes increasingly difficult to get all the nutrients we need for optimum brain health from food alone, so I do recommend supplementation.

"The best way to tell if your body is lacking key nutrients in this fight against premature brain aging and depression is to get tested for deficiency. Remember that we are all individuals, so a certain diet plan doesn't work for everyone. What we do know is that there is a direct link between vitamin and mineral deficiencies along with low levels of omega-3 fatty acids and depression. So by choosing nutrient-dense foods over junk foods, you are helping your mental health as well as your physical health."

Choosing St. John's Wort Wisely

St. John's Wort extracts can be as effective as standard antidepressant drugs for treating mild to moderate major depression with significantly fewer side effects. But recent ConsumerLab.com tests reveal that six out of ten supplements on the market contain far lower levels of key plant compounds than expected.

These compounds, hypericin and hyperforin, are associated with the herb's effectiveness. "The wide range of variation across the products we tested means that some St. John's Wort supplements may be helpful for treating depression, while others may not contain enough of the herb to have a meaningful effect," says ConsumerLab.com president and founder, Dr. Tod Cooperman.

He explains that the product is often adulterated with dyes that give the herb its characteristic reddish tinge when tested with outdated analytical methods but mask the fact that the pure herb has been "cut" with an inferior compound.

"We used a method that identifies the hypericin molecule and isn't 'tricked' by dyes," he says. "Supplements were also checked for potential contamination with the heavy metals arsenic, cadmium, and leads, and the pills were checked to ensure that they break apart to properly release their ingredients."

Sales of St. John's Wort top $57 million annually according to sales records, and it's one of the most popular herbal remedies on the market. Although the US Food and Drug Administration (FDA) regulates herbal supplements, Cooperman says that the "enforcement is loose and regulations lax."

"That's why I formed ConsumerLab.com in 1999 to become a leading provider of consumer information and provide independent evaluations of products that affect health and nutrition," he says. The company is supported by subscribers and provides information on more than one thousand products from more than four hundred brands.

St. John's Wort has been the subject of numerous double-blind, placebo-controlled studies that found the herb as effective as standard antidepressant drugs, including medication in the selective serotonin reuptake inhibitors (SSRI) family, such as Prozac.

"But you need to choose carefully," notes Cooperman, "since six out of the products we tested failed to make the grade."

Those that passed include

- Gaia Herbs St. John's Wort Flower Buds and Tops drops
- Nature's Way Perika St. John's Wort tablets
- Shaklee Moodlift Complex capsules
- Standard Process Mediherb St. John's Wort tablets

The products that didn't pass muster include

- Now St. John's Wort capsules
- Planetary Herbals Full Spectrum St. John's Wort Extract tablets
- Swanson St. John's Wort capsules

- Vitacost St. John's Wort Extract capsules
- The Vitamin Shoppe St. John's Wort capsules
- Whole Foods St. John's Wort capsules

As with conventional antidepressants, it appears that St. John's Wort takes several weeks to achieve its full effect, notes Cooperman. It's generally considered to be safe when taken in appropriate amounts and seldom causes more than occasional digestive distress, he says. "However, other reported side effects could include anxiety, fatigue, headache, insomnia, and skin rashes."

One long-term study found that the use of St. John's Wort can cause sexual difficulties and, like conventional antidepressants, might cause hair loss. In addition, Cooperman warns that St. John's Wort might interact with several common medications, reducing their effectiveness. These include statin drugs, cancer chemotherapy drugs, oral contraceptives, warfarin, and medications like Prilosec that treat esophageal reflux symptoms.

"Always check with your health care provider before taking St. John's Wort to ensure that it won't interfere with your medications to get the maximum benefits," says Cooperman. "This is an exceptionally well-studied herb, so the risks are known, but it's always wise to check with your physician before taking the herb, and never suddenly stop taking the supplement without supervision."

Ten Ways to Beat Anxiety Naturally

An estimated fifteen million American adults take anxiety medications, even though they pose serious mental and physical health risks.

Benzodiazepines such as Xanax, Ativan, Klonopin, and Valium work by depressing the central nervous system (CNS), which takes the edge off anxiety but can also put people into a mental fog. The drugs are also addictive, come with some brain-numbing side effects, and are responsible for some eight thousand overdose deaths every year.

"People have anxiety and they are thinking about functioning, and [asking themselves] 'What's the best way I can get through life?'" says Maryland-based addiction specialist Dr. Peter Cohen. "It's human nature to take the path of least resistance."

But the easy way might not be the best in the long run. Here are ten proven ways to reduce anxiety without taking drugs:

1. **Have a sip of bliss.** Studies show that compounds in chamomile and green tea have soothing effects.

2. **Don't worry, be hoppy.** Hops, the same compounds that give beer its bitterness, also have tranquilizing properties.

3. **Try aromatherapy.** Some essential oils—lavender, rose, frankincense, ylang ylang, bergamot, and vetiver—are known for their calming capabilities.

4. **Take adaptogens.** Scientific research shows that adaptogenic herbs such as ginseng, rhodiola, ashwagandha, and eleuthera root help regulate levels of the stress-triggered hormone cortisol.

5. **Heat things up.** Saunas, steam rooms, Jacuzzis, lying in the sun, or sitting close to a campfire also help melt your cares away.

6. **Embrace Mother Nature.** A stroll through the local park is a great respite from the helter-skelter of modern life, and research shows that it can lower levels of stress hormones.

7. **Gut it out.** Studies show that keeping your gut flora robust, with the help of probiotics, reduces stress and anxiety levels.

8. **Get moving.** Exercise is one of the simplest, most convenient, and cheapest ways to bust stress.

9. **Breathe deep.** There are many therapeutic breathing techniques, but the key is to focus on each breath, which will naturally take your mind off things that might be causing you anxiety.

10. **Don't overreact.** How often do we worry about things that never come to pass? One study puts the figure at 85 percent. And when the study participants' fears did come true, a vast majority of them found that the catastrophe wasn't as bad as they imagined.

Best of Both Worlds

If you're trying to choose between an antidepressant and a nutritional supplement to treat depression, new research suggests that you might want to consider both options.

Medical investigators from Harvard University and the University of Melbourne found that omega-3 fish oils, S-adenosylmethionine (SAMe), methylfolate (a bioactive form of folate), and vitamin D might actually enhance the effectiveness of antidepressants in people who have been diagnosed with clinical depression.

To reach their conclusions, the researchers examined forty clinical trials that used nutritional supplements to treat depression in combination with common antidepressants such as SSRIs, serotonin-norepinephrine reuptake inhibitors (SNRIs), and tricyclics.

Although the most significant improvement was with omega-3 fatty acids, effectiveness was also improved by SAMe, folate, and vitamin D.

A Doctor's Perspective: Treating Seasonal Affective Disorder

Seasonal affective disorder (SAD) is a type of consistent depression that occurs during the winter season. People start to become depressed during the darkest days and gradually feel better when spring and summer arrive.

Dr. Kelly Rohan, a professor and director of clinical training in the department of psychological science at the University of Vermont, explains how common it is and the best ways to treat it.

Q: How common is SAD?

A: In the United States, it is estimated that between 4 and 6 percent of the population might have full-blown SAD, but 10 to 20 percent might suffer from milder winter blues.

Q: Who is at risk for developing SAD?

A: It's a condition that affects people in regions of the world farther away from the equator and strikes more women than men. Children and adolescents can also develop it, but it's much less common. We don't know exactly why more women than men suffer from SAD, but women in general are more likely to be affected by depression than men. Scientists think there might be a genetic predisposition for developing the condition, and the symptoms get triggered in particular ways.

Q: What are the symptoms?

A: Common symptoms include fatigue, sleeping more hours per day than usual, weight gain of at least 5 percent of body weight, sad moods, loss of interest in normal activities, and difficulty concentrating. At the extreme, the sufferer might experience suicidal thoughts. It's important to note that many people can have mild to moderate symptoms during winter months, and these people are considered to have subsyndromal SAD, or the winter blues.

Q: What can you tell us about your breakthrough study?

A: I was the principal investigator in a study published in the *American Journal of Psychiatry* comparing treatment options for SAD. We found that cognitive behavior therapy, or CBT, could be better in the long run than light therapy, which has been the gold standard of treatment for years. We studied two groups over a period of three winters. One group had light therapy while the other had CBT for six weeks the first winter. When we followed up with the subjects two years later, we discovered that 27.3 percent who received CBT had recurring depression while 45.6 percent of those who received light therapy had recurrences. They also had less severe symptoms.

Q: Why does CBT work so well?

A: CBT teaches people a set of skills that they can use forever, while you have to spend time with a light box for light therapy to work. While light therapy works by manipulating sluggish circadian rhythms back into the correct phase, evidence shows that CBT for SAD helps a person deal with negative thought patterns and turn them around. CBT teaches the patient skills to use in the future when faced with stress or feeling down. After CBT, the patient learns to be proactive about their mental health. Light therapy, on the other hand, is only effective when you use the lamp and does little to address the mindset. However, if you choose the lamp, invest in a full-sized light box that gives off 10,000 lux of cool white fluorescent and has a screen to filter out harmful ultraviolet rays. Other treatment options to consider are antidepressant medications used to treat nonseasonal depressions. Wellbutrin extended release is FDA-approved for SAD.

Medical Marijuana: Promising Treatment for Depression and PTSD?

Dr. Sue Sisley is not a military veteran, but she wears or carries a dog tag at all times. Stamped with the number "22," it is a constant reminder of how many American vets commit suicide each day—most suffering from depression or PTSD—based on federal estimates.

"Even though we all realize that is a falsely low number . . . it is a horrific number," she says, noting that veteran suicides far outnumber the national civilian average. "The fact is, the government is not doing anything tangible to find solutions to this. This is why I have this dog tag with me."

Sisley, a former Department of Veterans Affairs (VA) physician, has devoted her life to doing what federal health officials have failed to do—that is, come up with an effective treatment for PTSD. But her work, while promising, is controversial and not without detractors.

As perhaps the nation's foremost scientific expert on medical marijuana, Sisley is spearheading what many experts regard as groundbreaking research on the potential benefits of cannabis in treating PTSD and other maladies suffered by millions of veterans. If her research proves her right, it could lead to the first and only effective therapy for the debilitating condition, which increases suicide risk among military personnel and other Americans.

For the study, funded by a $2 million grant from the Colorado Health Department, Sisley is partnering with collaborators at three top-notch institutions: Johns Hopkins University, the University of Pennsylvania, and the University of Colorado Denver.

"If there is even a chance that cannabis could help reduce the suffering of our veterans' community, then we have a duty to these vets to find ways to change public policy—to bring the science forward and let the data speak for itself," she says.

Skeptic Turned Believer

Sisley first became interested in cannabis as an alternative medicine therapy for PTSD after several veterans she was treating as a VA physician and psychiatrist told her that it was easing their symptoms in ways that conventional drugs were not. As a practicing Scottsdale physician, Sisley was initially skeptical because of her training as a conventional doctor and her unfamiliarity with medicinal marijuana.

"I've never used cannabis personally, I'm not part of the industry, I don't own dispensaries . . . and I don't write [prescriptions] for patients," she notes. "Sadly, I was highly judgmental when [vets] first started disclosing this to me about ten years ago. I was immediately dismissive. I was trained in a really conservative medical model where you don't do anything in medicine unless it's been put through the FDA [approval] process."

But over time, the anecdotal evidence began piling up, with hundreds of veterans telling her that cannabis was helping control their symptoms of PTSD, depression, and anxiety.

"They would come in and say, 'This is helping me in some areas.' And I would really try to cajole them and say, you know, 'Let's give you another prescription, because you can't possibly be telling me that cannabis is helping with this,'" she notes. "But then I was also getting a lot of collateral information from their family members who would explain to me that they got their husband back, or kids would say, 'I got my dad back,' and it was so compelling."

Darker Reality Evident

Another darker reality was also becoming evident to Sisley: conventional treatments approved for PTSD—largely antidepressants and painkillers—were not working for many of her patients, often with tragic consequences. "One of the things that became clear to me was that I was losing a lot of veterans to suicide in my practice," she notes. "They weren't responding to conventional medicine."

For Sisley, the turning point came in early 2013, when the VA released its landmark study estimating that twenty-two vets commit suicide, on average, every day. As a professor at the University of Arizona, she decided the time was right for a clinical trial to evaluate cannabis. In March 2014, the US Health and Human Services Department (HHS) gave its approval for the study, and it was set to get under way within a year. But the project put her at odds with the university administration. Her supervisors terminated her in June 2014 after she unsuccessfully lobbied the Arizona legislature to use money from the state's medical marijuana revenues to fund her research.

"Our administration . . . was highly opposed to hosting that kind of work at a public university," she recalls. "They felt it would harm the federal funding, [and] they didn't like the notion of veterans smoking weed on campus."

University officials have declined to discuss why Sisley's faculty position was not renewed, calling it a "personnel matter," and denied politics were a factor. But Sisley spent little time grieving the job loss. Her dismissal drew national media attention and sparked a backlash that included many veterans' groups and medical scientists. Her supporters argued that her termination spotlighted barriers that have long blocked marijuana from mainstream medical research circles.

Meanwhile, Sisley moved forward with her study with help from the nonprofit Multidisciplinary Association for Psychedelic Studies, which will buy research-grade cannabis for the trial from the lone federal agency allowed to disperse it—the National Institute on Drug Abuse.

In April, the US Drug Enforcement Administration (DEA) gave its blessing to the project, making Sisley the first US researcher to win federal approval for a clinical trial to study smoked marijuana as a potential FDA-approved prescription medicine for PTSD. Sisley and her colleagues have begun recruiting participants, including seventy-six veterans who have treatment-resistant PTSD, and expect results within three years.

"This is a really nice comeback story," she says. "We ended up gaining . . . worldwide media coverage [of my termination], which helped shine a giant spotlight on the barriers to cannabis research."

Marijuana's Checkered History

The federal government first acknowledged cannabis as a potential treatment for a variety of ills—including drug addiction, alcoholism, PMS, and menopausal symptoms—in the 1800s. But allegations about the risks of marijuana—crystalized in the 1936 film *Refer Madness*—and passage of the 1970 Controlled Substances Act raised insurmountable hurdles to research into its potential benefits.

Under federal law, cannabis is lumped into the same "Schedule 1" classification as harder drugs such as heroin and LSD, "putting the nail in the coffin for cannabis research," Sisley notes. Meanwhile, the DEA falsely classifies many other drugs used off-label to treat PTSD as having little addiction potential, including opioid painkillers linked to a soaring increases in overdose deaths among vets and other Americans.

The FDA has approved only two medications for PTSD—Zoloft and Paxil, both antidepressants. "That's it," Sisley explains. "But when those fail, then I'm able to use all these other medications off-label"—including pain meds, antidepressants, sleep aids, bipolar-disorder drugs, anticonvulsives, and antipsychotics. "Most of these meds are no better than placebo and . . . so slowly it snowballs into twelve or thirteen different prescriptions to treat one syndrome—PTSD."

Yet at the same time, scientific studies have found that medical marijuana might help treat dozens of health conditions, including certain cancers, chronic pain, epilepsy, glaucoma, depression, and even dementia. Sisley says she is particularly interested in the potential use of cannabis to combat the growing national crisis of painkiller abuse, noting that veterans have a 33 percent higher rate of prescription drug overdoses.

Some research backs her up on this point. In 2015, a landmark study published in the *Journal of the American Medical Association* found states that legalized medical marijuana experienced dramatic reductions in prescription overdose deaths in the years after those laws passed.

Sisley says she has been cheered by the growing acceptance of cannabis as a legitimate potential alternative-medicine therapy. In particular, she hails CNN medical correspondent Dr. Sanjay Gupta's recent decision to come out in favor of medical marijuana and criticizing the DEA for claiming cannabis has no medical value.

"That was a real game changer for the [medical] cannabis movement," she says, saying it has helped open doors to new research into the benefits of marijuana, in addition to her own landmark study.

"This is exciting because, finally, we have government money going to look at the efficacy of cannabis all different illnesses [including] the potential for cannabis to be used for pain management," she adds. "So we are going to be answering all of these questions through these clinical trials and you'll have this data, you'll see this emerge, and [it will] get published over the next three years."

Medical Marijuana Research Findings

Many studies have suggested that compounds in marijuana have significant clinical properties, including cannabidiol (CBD), which has a positive impact on brain functions without causing a high, and tetrahydrocannabinol (THC), a proven pain reliever.

To date, scientific researchers have identified cannabis-based therapeutic applications for more than forty mental and physical health conditions. Among them are the following:

- anxiety
- Alzheimer's disease
- arthritis
- cancer
- chronic pain
- depression
- epilepsy
- glaucoma
- HIV/AIDS
- inflammatory bowel disease
- multiple sclerosis

Medical Marijuana Industry Projected to Top $40 Billion

Remember that scene from *The Graduate* when Dustin Hoffman's character is advised that "plastics" will become the next guaranteed US growth industry? If that classic 1967 film were remade today, the same projection might be made for cannabis.

Two recent economic analyses project the marijuana industry—for medical and recreational use—will top $40 billion over the next five to ten years. And if cannabis becomes legal nationwide, the industry could hit $100 billion by 2050.

- Ackrell Capital, an independent investment finance bank focused on emerging growth industries, estimates that the US consumer market for cannabis will rise from $4.4 billion today to $37 billion in five years and $50 billion in ten years.
- A second analysis, by *Marijuana Business Daily*, projects that the industry will earn $44 billion by the year 2020, regardless of changes in state or federal drug laws.

The primary drivers of industry growth are recreational sales in Colorado, Washington, and Oregon, which have legalized marijuana. But new markets are also sprouting up in the twenty-three states that have legalized medical cannabis and more than a dozen others that have decriminalized its use.

Larry Schnurmacher, managing partner with Phyto Partners—a private equity venture capital investment firm that specializes in helping businesses in the cannabis industry—says this growth is just the tip of the iceberg and that the market for medical marijuana is poised for exponential development.

"Yes, the industry is growing, very rapidly, especially the medicinal marijuana industry," he says. "I believe the biggest potential for growth for the industry is in the mostly untapped health, wellness, and pharmaceutical medicinal markets.

"New products are coming out daily that people are finding many uses for and replacements for their current drugs, which are toxic, addictive, and have other negative side effects. I believe that the medicinal marijuana industry is comparable to the biotech industry, as many new drugs will be discovered, and cures for currently incurable diseases will be found in medicines derived from the cannabis plant."

Iraq War Vet Turns Pain into Gain with Alternative Treatment for Psychological Wounds

In two tours of duty in Iraq, Stan Deland saw more than his share of war horrors. As a Marine Corps Infantry Company lieutenant in charge of casualty evacuation in Fallujah, he wasn't on the front lines of the fighting but saw the daily evidence of its bloody toll.

"I didn't have to pull the trigger and shoot anyone, I didn't kick in any doors . . . but I saw guys that definitely didn't make it," he recalls. "I saw guys cut in half."

Yet the memory that haunts him most might come as a surprise: the suicide of a fellow Marine shook Deland more profoundly than anything else he'd experienced. "He hung himself and I found him—me and another guy," Deland says, lowering his voice at the memory. "I basically watched him write his suicide note before he did it. I didn't know it at the time, but that's what he was doing. He'd been on Paxil and was having some problems. That was more intense for me than anything that happened in the war."

So when Deland returned to the states in 2004—and began experiencing the psychological fallout of military service himself—he sought out alternative treatments for the extreme mental and emotional pain many veterans experience.

His primary research laboratory? His own body and mind.

That four-year journey of discovery led him to try a host of therapies, including drugs, psychoanalysis, acupuncture, chiropractic medicine, and meditation. But in the end, the approach that worked best for him was homeopathic medicine—a traditional mind-body therapy dating to 400 BC, when Hippocrates first prescribed a small dose of mandrake root to treat anxiety.

Drawing on his own experiences, Deland founded his own Malibu-based company in 2008—Siddha Flower Essences Homeopathic Brand—which produces a line of alternative-medicine products to treat anxiety, depression, and PTSD. Today, they are sold in 650 stores across the United States, including Whole Foods, as well as online.

Deland says he felt compelled to help the millions of military vets—and others—who struggle with psychological wounds no one can see that conventional medicine can't heal. "I would love to be able to get this stuff to veterans because, as I said, I've tried all these things, and yet this subtle medicine has been the most impactful to me," he says. "If I can I explain how it works well enough, and people are willing to give it a shot, I'd even give it to vets for free."

Medical research confirms Deland's hunch about the need for effective treatments to help veterans suffering from postwar anxiety, depression, and PTSD—all of which raise the risk for suicide. A recent study noted that the US suicide rate has been rising sharply since 2003, with veterans—as well as police officers, farmers, and doctors—among those most at risk.

Hope Tiesman, an epidemiologist with the National Institute for Occupational Safety and Health who led the study, says individuals in high-pressure situations (such as vets) often struggle with mental health issues that can lead to suicidal thoughts. "Exposure to high-stress events can lead to negative mental health outcomes such as [PTSD], generalized anxiety disorders, and depression," noted Tiesman, whose research was published in the *American Journal of Preventive Medicine*.

Deland's experiences in Iraq certainly qualify as "high-stress events," to say the least. He had two different deployments—the first in 2003, the second in 2004—and spent a total of eighteen months in Iraq. In many ways, they were different experiences, but "fear of the unknown" was a common link between the two.

"For the initial invasion, we trained a lot with gas masks, as we were told the NBC threat—that is, nuclear, biological, and . . . the chemical warfare threat—was real," he recalls.

Still, he remembers his marine battalion being greeted by the Iraqis "as liberators": "We were deployed during peacetime, and it was like the old saying, we were last to know and the first to go . . . but reading between the lines, we had a sense of what was coming . . . and so we get to Bagdad and literally we were greeted as liberators, really. Women crying tears of joy and children . . . and so it was really an upbeat thing."

But his second deployment, outside Fallujah, was very different. By 2004, the war-torn city had become a magnet for anti-American jihadists, and his company's charge was to quell the insurgency.

"I can remember toward the end of those five months of counterinsurgency operations, [it was] death by a one thousand scratches, as we called it. . . . And it was a weekly thing where someone was getting close to blown up or getting blown up. So it was totally different—from being greeted as liberators initially to a completely different vibe, with guys standing on the corners glaring at you."

In the time Deland and his battalion were in Fallujah, the city's population dropped from a population of two hundred thousand to less than five thousand. "We used every piece of ordnance we had, and when we left, there was not much standing," he says. "So Fallujah became a [rallying point] for [the] jihadist call. If you wanted to participate in the jihad [against America], go to Fallujah. My commanding officer once told me [the unit had] killed people from fourteen countries there."

That level of constant stress and fear—and the struggle to simply survive the combat day to day—accounts for much of the mental distress many returning veterans suffer. "It's why PTSD happens," Deland notes. "For some, their nervous system simply gets overloaded and fries itself a bit."

Deland himself never suffered PTSD, debilitating flashbacks, or nightmares. But soon after returning to the states from Iraq, he began to experience a crushing sense of anxiety and panic attacks. He also felt a paralyzing sense of disorientation and disconnection.

"I remember sitting in the air-conditioned chow hall after three weeks in Fallujah without a shower or a hot meal. TVs were on. I was looking at these talking heads, talking about the experience that I was personally having, and there was a disconnect," he recalls. "Like my direct experience was somehow a video game or a theatrical production."

That burgeoning alienation led him to seek treatment—and a sense of peace—in a variety of practices. "Within a few months of being back from Fallujah, I went to an alternative health place and did every treatment they had to offer," he says. "It was time for me to recalibrate. I'd been deployed for something like eighteen out of the previous thirty-six months. Because I so quickly immersed myself in things like diets, cleansing, acupuncture, homeopathy, chiropractic—to name a few—I feel like PTSD did not have an opportunity to develop.

"However, I was dealing with ongoing social anxiety that had existed before the Marine Corps and was getting to a point that I had to do something about it."

Deland had tried medications but found them ineffective. His father—Michael Deland, chairman of the Council on Environmental Quality under President George H. W. Bush—had also had mixed experiences with painkillers he took to ease discomfort from a disability that required him to use a wheelchair for much of his life.

Stan says he spent years seeking alternatives to conventional medicine for healing. "I wound up going to India four years in a row on meditation retreats," he notes. "I didn't have PTSD, but I had social anxiety to the point where I didn't know what to do with myself. One reason I got out of the Marine Corps is [that] I couldn't imagine being an officer and doing briefings and sweating bullets. I didn't know what a panic attack was, but that's what I was experiencing. So for years, I was looking for the silver bullet."

Then came the true turning point in his life. A girlfriend took him to an alternative-medicine clinic in Beverly Hills, where he was introduced to homeo-pathic medicine. The treatments gave him immediate relief. To this day, he isn't sure how homeopathy works and acknowledges that there is little science to explain its benefits.

But he points to his own recovery as proof that it works. "It's definitely anec-dotal, and I know that because of my own experience," he says. "When I started taking [it], it felt like a huge dark cloud was lifted off my head. Is it a placebo [effect], or something else? I don't know. But no one can take that direct expe-rience away from me.

"It's been about ten years, and I'm finally at a place where I'm comfortable enough in my own being that [the panic attacks] don't happen to me that much anymore."

He adds that he's not opposed to drugs or other conventional therapies for anxiety, PTSD, depression, and other mental and physical ailments. "I think pharmaceuticals have their place," he says. "But for me personally, one of the things . . . I realized [was] that nature is such an easy thing to trust. The intelli-gence of the plant in its whole form is incredible.

"When pharmaceuticals pull out a certain portion of that species and then you extract something . . . you lose some of that potency. Western drugs and even herbs are really forcing the body to do something, but . . . homeopathy is working in some way, synergistically, with the body."

Homeopathy is based on the idea that extreme dilutions of certain substances—usually derived from plants—preserve a substance's therapeutic properties while removing its harmful effects. Flower essences, cell salts, and other homeopathic ingredients are diluted in water and used to treat stress and relieve other ailments such as muscle and joint pain, irregular sleep, and damaged skin.

Siddha Flower Essences is a contemporary take on the centuries-old Eastern practice of homeopathy, offering an array of products designed to alleviate stresses, aches, pains, anxieties, and emotional imbalances. Available online (http://www.siddhaflowers.com) and in a growing number of retail stores, the products are manufactured at an FDA-registered facility that operates according to OTC Drug and Good Manufacturing Practices (GMP) industry guidelines.

Looking back, Deland believes that his interest in homeopathy was largely fueled by his experiences in Iraq. "Going from the life-depleting experience of war right into the life-affirming realm of the ancient, time-tested methods of healing, I guess I was just a sponge for that new experience," he says. "The thing about homeopathy and flower essences is that while there is some research, it is more anecdotal. People have the experience, and it works for them or it does not. Perhaps one day, our science will be able to explain homeopathy.

"In the meantime . . . I'm finally getting to the point where I am comfortable enough with myself and have done enough work on myself that this becomes about sharing with others."

Adaptogens: Ancient Chinese Treatment Eases Anxiety

During the Cold War, Soviet Union research scientists discovered something that traditional Chinese and Indian medical practitioners had known about for thousands of years—namely, that a group of remarkable herbs can help the human body beat stress and anxiety.

At first, the research was done in secret with hopes that the herbs, dubbed adaptogens, could give the Soviets an edge in their battle with the West by boosting the strength, stamina, and overall performance of soldiers, athletes, cosmonauts, and others.

Eventually, the Soviets published more than one thousand studies about adaptogens, concluding that they were stress busters that helped balance the body's hormones. "As far as something with concrete evidence of promoting health across the board, there is nothing even in the same ballpark as adaptogens," says herbalist Donnie Yance, author of *Adaptogens in Medical Herbalism*.

There are just a handful of widely recognized adaptogenic plants, most of which grow in harsh climates. One of them, *Rhodiola rosea*, grows in the arctic highlands of Europe and Asia. The botanical compounds that protect it against cold, altitude, and other extremes also help humans deal with the rigors of their environment, whether it's a blizzard or a bad day at the office.

"They're called adaptogens because of their unique ability to 'adapt' their function according to your body's needs," explains Dr. Frank Lipman, a New York–based internist and renowned integrative medicine expert. "Adaptogens can calm you down and boost your energy at the same time without overstimulating. They can normalize body imbalances."

Stress causes a lot of physiological problems by sparking the release of the "fight or flight" stress hormone cortisol. While that comes in handy when you're trying to outrun a bear, experts say it does more harm than good when you're stuck in a traffic jam.

The hormonal imbalance created by stress can hogtie the immune system, cause digestive problems, and induce inflammation, which can lead to heart disease, cancer, obesity, Alzheimer's, and many other maladies.

Adaptogens normalize cortisol levels, so even if you start getting worked up over being late to your kid's soccer game, your body knows better and calms itself down.

Recent scientific research has given adaptogens a big thumbs-up. In one recent example, a randomized double-blind, placebo-controlled study found that the adaptogenic herb ashwagandha reduced cortisol levels, and test subjects reported feeling less stressed.

So, you might ask, if these herbs have incredible powers that have been known for thousands of years and their value has been supported scientifically, why have most people not even heard about them?

"That's true across the board when it comes to herbal medicine," notes Yance, founder of the Mederi Foundation, a natural health clinic and research center. "Adaptogens haven't been marketed much when compared to things like pharmaceutical drugs."

They also don't get a lot of respect from the established medical community. Because adaptogenic supplements are not regulated by the FDA, Yance warns that quality among products varies immensely. "Do your research and make sure to get good quality products from a reliable company," he says.

Here are some commonly used adaptogens:

Ashwagandha. Native to arid areas in India, North Africa, and the Middle East, ashwagandha has been used in Indian Ayurvedic medicine since ancient times to increase energy and endurance, boost the immune system, and promote longevity.

Rhodiola rosea. This cold-weather herb is a great at balancing cortisol levels and promoting brain function and heart health.

Ginseng (Asian or American). Asian ginseng is said to be more potent, but both help regulate the endocrine system, improve pancreatic function, and boost vitality.

Eleuthero root. Another Chinese native, this small woody shrub fights chronic fatigue and is good for folks with stressful jobs, such as emergency room workers.

Schizandra. Called the "five-flavor berry" because it is sweet, salty, sour, pungent, and bitter, schizandra is found in Northern China and Eastern Russia. Studies show that it helps with work accuracy and fights fatigue.

Do You Have Adult ADHD?

Do you have difficulty focusing or concentrating? Is it hard for you to get organized? Are you often restless and impulsive? If so, you might suffer from adult attention deficit hyperactivity disorder (ADHD)—and you're not alone.

"Today, one in twenty adults suffers from ADHD," says Dr. Gary Small, professor of psychiatry and aging at University of California, Los Angeles (UCLA), and director of the UCLA Center on Aging.

ADHD is mainly characterized by the inability to pay attention and focus, together with hyperactive and impulsive behavior. Many people assume that ADHD affects only children—up to 11 percent have been diagnosed with the condition—but ADHD doesn't always disappear as children mature.

"It's often thought of as a childhood disorder, and for some, the symptoms decline when they reach their twenties," Small says. "Others have lifelong issues with attention. Many adults suffering from ADHD go undiagnosed and untreated."

Debilitating Effects

ADHD can have devastating effects on adults. "It can impair work performance, disrupt relationships, and lead to anxiety, depression, and substance abuse," says Small.

Some undiagnosed adults learn to cope with their condition, becoming involved in fast-paced, creative jobs, and don't become concerned until later in life, when their symptoms make them fear that they are developing age-related mild cognitive impairment (MCI).

"Many patients with adult ADHD are assumed to be suffering from age-related memory decline or mild cognitive impairment, since many of the symptoms of ADHD overlap with this condition," says Small. "Forgetfulness, mood swings, and impatience, which are signs of MCI, are also associated with ADHD."

Symptoms of ADHD include the following:

- being easily distracted
- difficulty following instructions
- high frustration levels
- impulsiveness
- problems concentrating or focusing
- problems controlling anger
- relationship problems
- restlessness
- talking excessively and often interrupting
- trouble organizing and finishing tasks

When to Seek Help

Since almost all of us have some symptoms of ADHD at some point in our lives, when do we seek help?

"When symptoms seem to interfere with everyday life," says Small. "The good news is that treatments for ADHD can be very effective. Several strategies can diminish both the attention and the hyperactivity components of the condition. Both medications and psychotherapy are helpful and are often used together."

Stimulant medications improve attention and decrease hyperactivity. According to Small, "these medications increase and balance the levels of various brain neurotransmitters, such as dopamine and norepinephrine." (Some studies have found that adults with ADHD have fewer dopamine receptors, which are involved in many neurological processes, including pleasure and motivation.)

The following are a few of the drugs used to treat ADHD:

- dextroamphetamine (Dexedrine)
- dextroamphetamine-amphetamine (Adderall XR)
- lisdexamfetamine (Vyvanse)
- methylphenidate (Ritalin, Metadate, Concerta)

Psychotherapy and education are also helpful, teaching patients to control their temper, organize their lives, deal with their impulsiveness, and manage their time better. In addition, counseling can help patients improve marital and other relationships.

Coping Strategies

If you have adult ADHD, or just want to improve your mental focus, Small suggests the following strategies:

Use "to-do" lists. By making a list and prioritizing items, you can keep from overwhelming yourself with tasks and can make sure the most important ones are finished first.

Make tasks manageable. Break complex tasks into small jobs and complete them one by one.

Carry a calendar. Make a habit of writing down all appointments in a calendar—preferably one you can carry with you at all times, like an app on your phone or tablet.

Write notes. Keep notes of errands and tasks and put them in a place you're sure to see them, such as your computer monitor or refrigerator.

Stick to a routine. Make a schedule of daily tasks and adhere to it every day, making them easier to remember.

Don't be afraid to try alternative strategies to find methods that work for you.

Yoga, meditation, and other relaxation strategies ease anxiety in some patients. Others have found that eliminating certain foods, such as sugar, artificial food colorings, and additives, can help control their symptoms.

Even though ADHD isn't a problem most people welcome, it can have a positive side. "The hyperactive aspect of ADHD also reflects high energy, which can be a positive for someone who needs stamina," says Small. "In addition, even though patients have trouble paying attention, when they are interested in something, they become hyperfocused and may pick up on details others miss."

DIABETES

Fifty years ago, diabetes was a relatively rare condition, striking less than one in twenty Americans (0.93 percent of the population, or 1.6 million people in 1958, according to the US Centers for Disease Control and Prevention [CDC]).

Today, blood sugar problems are epidemic, with diabetes afflicting nearly thirty million Americans (more than 8 percent of the population), and a whopping eighty-six million more have prediabetes, according to the American Diabetes Association (ADA).

According to the National Institutes of Health (NIH), Americans spend at least $44 billion a year on prescription diabetes medicines, and the disorder is first on the list of the ten top contributors to rising drug costs.

Most cases of diabetes are the type 2 form of the disease, tied to obesity, inactivity, and poor diets. That's both bad news (since one-third of Americans is obese and another third is overweight, according to the CDC) and good news, since even modest changes in diet and activity levels can virtually cure diabetes without medication.

"Losing weight and exercising regularly are the best ways to prevent and control the disease," says Dr. Jacob Teitelbaum, author of *The Complete Guide to Beating Sugar Addiction*. "There's good evidence that these two simple lifestyle changes work."

Case in point: the landmark Diabetes Prevention Program (DPP) Study. Initiated in 1996, the federally run study tracked more than 3,200 overweight people with prediabetes to see whether lifestyle changes could combat diabetes.

Researchers divided the participants into three groups. The first took a placebo and received coaching about lifestyle modifications, diet, and exercise; a second group took the common diabetes medication metformin twice daily; and a third engaged in an intensive lifestyle modification program (such as eating well and getting fifty minutes of moderate-intensity exercise each week to lose weight).

After three years, the people who followed the lifestyle program (lower-calorie, low-fat diet and regular exercise) had a 58 percent lower rate of developing diabetes than those who did not. By comparison, those who took metformin had a 31 percent lower rate, while those who took the placebo experienced very little change in their condition.

The integrative approach emphasizes the following strategies to effectively reverse insulin resistance, the hallmark of diabetes:

- Avoid sweets and high-carb foods (it's no surprise that a high-sugar diet is a cause of diabetes).
- Check hormone levels (important for both men and women).
- Exercise regularly (which tones insulin receptors too).
- Get more fiber (by slowing digestion, fiber helps balance blood sugar).
- Lose weight (decrease body fat).
- Take supplements (herbal supplements are effective for balancing blood sugar).

The DPP, coordinated by the CDC, is now carried out in multiple programs across the United States. "The CDC aims for 5 to 7 percent weight loss," explains health educator Santina Jaronki, who uses the program as part of her work with the Fairfield Health Department in Fairfield, Connecticut. "And that is what we aim for. After fifteen weeks, we see each person for monthly follow-ups.

"The program is absolutely helpful. Our initial group lost over eighty pounds. Not everybody stayed; life gets in the way, but eight or nine made it through."

For the best results in working the program, experts suggest the following:

- Make being active a way of life. Put in at least 150 minutes of activity every week. Take the stairs instead of the elevator. Park a few blocks from your destination. Engage in yard work or play ball with a child.
- Pay attention to other healthy lifestyle modifications—don't smoke, don't drink to excess or overeat, get at least seven hours of sleep every night, and figure out ways to manage stress (through yoga, meditation, or simply listening to calming music you enjoy).
- Read nutrition labels to keep track of fat, calories, and sugar in the foods you eat. Aim to reduce your intake of sugary, high-carb foods, including not only sweets but also bread and pasta.

Diabetes: At a Glance

What Is Diabetes?

Diabetes is a condition in which the body does not properly process food for use as energy. Many foods we eat are converted into sugar (glucose) for our bodies to use for energy. The pancreas makes a hormone called insulin to help glucose get into the body's cells.

People with diabetes either don't make enough insulin (type 1) or don't use it as well as their bodies need to in order to stay healthy (type 2). This causes sugars to build up in your blood, which can cause serious health complications.

Can It Be Life Threatening?

Yes. In fact, diabetes is the seventh leading cause of death in the United States, according to the CDC. Left unchecked, it can cause heart disease, blindness, kidney failure, and lower-extremity amputations.

What Are the Signs and Symptoms?

Some people with diabetes or prediabetes, in which blood sugar levels are higher than normal but not sufficiently elevated to be diagnosed as diabetes, have no symptoms at all. But some people with the metabolic disorder experience the following:

- excessive thirst
- extreme hunger
- frequent infections
- frequent urination
- nausea, vomiting, or stomach pain
- severe fatigue
- sudden vision changes
- tingling or numbness in hands or feet
- unexplained weight loss
- very dry skin
- wounds or sores that are slow to heal

How Are the Two Types of Diabetes Different?

Type 1 diabetes, sometimes called insulin-dependent diabetes mellitus (IDDM) or juvenile-onset diabetes, accounts for about 5 to 10 percent of all diagnosed cases. People with this form of diabetes must check blood sugar levels regularly, through skin-prick tests, and usually take insulin shots because their bodies don't produce enough of the hormone. Scientists believe autoimmune, genetic, and environmental factors might be involved in the development of type 1 diabetes.

Type 2 diabetes, previously called noninsulin-dependent diabetes mellitus (NIDDM) or adult-onset diabetes, accounts for 90 to 95 percent of all diagnosed cases. People with this form of diabetes don't process glucose properly, must also use blood-glucose monitors, and might need to take medications, such as metformin (Glucophage, Glumetza), Avandia, and Januvia, among others, to help their bodies function well.

Risk factors for type 2 diabetes include older age, obesity, family history of diabetes, prior history of gestational diabetes (during pregnancy), impaired glucose tolerance, physical inactivity, and race/ethnicity (with African Americans, Hispanic/Latino Americans, American Indians, and some Asian Americans and Pacific Islanders facing higher risks than whites for reasons scientist don't entirely understand).

Type 2 diabetes sufferers can usually reverse the condition by losing weight, exercising regularly, and eating a healthy low-sugar, lower-carb diet, studies show. But up to 40 percent of Americans with type 2 diabetes require insulin shots or other medications.

Other specific types of diabetes can result from specific genetic syndromes, surgery, drugs, malnutrition, infections, and other illnesses.

Foods That Naturally Lower Your Blood Sugar

Millions of Americans take medications daily to keep blood sugar in check. But a wide variety of foods can naturally lower blood glucose. Some might even be as effective as medication for many people.

"You know that 'hangry' feeling when you want to bite somebody's head off? That feeling of fatigue and brain fog? Do you ever feel shaky, sweaty, and light-headed? These are often signs that your blood sugar levels are out of whack," notes Tara Gidus Collingwood, team dietitian for the Orlando Magic NBA team and author of *The Flat Belly Cookbook for Dummies*. "Eating light and eating often can help regulate blood sugar levels throughout the day. Eating three meals and two snacks daily can prevent the rollercoaster effect, when your blood sugar plummets if you leave too many hours between meals and goes up when you finally provide nutrition."

Eating Your Way to Health

What you eat also plays an important role in how your blood sugar spikes during the day, says Collingwood. And while sweets, pasta, bread, and potatoes are the most well-known culprits in high blood sugar, they're not the only ones.

"Carbohydrates turn into sugar in the body and can be found in grains, fruits, and starchy vegetables," she explains. "Aim to make half your plate nonstarchy vegetables, a quarter grain, and a quarter protein. This will help you balance your diet and control your blood sugar."

Certain foods, beverages, and supplements are particularly effective at stabilizing or lowering blood sugar. Among them are the following:

BLUEBERRIES. A groundbreaking study published in the *Journal of Nutrition* found that a daily dose of the active ingredients in blueberries increases sensitivity to insulin and might reduce the risk of developing diabetes in at-risk individuals. Collingwood explains that these tasty berries are high in phytochemicals and antioxidants as well as fiber and vitamin C.

AVOCADOS. These staples of Mexican foods are full of healthy monounsaturated fats, which slow the release of sugars into the bloodstream and reduce inflammation. They also provide protection for the heart.

CINNAMON. A study in the *Journal of Diabetes Cure* showed that this aromatic spice causes muscle and liver cells to respond more readily to insulin. Eating a mere ½ teaspoon daily for twenty days is enough to improve your insulin response and lower blood sugar levels up to 20 percent.

CHIA SEEDS. These ancient gluten-free grains might be small, but they pack a mighty wallop. Chia seeds stabilize blood sugar, manage the effects of diabetes, improve insulin sensitivity, and help deal with imbalances of blood pressure, cholesterol, and extreme rises in blood sugar after meals.

MANGOS. These sweet fruits are full of antioxidants, fiber, and vitamins to slow down blood sugar in the body, decreasing the frequency of spikes.

OLIVE OIL. This Mediterranean diet staple is rich in the same monounsaturated fats found in avocados. It prevents not only belly fat accumulation but insulin resistance. "Cooking with olive oil can set your meal up to increase insulin sensitivity through the day," says Collingwood.

EGGS. Long maligned in nutritional circles, eggs have made an extraordinary comeback and are now considered nutritional powerhouses. "They contain protein and healthy unsaturated fats," says the expert. "This combination of protein and healthy fats [increases] the feeling of fullness and maintains sugar levels in the body."

CHERRIES. These sweet fruits contain naturally occurring chemicals called anthocyanins, which could lower blood sugar levels in people with diabetes. A study published in the *Journal of Agricultural and Food Chemistry* found that anthocyanins reduce insulin resistance by as much as 50 percent. Cherries might also protect against heart disease and cancer, say experts.

BLACK TEA. Drinking 3 or more cups of black tea a day cuts the risk of type 2 diabetes and helps manage the disease in those who have it, new research shows. A study from Framingham State University extracted numerous types of antioxidants from black tea that have been found to block the enzymes that increase blood sugar caused by carbohydrates. The report, published in *Frontiers of Nutrition*, suggests that black tea might reduce blood sugar levels naturally.

INDIAN KINO TREE EXTRACT. This compound—taken from the bark, leaves, flowers, and wood of the *Pterocarpus marsupium* tree native to India, Nepal, and Sri Lanka—has been shown to lower blood sugar levels and prevent oxidative damage in the body. It also helps transport sugar from the bloodstream into the cells and has been used in a wide spectrum of healing practices. The tree is a major source of beneficial polyphenols and flavonoids that have strong antidiabetic and anti-inflammatory properties, studies show, according to the NIH.

GYMNEMA SYLVESTRE. Research shows that this natural compound can be nearly as effective as prescription medications when it comes to lowering blood sugar. Gymnema sylvestre has been used for more than two thousand years to help reverse diabetes and is one of nearly eight hundred natural substances that scientific research has found might naturally lower blood sugar.

ALOE VERA. A review of nine studies investigating the benefits of aloe vera found that it keeps blood sugar levels on an even keel. The study, which was published in the *Journal of Alternative and Complementary Medicine*, gave oral supplements of aloe vera to patients with prediabetes and type 2 diabetes for four to fourteen weeks. They found that aloe vera stimulated the secretion of insulin and significantly lowered glucose levels in the blood by 46.6 mg/dl. It also lowered levels of HbA1c, which indicate sugar levels over the preceding three months. Experts recommend supplements in the range of 200–300 mg daily.

BIOTIN. This vitamin helps with glucose management inside the cell through the enzyme glucokinase. Biotin is a coenzyme and a B vitamin often called vitamin H. Research shows that the combination of chromium and biotin might improve blood sugar levels for people with type 2 diabetes. This important vitamin, which also staves off hair loss and depression, is found naturally in wheat germ, whole-grain cereal, eggs, dairy products, Swiss chard, salmon, and chicken. Stagg recommends 3–16 mcg daily.

VITAMIN D. The "sunshine vitamin" improves the secretion of insulin from the pancreas. Studies have also shown that it improves glucose tolerance and insulin sensitivity. Despite the name, vitamin D is actually considered to be a prohormone because the body is capable of producing its own vitamin D through the action of sunlight on the skin, while vitamins are nutrients that cannot be synthesized by the body and are only acquired through diet and supplements. In type 2 diabetics, low vitamin D levels might have adverse effects on insulin secretion and glucose tolerance. In one study, infants who received 2,000 IU daily had an 88 percent lower risk of developing type 1 diabetes by the age of thirty-two. Stagg recommends 800–2,000 IU daily.

D-CHIRO-INOSITOL. This chemical variant of inositol, a B vitamin, helps insulin work better because it improves the glucose pathway after the insulin has bound its receptor on a cell. It might significantly lower the fasting glucose level, and since diabetics seem to excrete this compound more than others, supplementation—especially for women who also have polycystic ovarian syndrome (PCOS) and who are insulin resistant—might benefit from this complimentary addition. You can find this nutrient in its highest concentration in buckwheat, soy lecithin, and legumes such as lentils, chick peas, and garbanzo beans. The recommended dosage for supplementation is 600–1,200 mg daily.

BERBERINE. This natural alkaloid originated in China and India, where it was used in Ayurvedic medicine. It's found in the herbs goldenseal, goldthread, and tree turmeric. Research has shown that it lowers blood glucose levels, and in one study, those taking 500 mg of berberine daily for three months showed the same medical benefit as the drug metformin in diabetics. In other words, berberine was able to control blood sugar levels as effectively as the most commonly used prescription drug. Other studies point out that this alkaloid can improve insulin sensitivity. The recommended dosage is 500 mg three times daily.

Food Swaps That Lower Blood Sugar

Making a few small adjustments in your diet can have a big impact on your blood sugar as well as your weight. "Blood sugar rates are really high, and diet certainly plays a role in that," says naturopath physician Trevor Cates. "It doesn't have to be supercomplicated. You can do simple things on a day-to-day basis, and it will make a difference in your blood sugar over time. And you don't have to compromise your life and do without all the things you love. You just have to modify it a bit."

For instance, one can of Coke has 39 grams of sugar in the form of high fructose corn syrup. It not only has an extremely high glycemic index but it is also 140 empty calories that won't put a dent in your appetite. Instead of soda, you can drink sparkling water with flavored stevia, a no-calorie natural sugar substitute.

Here are some other food swaps that you can use to control your blood sugar:

BERRIES FOR BANANAS. Bananas might be loaded with potassium and other nutrients, but they also have a high GI and can make blood sugar spike. Berries are a better choice to put in your morning cereal or for snacking.

DARK GREENS FOR LIGHT GREENS. All greens provide a lot of nutrition packed into low-calorie packages. But the dark ones—kale, spinach, arugula, chard, and so on—have higher levels of magnesium and potassium. These minerals are vital in the metabolism of sugar, and both are associated with a reduced risk of diabetes.

BROWN RICE FOR WHITE RICE. Both are heavy on the carbs, but the white version is stripped of magnesium, potassium, and other nutrients. The brown variety also has a lot more fiber, which keeps blood sugar in check.

BEANS FOR POTATOES. Get your starch fix with beans instead of potatoes. Beans have a considerably lower GI, along with more fiber, protein, and blood sugar–balancing potassium. Kidney, garbanzo, soy, pinto, and black beans are best.

OATMEAL FOR CEREAL. Even "healthy" boxed cereal tends to be loaded with sugar, but plain oatmeal is just oats. Oatmeal also has a lot of soluble fiber that slows down the release of its natural sugars. But read the labels of instant oatmeal carefully because the flavored varieties often have a lot of added sugar and preservatives. You can always add some fruit or honey yourself to sweeten up plain oatmeal. Steel-cut oats are best.

WHOLE FRUIT FOR FRUIT JUICE. Both contain a lot of sugar, but the juice has no fiber to cushion the blow and can spike your blood sugar as quickly as soda.

CARROTS OR CELERY FOR CRACKERS. When it comes time to eat guacamole, spinach dip, or hummus, instead of piling it on a cracker or chip, use a stick of carrot or celery. Many brands of crackers are made with refined grains that have had most of their nutrients processed out, and they also contain added sugars, salt, and preservatives.

WHOLE GRAINS FOR REFINED GRAINS. This one is a no-brainer. When it comes to breads and pastas, why opt for bleached, flavorless stuff when you can have tastier versions with more nutrition, including fiber to counter the negative impact of the carbs? Grow up and graduate from white bread.

NUTS FOR GRANOLA BARS. Granola bars have a reputation for being a healthy snack, but many of them are just as high in carbs as candy bars. Grab a handful of raw organic nuts instead. They'll fill you up and are also mighty mites when it comes to healthy fats and nutrients.

SMALL PLATES FOR BIG PLATES. Although not technically a "food swap," research shows that people eat less when they use small plates. That's because a full small plate looks like more food than a half-empty big plate, and we eat with our eyes as much as our stomachs. Since portion size is a big factor in diabetes, go small and save yourself a bunch of calories.

Chromium: Surprising Key to Controlling Diabetes

Chromium is easy to overlook. It's one of several essential minerals in multivitamins, but beyond that, we don't usually hear much about it. Yet it represents the key to staying healthy and independent throughout a long life and has strong antidiabetes properties, according to the latest research.

"It overcomes insulin resistance, and that's a very important part of the aging process," says Dr. Harry Preuss, professor at Georgetown University and a researcher who has studied chromium for several decades. Insulin resistance, although not well understood, is a major driver of premature aging, weight gain, diabetes, and heart disease.

As we age, our ability to utilize sugar and starch decreases because our cells become less sensitive to insulin. As a result, levels of blood sugar rise, increasing risk for diabetes and heart disease, and more and more food is converted to fat instead of being used to generate energy and preserve muscle.

The all-too-common high-starch, high-sugar American diet adds insult to injury.

What Chromium Does

"It switches your metabolism," Preuss says. In other words, chromium restores the ability to utilize starches and sugars as energy and to maintain muscle, rather than storing more fat.

Studies have found that it does this by increasing sensitivity to insulin and keeping blood sugar to lower, healthier levels—which also helps prevent type 2 diabetes.

In one of his studies, Preuss found that on a reduced-calorie diet, people lost the same amount of weight with a placebo or a chromium supplement. But those taking chromium lost mainly fat, whereas placebo takers lost mostly muscle.

Studies have also found that by regulating blood sugar, chromium has reduced unhealthy levels of cholesterol. In one study, "bad" low-density lipoprotein (LDL) cholesterol dropped by 14 percent.

How Much Do You Need?

The federal government does not specify how much chromium we need for optimum health. Rather, it has developed an adequate intake (AI) guideline, which is an estimate of the amount of chromium the average American consumed in 2001, when it established AI. These amounts are 20–25 mcg for adult women and 30–35 mcg for adult men.

Consuming foods that are high in sugar and starch, intense exercise, infections, and injuries increase the amount of chromium that is excreted and reduce levels of the mineral. Pregnant women and the elderly are more likely to be deficient. Antacids, corticosteroids, and heartburn drugs also reduce chromium levels.

Based on the research, Preuss recommends that healthy people of all ages take at least 200 mcg of chromium daily. This amount, he says, can protect against premature aging by improving metabolism, maintaining muscle, and reducing the age-related tendency to gain fat.

If you take it on an ongoing basis, as time goes by, he says, "You can hold your own."

Chromium Sources

Our bodies require chromium in trace amounts. Quantities of the mineral are measured in micrograms (mcg; there are one thousand micrograms in one milligram). In food, it's difficult to identify amounts of chromium because it depends on the amount of chromium in the soil where plant foods are grown. In meat, levels are influenced by chromium content of animal feed, which varies.

As a rough guide, the government estimates these amounts of chromium in some of the top food sources:

- **broccoli, ½ cup:** 11 mcg
- **grape juice, 1 cup:** 8 mcg
- **one whole-wheat English muffin:** 4 mcg
- **mashed potatoes, 1 cup:** 3 mcg
- **dried garlic, 1 teaspoon:** 3 mcg

- **dried basil, 1 tablespoon:** 2 mcg
- **orange juice, 1 cup:** 2 mcg
- **turkey breast, 3 ounces:** 2 mcg

Chromium Supplements

These come in different forms. Chromium chloride is poorly absorbed. For good absorption and overall health, Preuss recommends taking 200 mcg of one of these forms: chromium polynicotinate, chromium picolinate, or chromium histadinate. If you are trying to lose weight, you might want to take up to 600 mcg daily. Be patient, take it consistently, and don't expect an instant result, he cautions, as change takes time.

DIGESTIVE DISORDERS

Celiac disease, irritable bowel syndrome (IBS), and gastroesophageal reflux disease (GERD) don't garner the same attention as heart disease, cancer, or diabetes when it comes to health headlines. But millions of Americans suffer from these and other digestive disorders in ways that can be equally debilitating.

The good news is that all three are largely preventable or treatable through lifestyle changes, healthy dietary habits, and other nondrug approaches. Here's what you need to know.

Celiac Disease: Causes and Cures
The gluten-free food craze is fueling a multibillion-dollar US growth industry.

- As many as one in three restaurant-goers are asking for gluten-free menu items in Los Angeles and New York, by some accounts.
- Facebook has more than one thousand groups with "gluten-free" in the name, and there's even a dating group called "Gluten-free singles."
- The trend has prompted the Russian maker of Stolichnaya vodka go so far as to introduce Stoli Gluten Free in 2016—made from 88 percent corn and 12 percent buckwheat.

But is going gluten-free the right choice for everyone, and are there any downsides to consider? These questions are driving a healthy debate pitting gluten-free advocates, who say such foods promote weight loss and lower inflammation, against health experts, who argue that there is no major benefit except for people with celiac disease, whose bodies can't process the protein in wheat, barley, rye, and other grains.

Until recently, most doctors took a dim view of gluten-free diets for people without celiac disease, noting that some contain fewer vitamins, less fiber, and more sugar. But that view is changing with a growing number of nutritionists and some doctors, who are now saying that gluten-free foods are nutritionally equal to or better than their gluten-containing counterparts—even for individuals without celiac disease.

Dr. Robert Newman, a certified nutritionist and wellness expert from East Northport, New York, notes that gluten-free diets aren't for everyone. But many people with gastrointestinal problems who have sensitivities to gluten (including some who have not been diagnosed with celiac disease) will benefit from eliminating the protein from their diet.

"Really what we're talking about is a spectrum—from celiac disease, a disease process, to just a sensitivity to gluten," he explains. "You can have a whole myriad of symptoms that [can be addressed] by going gluten free."

Newman notes that many products containing gluten from wheat, barley, rye, and other grains are high-calorie foods that can contribute to high blood sugar and obesity. He adds that a number of foods are naturally free of gluten, as are many ancient grains, such as quinoa, amaranth, teff, buckwheat groats, and millet.

For people who are having unexplained gastrointestinal (GI) problems, he recommends consulting a doctor. A blood test can indicate a strong possibility of gluten sensitivity or celiac disease. Going gluten-free for a period of time, and monitoring any changes in symptoms, can also provide a clue for people with gluten sensitivities.

"I really think you need to go to your physician to get diagnosed," he advises, noting that genetic and antibody blood testing is available. "If you're having that whole myriad of symptoms and you just can't solve it and all of a sudden you go gluten-free for, let's say, two weeks, and you feel so much better, that's a great response."

Gluten-free diets are a relatively new health trend. A decade ago, most Americans had never heard of gluten. Today, many restaurants and food manufacturers are recalibrating recipes to capitalize on the growing interest in gluten-free products. Global retail sales of gluten-free products have nearly doubled since 2007 to $2.1 billion, according to a recent analysis by the *Wall Street Journal*.

About three million Americans suffer from celiac disease and must avoid gluten. For those individuals, the protein triggers an autoimmune response that damages or destroys the tiny fingerlike outgrowths (called villi) that line the small intestine like a microscopic carpet. Villi absorb nutrients into the bloodstream, but when they are damaged, it can cause malnutrition, serious weight loss, deficiencies in many nutrients, and exhaustion.

The National Foundation for Celiac Awareness estimates another eighteen million Americans have gluten sensitivities and experience GI discomfort when they eat products containing the protein.

Part of what's driving the trend toward gluten-free diets is a growing interest, particularly among aging baby boomers, in adopting healthier eating habits. Food manufacturers have sought to capitalize on the trend over the past decade by producing not only gluten-free products but those labeled "low-carb," "all-natural," "organic," "non-GMO," "dairy-free," "probiotic," and "hormone-free."

Some health experts say we are focusing too much on what we eat and not enough on how much we eat—and the fact that Americans are becoming ever more sedentary. Federal health statistics show that Americans are consuming nearly five hundred more calories per day, on average, than in the 1970s. And over the last two decades, the number of sedentary Americans—those who say they get no regular physical activity at all each day—has risen about 50 percent.

Regardless of whether you have a gluten sensitivity or celiac disease, Newman and other nutrition experts say it's important for everyone to eat a balanced diet of foods with high-quality nutrients. "There are so many foods you can eat instead of gluten-free foods," he says.

Wheat flour–based foods can be replaced with nutrient-packed whole grains, such as quinoa, teff, or whole-grain rice (brown, red, black, or wild). Fresh fruits and vegetables, eggs, beans, and nuts are naturally gluten-free.

As the gluten-free craze takes hold, it is also likely to prompt food makers to reformulate popular foods that are now off-limits to some people. In fact, it's already happening. "There is gluten-free pizza . . . made out of corn foods, and it actually tastes decent," he notes. "You just have to get a very thin crust."

IBS: At a Glance

IBS and its multitude of gastrointestinal (GI) symptoms plague 10 to 15 percent of the US population, or between twenty-five and forty-eight million people.

The medical condition affects more women than men, and although it affects all ages, most people diagnosed are under age fifty, according to the International Foundation for Functional Gastrointestinal Disorders (IFFGD). Doctors have not determined exactly what causes IBS, but IFFGD said it has "well-defined clinical features" and "specific diagnostic criteria."

The primary symptoms of IBS include the following:

- abdominal pain or discomfort
- constipation
- diarrhea
- irregularity

Other symptoms might be a problem for people with IBS, according to the IFFGD:

- anxiety
- chest pain
- depression
- fibromyalgia
- headaches
- insomnia
- urinary or gynecological symptoms

Doctors typically diagnose IBS in people who experience symptoms at least three days a month for a period of six months or more.

Gut-Brain Link?

While scientists don't know what causes IBS, some research suggests that there might be a link between the brain and gut in its development. New Australian research suggests that anxiety might increase the risk of developing the condition by up to 50 percent.

Conversely, two-thirds of suffers reported gut troubles before the onset of anxiety symptoms. For the study, the researchers from the University of Newcastle, Australia, tracked 1,900 people for one year, checking their levels of depression, anxiety, and IBS symptoms.

The results showed that those with the highest levels of anxiety and depression when the study began had a greater risk of developing IBS within one year. "We found that higher levels of anxiety and depression at baseline were significant predictors of developing IBS," noted the researchers, who published their findings in the journal *Alimentary, Pharmacology & Therapeutics*.

A similar relationship between the gut and the brain has been identified in other studies of Crohn's disease—an inflammatory bowel disease (IBD)—and brain function. It's common for Crohn's sufferers to have subtle cognitive impairment, difficulty concentrating, sleep disorders, and memory problems.

Stress and diet are well-known factors for triggering IBS. The good news is that both can be managed and controlled to combat IBS and other digestive disorders. In fact, the Newcastle researchers noted that the risk of developing IBS was reduced by 60–70 percent for participants with low levels of anxiety and depression at the start of the study.

How to Ease IBS

For years, doctors treated IBS with laxatives, over-the-counter (OTC) stomach medicines, avoidance of certain trigger foods, and other Band-Aid approaches. But the latest research has shown that people with IBS who follow certain diets—including consuming probiotics, which are "healthy bacteria" found in yogurt, aged cheeses, and other fermented foods—can virtually cure the condition without resorting to medication:

- A recent review of forty-three studies of probiotics for IBS symptoms, conducted by the National Institutes of Health (NIH), found that "probiotics had beneficial effects on global IBS symptoms, abdominal pain, bloating, and flatulence scores; however, the species and strains that provide the most beneficial effects are unclear."
- A landmark study published in the journal *Gastroenterology* clarified the uncertainties by finding that a specific probiotics strain, *Bifidobacterium infantis 35624*, alleviated IBS symptoms in sufferers who took one billion live *B. infantis* cells once a day.
- Another clinical trial, examining the effects of *Bifidobacterium animalis (regularis) DN-173 010*, found that IBS patients given the probiotics reported improved regularity and alleviation of bloating symptoms, according to the NIH. This particular strain of probiotics is contained in such products as Activia and Dannon yogurt.

In addition to the promising research on probiotics, a 2016 study found that the so-called low-FODMAP diet—which restricts foods that are high in fermentable oligo-, di-, and monosaccharides and polyols (FODMAPs)—also has the potential to alleviate IBS symptoms.

FODMAPs are short-chain carbohydrates that are poorly absorbed by the body but quickly fermented by intestinal bacteria, which leads to gas and diarrhea—underlying the symptoms of IBS, the University of Michigan researchers noted in the *American Journal of Gastroenterology*.

FODMAPs include high-fiber foods and simple sugars that certain intestinal bacteria thrive on fermenting. The low-FODMAP diet limits many high-carb vegetables, fruits, and all wheat products while allowing some low-carb vegetables and fruits, protein, oats, rice, and quinoa.

For the Michigan study, researchers compared IBS patients following a low-FODMAP diet to others following dietary recommendations for IBS from the National Institute for Health and Care Excellence, which advises smaller, frequent meals; avoiding trigger foods like wheat products and starches; limiting fresh fruit; avoiding the artificial sweetener sorbitol; and steering clear of excess alcohol and caffeine.

After four weeks, more than half of the patients on the low-FODMAP diet reported feeling better compared to 41 percent of those who followed the National Institute for Health and Care Excellence diet.

Should You Be Taking Probiotic Supplements?

You've no doubt heard about the benefits of probiotics—those good-for-you bacteria and yeasts that have been shown to aid digestion, boost immunity, combat a host of ailments, and improve your overall mental and physical health.

But there's only so much yogurt, sauerkraut, aged cheeses, pickles, and other probiotic-laden foods you can pack into your diet, right? Well, here's the good news: taking a probiotics supplement can increase your consumption of these healthy microbes easily without resorting to a major overhaul of your daily meals.

Dr. Robert Newsman—a certified nutritionist, chiropractor, and wellness expert from East Northport, New York—says it's important to know what to look for when choosing a supplement. One key factor is that the most effective formulations are refrigerated to keep the live cultures active.

"Generally speaking, the most active formulas are found in the refrigerated section at your health food store," says Newman. "Always store the container in the refrigerator for increased viability."

Newman also recommends choosing products that contain high "therapeutic counts" of certain healthy-bacterial strains and colonies. "I like to look for a varied five to ten strains of *Bifido* and *Lactobacillus* bacterium and a therapeutic count of thirty to fifty billion," he explains. "For very severe intestinal dysbiosis, I will dose up to one hundred to two hundred billion, and a probiotic yeast named *Saccharomyces boulardii* has proven to be most effective for diarrhea symptoms."

Nearly 2 percent of Americans take probiotic supplements, and their popularity is growing. In fact, the use of probiotics quadrupled between 2007 and 2012, according to the most recent National Health Interview Survey, a long-running poll of Americans health habits by the US Centers for Disease Control and Prevention (CDC).

Scientific studies have linked probiotics to a wide range of health benefits and fueled public interest. The following represent a few of these:

Digestive health. Probiotics are a frontline treatment for IBS, chronic constipation, abdominal pain, gas, bloating, and other GI disorders. They're also helpful for maintaining healthy levels of "good" bacteria in the GI tracts of people taking broad-spectrum antibiotics, which kill bacteria of all kinds.

Cancer. University of California, Los Angeles (UCLA) researchers found that mice that were fed healthy, anti-inflammatory gut bacteria produced microbes known to prevent cancer and reduce gene damage. This suggests that probiotic supplements might help prevent cancer from developing. A second study, published in the *Proceedings of the National Academy of Sciences*, found that probiotics might help block tumor growth. Mice designed to develop liver cancer that were fed probiotics had a 42 percent reduction in tumor size and a 52 percent reduction in the growth of the blood vessels tumors use to grow and spread.

Weight loss. A study published in the *British Journal of Nutrition* found that probiotics might help women lose weight and keep it off. Over a three-month period, overweight women who took two pills containing probiotics from the *Lactobacillus rhamnosus* family daily lost almost twice as much weight as those who did not take the supplements. Researchers from Washington University School of Medicine have also found that certain healthy bacteria are more common in thin people than overweight folks.

Heavy metal poisoning. A study at Lawson Health Research Institute's Canadian Centre for Human Microbiome and Probiotic Research found that pregnant women taking probiotics absorbed 78 percent less arsenic and 36 percent less mercury. Both are common environmental toxins found in water and food, and exposure is associated with some cancers and lowered IQs in children.

Allergies. An analysis of twenty-three studies at Vanderbilt University Medical Center found that probiotics improved the symptoms of people with seasonal allergies, such as sneezing and stuffy nose, in seventeen of the studies. Researchers believe probiotics change the composition of bacteria in the intestines in ways that modulate the body's immune response and stop it from reacting to pollen and other allergens. The study was published in the journal *International Forum of Allergy & Rhinology*. Probiotics have also been shown to eliminate cow's milk and peanut allergies in some children.

High blood pressure. Researcher published in the journal *Hypertension* found that people who took probiotics daily for more than two months experienced an average drop of 3.6 mmHg in systolic blood pressure (the top number) and a 2.4 mmHg drop in diastolic blood pressure (the bottom number). "We believe probiotics might help lower blood pressure by having other positive effects on health, including improving total cholesterol and low-density lipoprotein, or LDL, cholesterol; reducing blood glucose and insulin resistance; and by helping to regulate the hormone system that regulates blood pressure and fluid balance," said researcher Jing Sun.

Depression. A University of Toronto study found that patients suffering from chronic fatigue syndrome (CFS) who went on a two-month course of probiotics significantly reduced their depression and anxiety. Experts said the healthy bacteria encouraged by the probiotics boosted the production of L-tryptophan, a "feel-good" neurotransmitter. A second study, from Leiden University in the Netherlands, found that healthy people who took probiotics, which included *Bifidobacterium* and *Lactobacillus*, were significantly less prone to sad moods than those who did not.

GERD: What You Need Know

Heartburn. Agita. Acid indigestion. All are nicknames GERD, the backward flow of stomach acid into the esophagus—the tube that connects the throat and stomach. GERD strikes about sixty million Americans, who typically experience a burning sensation in the chest known as heartburn. But symptoms can also include regurgitated food or a sour taste at the back of the mouth. Untreated, it can lead to esophageal cancer, which has been rising in recent decades.

Millions of people who suffer from GERD take medication, including OTC antacids. Others are prescribed powerful prescription drugs to control and neutralize stomach acid. In fact, consumers spend an estimated $24 billion worldwide each year on prescription heartburn drugs. But if you're one of the millions of Americans who regularly take a pill for reflux, you might unwittingly be setting yourself up for serious health problems, many studies show.

"Millions of people are dealing with acid reflux and indigestion every day, but those that seek help from their doctors are stuck in a never-ending cycle of dangerous—and sometimes even deadly—medications and procedures," says Kevin Passero, ND, one of America's leading naturopathic physicians.

The top-selling prescription and OTC drugs used to treat acid reflux disorder fall into two main types: proton pump inhibitors (PPIs), such as Prilosec, Prevacid, and Nexium; and H2 receptor antagonists like Tagamet, Pepcid, and Zantac. Since their introduction in 1990, PPIs have become the primary way that acid reflux disease is treated, and they are so popular that Nexium is now the third top-selling drug in the United States, according to Intercontinental Marketing Services Health.

But these drugs can be dangerous and might not be as effective as nonmedication alternatives, says Passero, author of the book *The Drug-Free Acid Reflux Solution*. For example,

- The US Food and Drug Administration (FDA) has issued many warnings against PPIs and acid-blocking drugs, saying that they increase the risk of bone fractures, infection, and nutritional deficiencies. Some studies have also linked pneumonia, osteoporosis, low magnesium levels, and weight gain to these drugs.

- PPIs might hike heart disease risks in some people because they constrict blood vessels, which can lead to high blood pressure and a weakened heart, according to a new study from Houston Methodist Hospital. In addition, PPIs can interact with other drugs, including Plavix, a blood thinner used to prevent heart attacks and strokes. Other heartburn drugs—known as H2 receptor antagonists—also block production of stomach acid. While they are older and their effect is not as pronounced as PPIs, their side effects are not considered as problematic.

- Recent research published in the Public Library of Science journal *PLOS ONE* suggests that PPIs might increase heart attack risk by up to 21 percent, building on past studies that have suggested that PPIs might cause possible cardiovascular drug interactions.

- Johns Hopkins University researchers have found troubling links between PPIs and kidney disease. A study of more than 260,000 patients in five states, published in 2016 in the journal *JAMA Internal Medicine*, indicated that those who took prescription PPIs were 20 to 50 percent more likely to develop chronic kidney disease than nonusers.

- A Mayo Clinic study found that PPIs can disrupt the makeup of bacteria in the digestive system, potentially boosting the risk of infections, like pneumonia and the stubborn *Clostridium difficile* that plagues many hospital patients. Scientists believe that by reducing the acidity of the stomach, PPIs allow bacteria to thrive and then spread to other organs like the lungs and intestines.

- Older people might be particularly at risk because they are more likely to have reflux, in part because the muscle that prevents stomach acid from rising into the esophagus weakens with age, research shows. As a result, seniors are more vulnerable to the diseases and disorders associated with them in the long run.

- Heartburn drugs might interfere with body's absorption of protein and calcium, critical to the development and maintenance of strong, healthy bones, several studies have found. This might increase the risks of osteoporosis, particularly in seniors.

Despite the growing evidence of heartburn drug risks, Dr. Lani Simpson, author of *Dr. Lani's No-Nonsense Bone Health Guide*, notes that many people have no idea they might be doing themselves more harm than good and that safer alternatives can alleviate problems.

"I'm not telling anyone to stop taking these medications," she explains. "But what I am saying is that a lot of people, in fact, can get off of them with the right guidance in working with a nutritionist, because a lot of times when people have GERD or gastric reflux or acid problems, it's because of their horrendous diet."

Dr. Chad Larson, a naturopathic doctor in in the San Diego area, adds that the big problem with PPIs is that they're often prescribed and taken over a lifetime, which significantly increases the risks they pose. "They're only supposed to be prescribed for a very short period of time for a specific situation, and unfortunately, they're prescribed and forgotten about, and the patient keeps getting refill after refill after refill," he notes.

He sees too many patients in this situation and says the real solution is to identify and correct the cause of the heartburn, rather than medicating symptoms.

Stomach Acid Is Essential

Heartburn drugs suppress stomach acid for quick relief. But over the long term, lack of acid can be a problem because it's needed to break down and digest food, kill food-borne pathogens, and trigger production of digestive enzymes by the pancreas. It can also interfere with the effectiveness of some medications. Without enough stomach acid, we can't properly digest food and absorb nutrients.

With heartburn, discomfort is caused by partially digested foods and stomach acid backing up into the esophagus instead of moving downward. There's a muscle that works like a valve to seal food in the stomach—the lower esophageal sphincter (LES)—and it can relax and open at the wrong time.

Then acidic stomach contents gurgle upward and produce a burning sensation. The acid in the stomach might not be abnormally high, but it's in the wrong place, hence the irritation. These, says Larson, are some common reasons this happens:

- Obesity, especially a big belly, puts pressure on the stomach, forcing food up into the esophagus. (This is also common in pregnancy.)
- A hiatal hernia (easily corrected, often without surgery) can exert a similar type of pressure.
- Too much food in the stomach forces the LES muscle to open. Eating smaller, more frequent meals will avoid pressure and might curb overeating and lead to weight loss.

Controlling the Key Muscle

Certain foods and drinks tend to relax the LES, says Larson, making it more likely that food will move in the wrong direction. These include mint, onions, spices, citrus fruits, alcohol, and coffee. Avoiding these at meal times can help.

Some medications can have a similar effect. These include benzodiazepines for anxiety, calcium-channel blockers for heart disease, beta-blockers for blood pressure, and ibuprofen and other nonsteroidal anti-inflammatory (NSAID) drugs for pain.

Sometimes heartburn can be a symptom of *H. pylori* infection. Food sensitivities can also relax the LES, allowing food to escape into the esophagus. Dairy is the most common culprit, but individuals can be sensitive to virtually any food. A blood test can identify individual sensitivities.

Natural Heartburn Remedies

Although they are not a substitute for finding and addressing an underlying cause of heartburn, natural remedies will enhance digestion and soothe the esophagus. If you're taking a PPI, stopping suddenly can cause a rebound reaction, worsening heartburn, says Larson.

He recommends gradually tapering off (work with your doctor if you're taking a prescription version) while using one or more of these:

Slippery elm tea. This tea creates a soothing coating in the digestive tract. Drink it before eating or add slippery elm powder to oatmeal and chew thoroughly.

Deglycyrrhizinated licorice (DGL). Thoroughly chew DGL wafers before and after meals.

Apple cider vinegar. Mix 1 tablespoon in ¼ cup of water and drink fifteen minutes before each meal.

Digestive enzymes. Take a formula with enzymes that break down proteins, fats, and carbohydrates at the start of each meal.

In addition, Simpson suggests that the following lifestyle changes can ease GERD without the use of drugs:

- **Exercise.** Working out regularly, at least thirty minutes daily, can help keep you lean. Obesity has been shown to double the risk for heartburn.
- **Change Your Diet.** GERD can be held in check by eating a healthy diet rich in fruits, vegetables, and lean protein and low in foods that have high levels of acidity.

- **Limit alcohol.** Drinking weakens the LES, which keeps stomach acid out of the food pipe.
- **Kick the habit.** Quit smoking if you use tobacco, which also increases the risk for GERD.
- **Talk to your doctor.** Consult your physician about safely halting the use of antacids and PPIs if you take them. He or she can also help you address any GI problems, including GERD, which can be managed through diet.

Experts note that it can take a few months for a digestive tract to heal and to taper off PPIs if you're taking the drugs. During the process, natural remedies and healthy lifestyle changes can alleviate symptoms. "Nutrition, gastrointestinal health, and exercise should be the core treatment program," Simpson says.

Passero agrees and recommends a similar treatment plan that includes his Reflux Recovery Diet (RRD) as well as a program of supplements and vitamins. The RRD diet includes these principles:

- Avoid alcohol and caffeine.
- Avoid spicy and acidic foods.
- Focus on whole foods and increase fruits, vegetables, and other sources of fiber (with the exception of acidic fruits like citrus and tomatoes).
- Increase your intake of culture, probiotic-rich foods and beverages, like kombucha (a fermented black or green tea), as well as yogurt and kefir.
- Reduce or eliminate all processed sugars, most dairy products, and gluten.
- Substitute "healthy fats" for fried foods and saturated fats.

Overeating: The New National Pastime?

For many people, overeating (technically known as dyspepsia) is simply a habit—something they do without thinking. Do you typically open a bag of chips while watching TV, eat whenever you're reading something (like a newspaper or magazine), or expect food to accompany certain times of the day—breakfast, lunch, dinner, afternoon snack, late-night bite?

If so, you might be eating simply out of habit and not because you're hungry or needing nourishment. But doing so can boost your risk for obesity, heartburn, and a host of chronic health conditions. Overeating is often fueled by a handful of factors. Among them are the following:

Emotions. There is some science behind the clichéd images of a woman diving into a pint of ice cream after a breakup or a man "drowning his sorrows" in beer and nachos after a stressful day at the office. In fact, many people overeat to deal with underlying emotional problems that would be best addressed in healthier ways. If you're first instinct when you're feeling down is to reach for junk food, you might be an "emotional overeater."

Food addiction. An emerging body of medical research has found that sugary, fat-laden, and salty foods might trigger a kind of addiction by changing signals between the gut and the brain—changing neurochemistry in ways similar to drug addiction. Studies in animals have shown, for instance, that laboratory rats that binge on sugar develop signs of dependency. Other studies have shown that junk foods stimulate the release of "feel-good" chemicals in the brain that can prompt overeating.

Yo-yo dieting. Sometimes an overly restrictive diet can begin a cycle of yo-yo dieting. In such cases, people starve themselves for some set period of time to lose weight and then compulsively overeat or go on food binges—a pattern some experts have dubbed the "eat, repent, repeat" cycle. If you find yourself frequently going on a restrictive diet because you feel bad about your weight but then binge on junk foods because you can't stick to it, you might be at risk of falling into this pattern.

How to Break the Cycle

Exercise. Working out might boost your appetite, but it also helps you burn off any excess calories you consume when you overeat. To compensate for occasional binge eating during the holidays or other times of year, increase your exercise regimen.

Calculate calories. It might help to think about the amount of exercise you'll need to burn off any extra foods you consume. For instance, about fifty minutes of vigorous exercise or a five-mile walk will burn off the same amount of calories contained in a single soda or piece of cake. If you think of the foods you eat in terms of exercise required to compensate for them, you might find yourself eating less.

Have a plan. Developing a healthy eating plan can keep you from overeating during special occasions. For instance, if you're going to a holiday party or a family meal with a buffet table, load your plate with vegetables, salad, and other healthier items first—that will leave less space for mashed potatoes, gravy, fatty foods, and sweets.

Don't go on a diet. The yo-yo diet cycle can be hard to break. But try to build into your daily life and lifestyle regular patterns of healthy eating to last a life-time. Don't skip breakfast; research shows eating a healthy breakfast cuts the risk of overeating throughout the day. Eat only when you're hungry (usually four to five hours after your last meal) and not just because it's lunchtime or dinner time. Stop eating when you feel full or satisfied. And resolve to eat at least five servings of fruits and vegetables, as well as lean protein and whole grains, every day—limiting sweets and high-carb processed foods.

Develop coping skills. Compulsive overeaters who use food as their only way of coping with negative emotions should develop healthier methods of dealing with stress, loneliness, and depression. Options can include meditation, yoga, listening to quiet music, and getting professional help.

Give yourself a break. Giving into food cravings on occasion is not a big deal. If you overindulge during the holidays or in celebrating a friend's birthday, give yourself a break. Just get back on your regular healthy diet afterward and move on.

Seek professional help. For some people, willpower alone isn't enough to stop overeating. That's particularly true for people with deep-rooted emotional connections to food. Working with a therapist, dietitian, or counselor can help you uncover and avoid the psychological triggers behind overeating so you can replace old, unhealthy habits with new and better alternatives.

EYE DISORDERS

Americans are living longer than ever, with life expectancy stretching into the high seventies and low eighties for many people. But an unfortunate side effect of that longevity is an increase in vision problems. As many as sixty-one million adults in the United States are at high risk for serious vision loss, especially after age sixty-five.

Hereditary diseases and age-related deterioration of vision can rob us of the most basic human sense of sight. But high-tech gadgets, gene transplants, stem cell therapies, and natural healing practices are paving the way to cures. Here's a primer on the latest advances.

Gene Therapy

For inherited eye diseases that rob vision, there are many studies under way that are testing gene therapy to correct mutated genes that lead to common causes of blindness.

"The idea is simply to replace the defective component with a working component," says Michael Redmond, chief of the Laboratory of Retinal Cell and Molecular Biology at the National Eye Institute.

In the therapy, the working gene is attached to a harmless virus as a means of transportation, and the combination is injected into a patient's eye. "The viruses being used are viruses that everybody carries every day—they're common in human cells, and they don't cause any known disease," Redmond explains.

The RPE65 gene is the most studied so far. Its mutation underlies some 10 percent of Leber's congenital amaurosis type 2 (LCA2), the most common cause of blindness in infants and children. Small human trials of RPE65 treatment began about eight years ago and produced some remarkable improvements. Some of the patients did not retain their improved vision, but others did, and it's possible that RPE65 will become the first US Food and Drug Administration (FDA)–approved gene therapy for LCA2 patients with this specific mutation.

Other hereditary diseases that might respond to gene therapy include retinitis pigmentosa (RP) and Stargardt's disease, a juvenile form of macular degeneration. Age-related vision loss involves a more complex set of factors, but researchers are also testing a new form of a gene therapy—called RetinoStat—for advanced age-related macular degeneration (AMD) that has had promising early results.

One of the leading causes of vision loss, the two forms of the disease (known as "wet" and "dry" AMD) affect more than two million Americans age fifty or older.

Stem Cells

Stem cell treatments show promise for treating early stages of both AMD and diabetic retinopathy, which affects more than seven million Americans. So far, a few small human trials have had some success treating AMD patients.

"The majority of people showed some improvement," says Alexander Ljubimov, director of the Eye Program at the Cedars-Sinai Regenerative Medicine Institute in Los Angeles. "The problem is whether the improvement is a lasting one." But he's optimistic about the prospects.

A groundbreaking discovery—which won the 2012 Nobel Prize in Physiology or Medicine—is opening the door to more effective and widespread use of stem cells. The new technology enables researchers to use the patient's own cells, rather than stem cells from another person.

For example, cells can be taken from the patient's skin or fat and then transplanted back into the patient. This eliminates a major obstacle—namely, rejection of foreign cells, much like rejection of transplanted organs, which can require lifelong immune-suppression treatment. "I think this new technology will produce better and more impactful results," says Ljubimov.

For diabetic retinopathy, stem cell research has not yet advanced to human trials, but the treatment could potentially slow down or even reverse degeneration of cells in the retina. Because diabetes affects eyes in multiple ways, says Ljubimov, "combined therapies might work better."

That could mean various combinations of stem cells, gene therapy, and/or drugs—much like cancer treatment often consists of more than one type of treatment.

The Bionic Eye

RP, an inherited eye disease that affects about one in four thousand Americans, can cause vision to start deteriorating as early as childhood and eventually lead to complete blindness. There is no cure, but a high-tech implanted device is restoring some vision to those who have been blinded by the disease.

The retina is light-sensitive tissue in the back of the eye. It translates light signals so that these can be passed along through other tissues to the brain, where they are interpreted as images, like a satellite dish converts signals into a picture on a TV. In RP, cells in the retina don't function as they should, blocking the transmission of light.

A new device, called the Argus II, has three components designed to restore sight: a set of electrodes implanted in and around the eye, special dark glasses with a built-in video camera, and a very small computer that looks somewhat like a large pager. As the camera captures images, they are converted into tiny electrical pulses. These are transmitted wirelessly to the electrodes, enabling the person to see patterns of light, contours, and shapes in their environment.

For patients who have been blinded by RP, using the Argus II is life-changing. So far, the device transmits only light, not clearly delineated images or color, but that might change.

"The product is software-based, and it's upgradable, just like your iPhone," says Dr. Robert Greenberg, founder and chairman of Second Sight, the company that makes the Argus II. "We believe that with the software changes, we'll be able to improve the resolution and the quality of the vision."

The Argus II system costs around $145,000, but because it is approved by the FDA, it might be covered by Medicare or some private insurers for patients with advanced RP. Second Sight (http://www.secondsight.com) can help locate a hospital to provide the device.

The company is now testing a similar device to improve vision among people with early stage (also called "dry") AMD. The initial study is being done in England.

Tiny Chip Lets Blind Woman Read

Scientific researchers are also reporting progress in developing new electronic microchips, implanted in the eyes of blind individuals, that can help them regain their site.

Surgeons at the Oxford Eye Hospital at Oxford's John Radcliffe Hospital have been in the vanguard of such efforts. In 2016, they reported implanting a tiny chip in the right eye of a blind British woman that has allowed her to read again—for the first time in more than five years.

The implant, which was developed as part of ongoing UK-funded research of the technology, was placed at the back of Rhian Lewis's retina. The forty-nine-year-old mother of two was diagnosed with RP when she was five years old. In a delicate operation, the wafer-thin retinal implant chip was inserted into the back of her eye to replace damaged photoreceptors.

The chip was developed by German engineering firm Retina Implant AG and captures the light entering the eye to stimulate the nerve cells of the inner retina to deliver signals to the brain through the optic nerve. The device is connected to a tiny computer placed under the skin behind the ear that looks like a hearing aid.

Lewis says the device has changed her life in countless positive ways. "It's simple things like shopping—clothes shopping—you don't know what you look like," she told *Medical Xpress*. "It's been maybe eight years that I've had any sort of idea of what my children look like. And I've got friends now where I've got no idea what they look like. And I certainly don't know how I've aged."

Foods and Nutrients That Preserve Vision

In addition to treating vision after it has been lost, scientific researchers have identified a range of prevention strategies—involving foods, nutrients, dietary supplements, and other natural remedies—that can preserve eyesight.

Many studies have found, for instance, that a healthy diet can lower the risk of developing cataracts, a clouding of the clear lens of the eye that focuses light on the retina. Cataracts are a common cause of blindness, especially in older people, and greatly increase the risk for developing AMD. Removing cataracts is the most common elective operation for adults, and by the age of eighty, more than half of Americans have cataracts or have had cataract surgery.

While sunlight is the major source of the lens damage that causes cataracts, there is growing evidence that poor overall nutrition and chronic inflammation in other parts of the body damage the eyes, according to neurosurgeon Dr. Russell Blaylock. "This explains why diabetics have such a high incidence of cataracts, and it also clarifies the strong link between cataracts and cardiovascular disease," he says.

The good news is that a handful of healthy foods are loaded with nutrients that can help prevent cataracts and keep your eyesight sharp. Among them are the following:

CARROTS. The old wives' tale is true: carrots are good for your eyes. One of the powerful nutrients in carrots is lutein, which is a major component of many yellow and orange fruits and vegetables. Lutein, along with another carotenoid called zeaxanthin, absorbs the harmful ultraviolet blue light found in sunlight.

BROCCOLI. This cruciferous vegetable is loaded with both lutein and zeaxanthin, powerful nutrients that lower inflammation and prevent free radicals from damaging sight. Broccoli also contains sulforaphane, an antioxidant that protects eyes from the sun's damaging rays.

Another compound found in broccoli called indole-3-carbitol (I3C) helps maintain a healthy retina in aging eyes and fights blindness. I3C activates the aryl hydrocarbon receptor (AhR) protein involved in clearing cells of environmental toxins. When researchers at Buck University boosted the potency of I3C ten times—creating 2,2-aminophenyl indole (2AI)—they found that it protected retinal cells from the damage caused by light that leads to AMD.

SALMON. This fish is rich in astaxanthin, a carotenoid that gives salmon and lobster their reddish color. It protects the eyes from free radical damage and retards the formation of cataracts, notes Dr. Joseph Mercola, author of the best-selling *The No-Grain Diet*. Salmon is also loaded with docosahexaenoic acid (DHA), an omega-3 fatty acid. One study found that women who ate fish three times a week reduced their risk of cataracts by 11 percent when compared to women who only ate fish once a month.

ORANGE JUICE. Orange juice contains liberal amounts of vitamin C, and studies have suggested that vitamin C can reduce the risk of cataracts. A study by scientists at Oregon Health & Science University found that nerve cells in the eye need vitamin C in order to function properly. A study published in the *Journal of Nutrition* found that high levels of vitamin C reduced the risk of cataracts by 64 percent.

GREEN TEA. Researchers from the University of Scranton found that tea, both black and green, reduced glucose levels in the eye lens of rats and cut their risk of cataracts in half. In addition, Chinese researchers found that catechins, powerful antioxidants found in green tea, protect eyes from glaucoma. The study, which was published in the American Chemical Society's *Journal of Agricultural and Food Chemistry*, found that the effects of a single cup of green tea last for up to twenty hours.

WALNUTS. Walnuts contain antioxidants and vitamin E, which fight inflammation. Walnuts also lower a specific protein called C-reactive protein (CRP), which is a measure of inflammation in the body. Walnuts also contain omega-3 fatty acids that are converted into sight-saving eicosapentaenoic acid (EPA) as well as DHA.

BILBERRIES. These fruits resemble and are closely related to blueberries and huckleberries. Bilberries, blueberries, and blackberries all contain anthocyanins, the chemicals that give the berries their dark-purple color. Anthocyanins fight inflammation and keep the arteries and vessels that feed the eyes from narrowing. A Russian study found that bilberry extract completely prevented cataracts in rats genetically modified to have a 70 percent risk of developing them. A dose of 160 mg daily is recommended.

EGGS. The yolks in eggs contain generous amounts of both leutein and zeanxanthin, both of which protect against the sun's harmful rays. They also contain the omega-3 fatty acid DHA.

AVOCADOS. Dense in nutrients, avocadoes contain lutein, beta-carotene, vitamin C, vitamin B6, and vitamin E—all great allies in preventing cataracts.

LOW-CARB FOODS. You can also lower your risk of cataracts by limiting your intake of carbohydrates. An Australian study published in *Investigative Ophthalmology & Visual Science* found that people who ate the most carbohydrates had three times the risk of cataracts than those who ate the fewest.

Dry Eye Epidemic: Remedies That Really Work

Dry eye syndrome has become something of an epidemic, often striking older Americans. It's an uncomfortable condition in which, for various reasons, the eyes don't produce enough tears, and millions of Americans are struggling to find ways to cope.

The good news is that depending on the cause of dry eyes, a number of solutions are available, and some are very simple. Treatment is usually based on how severe the problem is but can include lubricating drops, cyclosporine, antibiotics, massaging the corner of the eye, and omega-3 oil supplementation.

"We normally blink sixteen times per minute," explains ophthalmologist Dr. Jeffrey Oberman, who practices in Fairfield County, Connecticut. "When your blink rate decreases, the eye isn't remoistened, and there will be dryness associated with it. And you can't increase your blink rate. It is involuntary and automatic. Trying to alter that is impossible."

What Causes Dry Eyes?

Tears incessantly bathe and protect the surface of the eye. They are a response to bits of dust, infection, inflammation, or strong emotion. Without tears, your eyes might feel irritated, gritty, and dry. It might feel like you have something in your eye—a sensation that most of us have experienced.

Part of the reason the number of dry eye patients is growing is because we are all spending more time using computers, smartphones, tablets, and televisions. Dry eyes is also a result of aging, so between an aging population and the time spent staring at some sort of monitor, the problem is only growing.

Many people over age sixty-five have this issue. Here are other things that can trigger difficulties:

- Tear-deficient dry eye occurs when the lacrimal glands fail to produce enough fluid to make tears.
- Evaporative dry eye is a result of inflammation of the meibomian glands. Environmental factors, like global warming, can contribute to this.
- Medication side effects from antihistamines or antidepressants can also cause dry eye.
- Autoimmune diseases such as Sjogren's syndrome, lupus, and rheumatoid arthritis, as well as diabetes, can also be responsible.

Vision correcting surgery can also lead to dry eyes. During a procedure called LASIK surgery, Oberman explains, the corneal nerves are cut, which can affect tear production. "They are part of elaborate, sophisticated feedback signaling, and the loop is interrupted," he said. Once the nerves have a chance to regrow, the eyes return to normal, usually within a few weeks to a few months.

For diabetic patients, the nerve endings might be altered, and this interrupts the feedback loop as well. There is also a predisposition to blepharitis, which feels like dry eye. And with autoimmune disorders, the body's immune system attacks the glands that make tears and saliva, resulting in both dry eyes and dry mouth.

For most of us, a prompt response to dry eyes is best. Don't just wait to see if things improve. Some damage can be permanent, and anyway, dry eyes are uncomfortable. See your ophthalmologist and find out what you can do. An eye exam might include studying how often a person blinks, evaluating the eyelids and cornea, and measuring the quantity and quality of tears.

If you are experiencing dry eye syndrome, the following tips might help you cope:

Avoid dry environments. Increase the level of humidity in your home, if you can, and avoid spending long hours outdoors during dry, cold, winter months. Hot, dry, or windy weather can also exacerbate symptoms.

Cover up. Wear sunglasses outdoors to reduce exposure to sun and wind. Glasses that wrap around the side of your head can offer even more protection.

Use artificial tears. Such products are commonly sold over the counter.

Give your eyes a rest. Break up long periods of extended work in front of a monitor with a few minutes when you might close your eyes or move away from the computer.

HEADACHES

Nearly everyone experiences occasional headaches, but for forty-five million Americans, they are a chronic problem that requires more than an aspirin or good night's sleep to address. In fact, headaches are a leading cause of doctor visits in the United States. About twelve million Americans seek a doctor's care each year for headaches, and one in four suffers from recurrent severe tension headaches or more serious migraines.

Scores of prescription and over-the-counter (OTC) drugs are available to treat headaches, making painkillers among the most commonly used medications in the nation. According to the US Centers for Disease Control and Prevention (CDC), Americans spend $72.5 billion a year on painkillers, plus another $1 billion on brain scans that do little to ease their suffering.

But popping a pill doesn't always help and might even do more harm than good, depending on what type of headache you have. The good news is that many studies show that natural remedies and lifestyle changes involving diet, exercise, and relaxation techniques are often better than costly medical treatments for headaches. Here's a primer.

Tension Headaches

Tension headaches are the most common type of headache, affecting up to 78 percent of people. They can be set off by any number of triggers, including stress, too little sleep, missing meals, or by a tightening of your neck and scalp muscles while reading, sitting at a computer, or watching TV for long hours.

If half of your days are marred by tension headaches, they're considered to be a chronic problem. Even though they are painful, tension headaches are usually not a sign of a more serious problem. OTC painkillers, such as aspirin, acetaminophen (Tylenol), and ibuprofen (Advil) usually alleviate the pain, but they can carry health risks:

- Acetaminophen can cause liver damage when used in large amounts or over a long period of time.
- Aspirin and ibuprofen can cause stomach upset and bleeding.
- Recent studies have indicated that ibuprofen can raise your risk of heart problems.

Fortunately, you can control your tension with a wide variety of natural remedies. For instance, in 2015, a team of Boston-based researchers found that lifestyle changes involving diet, exercise, and relaxation techniques are better than costly medical treatments for headaches. But doctors are increasingly ordering expensive tests and therapies that don't offer clear benefits.

"Contrary to numerous guidelines, clinicians are increasingly ordering advanced imaging and referring to other physicians and less frequently offering lifestyle counseling to their patients," says lead researcher Dr. John Mafi of Beth Israel Deaconess Medical Center in Boston. "The management of headache represents an important opportunity to improve the value of US health care."

Mafi's research found that millions of Americans who see a doctor each year for headaches often end up paying too much for painkillers, brain scans, and other care that isn't any better than inexpensive lifestyle changes proven to ease pain. Much of that advance treatment is unnecessary, expensive, and even be harmful, he says.

For instance, contrast dyes used in some scans can provoke allergies or kidney problems. In addition, unnecessary exposure to radiation is believed to cause about four thousand cancer cases among the eighteen million Americans who receive head computed tomography (CT) scans each year, the researchers noted.

To reach his conclusions, Mafi examined rates of advanced imaging like CT scans and magnetic resonance imaging (MRI) tests in nearly ten thousand patients who sought treatment for headaches and referrals to specialists.

From 1999 to 2010, the number of diagnostic tests rose from 6.7 percent of all doctor visits to 13.9 percent, while referrals to other doctors increased from 6.9 to 13.2 percent.

Don't Just Take Two Aspirin and Call Your Doc in the Morning

Mafi says the increase isn't because people are suffering more headaches. He linked the trend to doctors being more likely to order more tests and referrals, the advent of more advanced diagnostic machines, and a growing number of patients who press for more than the traditional doctor's advice: "Take two aspirin and call me in the morning."

But whether you suffer from occasional tension headaches, a throbbing hangover, or even debilitating migraines, you don't always have to reach for the medicine cabinet or seek out a specialist or costly treat or treatment, Mafi notes.

A number of natural methods have been clinically proven to ease pain as effectively as OTC medicines and more costly treatments. These include getting enough sleep; eating small, frequent meals; applying cold compresses to the head; taking a hot shower; getting a massage; or engaging in some type of relaxation practice.

Dawn C. Buse, director of behavioral medicine at the Montefiore Headache Center, adds that scientific research shows a variety of stress-busting psychological and behavioral practices can ease headache pain.

"These approaches can be very helpful," notes Buse, an associate professor with the department of neurology at Albert Einstein College of Medicine of Yeshiva University. "Once they are learned, they can be practiced almost anytime and anywhere for the rest of one's life."

Here are eight of the most effective drug-free ways to stop headaches, based on the latest health research:

1. **Get a good night's sleep.** Headaches can indicate that you are not getting enough rest, which can fuel head pain. Most experts recommend getting between seven and nine hours each day. Even a fifteen-minute "power nap" when you feel a headache coming on can head it off, research shows.

2. **Eat a healthy diet.** Going long periods without eating can bring on a headache. Eat healthy foods throughout the day to stave off headache pain. Magnesium—in green leafy vegetables, olive oil, and tofu—might also ease pain by combatting inflammation. A Scottish study at the Rowett Research Institute in Aberdeen has also found that common Indian spices are rich sources of salicylate, a natural painkiller that is the active ingredient in aspirin. In fact, a single serving of certain hot curries contain much higher amounts of salicylates than an aspirin tablet.

3. **Avoid trigger foods.** Certain foods can trigger tension headaches in sensitive people. They include monosodium glutamate (MSG), chocolate, cheese, red wine, nitrates, and caffeine. If you suspect a food is the cause of your headaches, try an elimination diet.

4. **Drink more water.** The Mayo Clinic says that headaches can be caused by dehydration. While thirst is a good indicator that your body needs more water, experts recommend looking at the color of your urine instead. If it's clear, you're drinking enough; if it's yellow, you might be dehydrated. The

darker the shade of yellow, the more dehydrated you are. Aim to drink at least eight tall glasses of water each day—more if you're exercising.

5. **Ice your forehead.** Scientific studies have proven that putting a cold compress on your forehead can provide relief from throbbing pain, possibly by reducing inflammation and slowing blood flow.

6. **Take a hot shower.** Headaches from sinus pressure or congestion can be alleviated by taking a hot shower, which might increase blood flow. Research suggests that finding a warm, moist environment—such as a sauna or steam bath—might also reduce headache pain.

7. **Try a massage or acupressure.** Massages ease stress and tension, stopping or preventing headaches. The traditional Chinese practices of acupressure and acupuncture have also been shown to work for some headache sufferers.

8. **Relax.** Mental, physical, and emotional stresses can all contribute to headaches. Consequently, a great way to ease the pain is by engaging in relaxation techniques (such as yoga or meditation) or cognitive behavioral therapy (CBT) and biofeedback—two techniques that involve learning to monitor your pain and address it through relaxation and changing behaviors to relieve stress.

Pain-Killing Supplements

The latest headache research has found that a handful of nutritious foods, calming beverages, and nutritional supplements can alleviate pain.

TRY PEPPERMINT OIL. One randomized, placebo-controlled German study applied 10 percent peppermint oil (mixed with 90 percent ethanol) to the temples or forehead of volunteers who were suffering from stress headaches. They found that in fifteen minutes, peppermint oil relieved pain just as well as 1,000 mg of acetaminophen with no side effects. In addition, breathing in the soothing aroma of peppermint tea can ease symptoms, especially if your headache is caused by sinus pressure. A recent placebo-controlled study found that migraine headache patients who used oil of peppermint and menthol applied topically had less pain or were pain-free more often than those who were given a placebo.

TAKE FEVERFEW. This herbal remedy has been used for hundreds of years to treat headaches. A recent British placebo-controlled study published in *The Lancet* found that one capsule of powdered, freeze-dried feverfew daily eliminated the symptoms of migraine headaches in 24 percent of patients and reduced the symptoms in other patients. In another study, 70 percent of the patients taking feverfew reported that the herb reduced the number and intensity of their headaches. Experts believe feverfew increases blood flow by relaxing blood vessels. (Note: Don't take feverfew if you're allergic to ragweed.)

GIVE WILLOW BARK A SHOT. Extract of willow bark has been used for thousands of years to ease headaches. It contains salacin, a chemical used to develop aspirin. A study at the University of Maryland found that it reduces inflammation as well as relieves pain, and other studies have found that it is as effective as aspirin. Researchers in Germany have likewise found that it is as effective as acetaminophen in easing headache pain. Willow bark can be bought in capsules or as a tea.

TRY BUTTERBUR EXTRACT. A double-blind study published in the journal *Neurology* found that migraine patients who took 150 mg of butterbur daily reported a 48 percent drop in migraines, and those taking 100 mg of the herb experienced 26 percent fewer migraines than the placebo group. Another double-blind study found that patients who took 50 mg of butterbur twice daily had a 50 percent reduction in migraines over those taking placebo.

GO FOR GINKGO. Several French studies have found ginkgo to be effective in reducing both migraine and severe headaches. In one study, ginkgo reduced headaches in 80 percent of migraine sufferers, and the researchers concluded that ginkgo could be one of the most effective remedies for migraine.

GIVE ACUPRESSURE A TRY. This ancient Chinese remedy has been used for centuries to ease pain and promote healing. Try this technique: Locate the two indentations on either side at the base of your skull (about two inches from the middle) with your thumbs. Press your thumbs in and slightly upwards until you feel a comfortable pain and knead the areas in a tiny circular motion for one to two minutes.

GET ENOUGH MAGNESIUM. Studies have shown that people who have tension headaches tend to have lower levels of magnesium in the blood and brain than those who are headache-free, and supplementing with magnesium (up to 250 mg three times a day) has been shown to significantly reduce tension headaches. Magnesium can be found in almonds, bananas, and avocados.

ENJOY COFFEE, TEA, OR AN ENERGY DRINK. The effective component is caffeine, so be sure to drink caffeinated versions. Caffeine reduces the swelling of blood vessels, which helps relieve headaches. Caffeine's ability to reduce swelling is why it's included as an ingredient in some extrastrength painkillers.

Migraine Treatments That Really Work

Migraines are not simply bad headaches. For many of the thirty-six million Americans who get migraines, they can be debilitating—causing not just crushing pain but also nausea, vomiting, sensitivity to light, or even a frightening blurring of vision and flashes of what appear to be bright lights.

Each year, Americans spend some $17 billion on migraine medication, outpatient services, doctor visits, and diagnostic services. Treatment typically includes a class of drugs called triptans, but they are expensive and don't work for everyone. But health experts from the Montefiore Headache Center of New York say there is a better way to treat migraines without drugs. Dawn C. Buse, a psychologist and director of behavioral medicine at Montefiore, notes that three scientifically proven techniques are as effective as medication in treating and preventing chronic migraines: biofeedback, CBT, and relaxation training.

The key, Buse says, is for migraine sufferers to learn how to avoid what triggers his or her headaches, and that includes managing stress levels that can lead to attacks. "Someone with migraine has a sensitive nervous system that reacts to changes in the external environment or inside their body. Those can be changes in hormonal cycles; changes in the weather, actually; [or] changes in stress level," she explains. "So what we try to do is teach people how to really keep a calm and steady nervous system by keeping a healthy lifestyle. And there are three very well proven, scientifically studied approaches that are nonpharmacologic, so not medicine. They are biofeedback, cognitive behavioral therapy, and relaxation training."

1. **Biofeedback** is a mental discipline that involves learning how to control the body's functions. With biofeedback, patients are typically connected to electrical sensors that help them receive information (feedback) about their bodies (such as heart rate). That helps them focus on making changes in the body, such as relaxing their minds and their muscles.
2. **CBT** is a type of treatment that helps patients understand that their thoughts and feelings influence their moods, behaviors, and ultimately, their health. It is used to treat depression, anxiety, and addictions, as well as migraines. CBT therapists teach patients to identify and change thought patterns and behaviors that lead to stress, which can trigger migraines and other health problems.
3. **Relaxation training techniques**—including meditation, yoga, or just making time for silent reflection or listening to soft music every day—aim to ease stress, which is linked to everything from cancer and heart disease to chronic pain and migraines. As Buse explains, "When I say relaxation training, I don't mean just kicking back on the couch.

Meditation can get you there, doing a guided visual imagery can get you there, yoga can do this. But basically we spend a lot of our lives in the fight-flight-or-freeze response—the activated stress response—and that is the sympathetic branch of the nervous system, and when we're in that activated response, people who are prone to migraine—people who have migraine—that might trigger an attack."

Buse notes that stress is a key trigger for migraines, but the hormones and chemicals stress produces in the body can linger after a taxing event in one's life. "We actually found after someone's been in a stressful period for a while and then the stress is over, many people will have their attack as they start to relax," she says. "And what may be happening there is they've had these activated hormones and neurochemicals from the stress response for a period of time—that relaxes, and again their body goes through a change, and then they have their attack."

Dr. Brian Grosberg, a neurologist and director of Montefiore Headache Center, adds that migraines are caused by a brain disorder, which distinguishes them from the simple headaches that nearly everyone experiences. "Migraine isn't just a headache; [it] is a brain disorder where there are a number of events that occur that lead to a cascade of changes that occur in the brain," he says. "Headache is one of the symptoms of a syndrome of a brain condition."

A number of new treatments have become available in recent years, including painkilling drugs and Botox, which the US Food and Drug Administration (FDA) has approved for treating people who have migraines at least fifteen days a month, he explains. The FDA also recently approved a nerve-stimulating headband—the Cefaly device—to treat migraines.

But Grosberg adds that the best way to combat migraines is to identify what triggers them—including stress, alcohol, anxiety, certain odors, caffeine withdrawal, loud noises, bright lights, and changes in regular eating, sleeping, and drinking habits. A number of foods have also been linked to migraines, including chocolate, peanut butter, wine, and others containing MSG and nitrates.

Both he and Buse stress that effective treatments often require a patient-centered combination of medication, lifestyle changes (to avoid migraine triggers), and nonmedical approaches, including biofeedback, CBT, and relaxation training.

"No two people with migraine have the same exact type of migraine, and I think that's the important thing to end up understanding—that each [treatment] plan needs to be tailored to that individual," Grosberg says. "It's employing a multidisciplinary approach, [including] nonmedication [and] paying attention to lifestyle modifications, which are just as important as medication approaches."

Migraines: At a Glance
What Causes Migraines?

Migraines are not simply bad headaches. For many of the thirty-six million Americans who get them, they can be debilitating—causing not just crushing pain but also nausea, vomiting, light sensitivity, or even a frightening vision disturbance.

To use an analogy to car accidents, if a typical headache is like a fender-bender, a migraine is like being blindsided by a Mack truck. Medical science has yet to determine exactly what causes migraines, but they often run in families, suggesting a genetic component at work.

Experts believe that migraines are brain disorders, which distinguishes them from a typical headache. Several key triggers—many of them manageable through lifestyle changes—can bring them on:

Foods. A number of foods have been linked to migraines. Among the most common are chocolate, peanut butter, nuts, alcoholic beverages (especially wine), caffeinated drinks, cheese, processed meats, and other items that contain MSG, gluten, and nitrates.

Stress. Migraines are often triggered by stressful situations, possibly because they lead to changes in stress hormones (such as adrenaline and cortisol) and biochemicals that might cause them. Stress-related chemicals can linger in the body after a taxing event in one's life, leading to migraines later on.

Menstruation. For many women, menstrual cycles can trigger migraines. A likely culprit is fluctuations in estrogen. As women near menopause, changes in estrogen levels might also trigger migraines.

Environmental factors. Flickering lights, strong perfume, loud noises, changes in the weather, and other environmental factors are known to trigger migraines in some individuals. That can make something as simple as a sudden flash of headlights on a dark road, bright images and loud explosions on a movie screen in a theater, or even a visit to the beauty counter of a department store a potential hazard for migraine sufferers.

What to Do?

The best way to combat migraines is to identify what triggers them and then avoid those triggers. It's important to recognize that what triggers migraines in some people doesn't cause a problem in others and that not all treatment options work for everyone. What follows are some nonmedical migraine remedies:

Keep a food diary. Tracking what foods trigger migraines can help you determine what to avoid. In general, experts recommend migraine sufferers limit consumption of processed foods, sodium, sugar, and caffeinated and carbonated drinks. Skipping or missing meals can also be a common trigger of migraines.

Maintain healthy habits. Getting regular exercise, getting sufficient sleep (seven to eight hours a night), and eating a nutritious diet (heavy on fruits, vegetables, and whole grains) can all help stave off migraines, research shows.

Manage stress. It's impossible to avoid stress, but it's important to develop a way to manage it. One way is to practice some form of relaxation training—including meditation, yoga, or just making time for silent reflection or listening to soft music every day. Doing so can ease stress, which is linked not only to migraines but also to cancer and heart disease.

Use biofeedback. This mental discipline involves learning how to control the body's functions. With biofeedback, patients are typically connected to electrical sensors that help them receive information (feedback) about their bodies (such as heart rate). That helps them focus on making changes in the body, such as relaxing their minds and their muscles.

Try CBT. This is a type of treatment that helps patients understand that their thoughts and feelings influence their moods, behaviors, and ultimately, their health. It is used to treat depression, anxiety, and addictions, as well as migraines. CBT therapists teach patients to identify and change thought patterns and behaviors that lead to stress.

Consider drug treatment. When all else fails, migraine medication might be worth discussing with your doctor. Treatment typically includes a class of drugs called triptans, but a number of other new therapies have become available in recent years, including painkilling drugs, Botox, and a nerve-stimulating headband called the Cefaly device.

Try combining therapies. Experts say that the best way to combat migraines often requires a combination of personalized lifestyle changes to avoid migraine triggers and medical and nonmedical approaches.

When Is Headache a Sign of Bigger Problems?

A minor headache—or even a migraine—is a manageable condition for most people. But some head pain can be a sign of a more serious condition, including a stroke, tumor, or blood clot. Any head pain that is sudden or unusually severe or unusual requires urgent care. Here are other warning signs that should prompt immediate medical attention:

- headaches that first develop after age fifty or following a blow to the head
- a major change in the pattern of your pain
- discomfort that increases with coughing or movement
- pain that gets steadily worse
- a headache that is accompanied by changes in personality, confusion, fever, stiff neck, memory loss, visual disturbances, slurred speech, weakness, numbness, or seizures

HEART DISEASE

Every forty seconds.

That's how often someone *somewhere* in the United States dies from heart disease. All told, that adds up to nearly 610,000 American deaths every year, making cardiovascular problems the nation's number-one killer.

To combat the threat, Americans spend billions of dollars on heart medications, drugs that lower cholesterol and blood pressure, surgery, and other expensive procedures designed to diagnose and treat cardiovascular disease.

But the truth is that heart problems are often preventable through diet, exercise, stress-reduction strategies, and other lifestyle modifications. In addition a wide variety of natural remedies can manage or even reverse heart disease in those it afflicts without the risks that heart pills and medications sometimes carry.

Here's an overview of what the latest research shows on alternative ways to boost your cardiovascular health and lower cholesterol, blood pressure, and other factors that contribute to heart disease.

Lower Your Cholesterol Naturally

More Americans than ever are taking statins and other cholesterol-lowering medications, with the percentage of folks taking statins rising from 20 percent to nearly 33 percent in people aged forty and older since 2003, according to the US Centers for Disease Control and Prevention (CDC).

CDC officials also say that the use of cholesterol-lowering drugs called statins to lower the risk of heart attack, stroke, and premature death in those at risk increases with age. The following groups take such drugs:

- 17 percent of those aged forty to fifty-nine
- 48 percent of those seventy-five and older
- 71 percent of adults with heart disease and 54 percent of adults with high cholesterol

But statins don't work for everyone and can have serious downsides. The good news is that they aren't the only way to lower your cholesterol. For some people, losing weight, eating a healthy diet, and getting regular exercise can all cut cholesterol as effectively—or more so—than medications.

So how do you decide what is best for you and, if you're already taking a statin, whether you should you continue to do so? First, it's important to understand what cholesterol is and how it can increase your risk for cardiovascular disease.

What Is Cholesterol?
Cholesterol is the waxy fat found in all the body's cells. It is crucial to many body processes. It travels through the blood stream in tiny particles called lipoproteins. But too much of it can cause plaque deposits that can clog your arteries like a blocked pipe, reducing blood flow and leading to a stroke or heart attack.

There are several main types of cholesterol:

- Low-density lipoproteins (LDL) are sometimes called "bad" cholesterol. High levels of LDL cholesterol can build up in your arteries, causing heart disease or stroke, and can be controlled by statins.
- High-density lipoproteins (HDL) are smaller particles than LDL and are sometimes referred to as "good" cholesterol because they don't raise cardiovascular risks.
- Triglycerides are another type of blood fat that, at high concentrations in the blood, can increase the risk for heart disease.

Many people in their midforties to fifties have dangerous plaque deposits in their blood vessels caused by high LDL cholesterol, which can be controlled by statins. The American diet is high in fat and inflammatory foods that can cause plaque to build up. But it's essential to stabilize these vulnerable plaques to avoid heart attacks and strokes.

How Do Statins Combat Cholesterol?
Statins are anti-inflammatory and cholesterol-lowering drugs that can reduce the likelihood of heart attacks caused by plaque deposits.

Popular statins include Altoprev (lovastatin extended-release), Crestor (rosuvastatin), Lescol (fluvastatin), Lipitor (atorvastatin), Livalo (pitavastatin), Mevacor (locastatin), Pravachol (pravastatin), and Zocor (simvastatin). Advicor, Simcor, and Vytorin also combine statins with other drugs.

While they are effective at cutting cholesterol, statins do carry some risks of side effects. According to the US Food and Drug Administration (FDA), some medications can interact with statins and increase the risk of muscle damage. There is a possibility of raised blood sugar levels and the development of diabetes for people on statins. Memory loss, confusion, and forgetfulness have been reported by some statin users, and liver injury, though rare, can occur.

If you have symptoms of liver damage—unusual fatigue, loss of appetite, right upper abdominal discomfort, dark urine, or yellowing of the skin or whites of the eyes—then liver enzyme tests might be warranted. People have reported memory loss, some immediately after starting statins, and others after long-term use. The symptoms are reversed after discontinuing the medication, but it isn't advisable to stop on your own. This is a situation where you need to consult with your physician.

The risk of developing type 2 diabetes might be somewhat increased for statin users, although the cardiovascular risk of not taking statins might outweigh this. Discuss with your doctor whether regular testing for high blood sugar levels is appropriate.

Some drugs interact with statins and can increase the risk of a muscle disorder called myopathy. This might manifest as muscle pain or weakness. Be wary of taking Lovastatin along with particular drugs that are listed on the Lovastatin label and adhere to the maximum dose of this drug.

Because of these risks, some health experts believe that statins should be a last resort and not a first line of defense against high cholesterol. Experts also say it's possible to get off cholesterol medicine if you have been taking a statin and have been able bring your numbers down to a total cholesterol count of less than 150 or an LDL level of less than 70.

But in order to stay off medication, it's important to keep your numbers low through other lifestyle changes, including diet and healthy habits.

What Causes Cholesterol to Rise?
High cholesterol is largely driven by diet, stress, and genetics. Someone who is working to reduce cholesterol levels in his or her forties or fifties has likely been eating a high-fat diet for decades, and trying to reduce cholesterol levels without statins might not be wise. A completely plant-based diet (difficult for most of us to pull off) or statins are probably the best course to take—at least initially.

How do you decide what you should do?

- Be aware of the risks of taking statins, even though some of them are rare.
- Follow your doctor's advice first; it is hard to know who might have vulnerable plaques that pose a significant risk for a heart attack.
- Don't stop taking your statins without discussing it with your physician.
- Remember that statins can impact your liver (rarely) and have been linked to high blood sugar, resulting in diabetes.

But if you're looking for a way to lower cholesterol and boost your heart health without the potential negative side effects of statins or other drugs, there are natural alternatives. Among them are dietary nutrients, natural cholesterol-lowering compounds, supplements, and exercise.

Eating Your Way to Heart Health
Many foods can boost levels of "bad" LDL cholesterol (although not as much as scientists once believed, which is why such high-cholesterol foods as eggs, shrimp, and even avocados are now seen as healthy dietary staples).

At the same time, some foods contain compounds that have been shown to lower LDL cholesterol without the side effects some people experience with statins. Among the best studied are plant-derived compounds called phytosterols, which are similar in structure and function to human cholesterol.

Foods rich in phytosterols include unrefined vegetable oils, nuts, legumes, and whole grains such as corn, rye, and wheat. According to the prestigious Linus Pauling Institute at Oregon State University, such plant sterols were staples in early human diets, but that is no longer true today. That's why phytosterol supplements might be a good option for many Americans, experts say. They can be taken in combination with other heart-healthy vitamins such as niacin, thiamine, and coenzyme Q10 (CoQ10).

When plant sterols are consumed in sufficient amounts, they block the absorption of cholesterol in the small intestine. A 2012 study published in the *Journal of the American Medical Association* showed that plant sterols lower bad cholesterol by 14 percent—an amount that is similar to using a statin drug. Research suggests that two grams of plant sterols a day delivers a potent cholesterol-lowering effect.

Unfortunately, the typical American diet—which is high in sugary, high-carb, processed foods—is relatively low in phytosterols and doesn't come close to hitting that mark. The average American diet contains only about 10 percent of that amount, by some estimates. The food industry has created many products, such as margarines, that contain plant sterols. But these products also contain unwanted ingredients (artificial flavorings and chemicals), so a supplement might be the better option for many people.

Clinical trials have demonstrated that daily consumption of foods enriched with these compounds lower LDL cholesterol and also have other health benefits:

- A recent analysis cited by the Linus Pauling Institute that reviewed eighteen studies found that the consumption of phytosterols lowered LDL cholesterol concentrations by up to 14 percent.
- A second analysis, tracking the results of twenty-three controlled clinical trials, found that the consumption of sterol-rich plant foods decreased LDL cholesterol concentrations by about 11 percent.
- Several studies have also suggested that phytosterol supplementation at relatively low doses can improve urinary tract symptoms related to benign prostatic hyperplasia.

Phytosterols are just one class of dietary supplements that have been shown to reduce LDL cholesterol levels. Others include the following:

- Red yeast rice is a natural compound that lowers cholesterol as effectively as statins, studies show.
- Probiotics (two to four capsules a day) are natural "good" bacteria that maintain a healthy balance of beneficial gut bacteria and promote heart health.
- Garlic (one to two capsules daily) and vitamin C (2,000 IU daily) are proven cholesterol-lowering agents. Aged garlic can reduce the buildup of plaque in arteries by 80 percent in one year, according to researchers at the Los Angeles Biomedical Institute.
- Plaquex is a mix of phospholipids made from soybeans and developed in Europe that has been found to decrease LDL cholesterol, increase "good" HDL cholesterol, reduce angina, improve sexual potency, lower high blood pressure, improve kidney function, and reduce homocysteine levels associated with heart disease. It is delivered in one IV treatment that takes about one hour.
- Drinking cherry juice can lower blood pressure as much as prescription medications, according to a study from England's Northumbria University. Researchers believe that the heart-healthy benefit comes from the high amount of phenolic acid—a powerful antioxidant—found in the juice.

Diet Only One Factor in Cholesterol

Diet isn't the only factor that contributes to high cholesterol levels and heart disease risks. Three other big ones are stress, sleep deprivation, and inadequate exercise.

Phytoesterols and the following strategies can combat the impact of these hazards while also lowering cholesterol and boosting your heart health naturally:

INCREASE NUTRIENT LEVELS. Eating a healthy diet will provide most vitamins and nutrients but not necessarily all that your heart needs. That's where supplements—including phytosterols—can help. Many experts recommend taking a daily well-balanced multivitamin that contains magnesium (400 mg), vitamin D (2,000 mg), and vitamin K (250 mcg).

BOOST YOUR FIBER INTAKE. If you want to reverse existing heart disease, increasing the amount of fiber you eat is the most critical factor. Soluble fiber is found in beans, nuts, oats, vegetables, and fruits. Aim to eat 5 cups of fruits and vegetables daily, along with beans and nuts. Doing so can cut LDL cholesterol and raise levels of HDL cholesterol.

CHOOSE FISH. Eating fish is important because it is rich in omega-3 fatty acids that reduce dangerous blood fats known as triglycerides. Most experts recommend cold-water, small-mouth fish—like salmon, sole, and trout—at least three times a week because they are highest in "good fats" and less likely to be contaminated with mercury. High-quality fish oil capsules taken daily are fine if you can't eat enough fish.

REDUCE BODY FAT. Obesity is an obvious heart risk factor. Therefore, reversing body fat can reverse disease. Excess body fat not only raises cholesterol, blood pressure, and blood sugar levels, but fat calls produce inflammatory compounds that accelerate the formation of plaque in coronary arteries. Losing even 10 percent of your body weight can pay significant health dividends.

INCREASE YOUR FITNESS. Strenuous exercise is crucial to heart disease prevention. Most experts recommend getting at least thirty minutes of moderately intense exercise every day—enough to make you break a sweat and raise your heart rate. Engage in aerobic exercise, strength training, and stretching, with intensity and duration tailored to your personal fitness level.

GET SUFFICIENT SLEEP. Aim to sleep seven to nine hours each night, which helps restore your mind and body and significantly reduces the risk for heart disease. It's a good idea to go to bed and wake at the same time every day, make sure your bedroom is as dark as possible, and avoid watching TV and using your smart phone, tablet, or laptop close to bedtime, which can disrupt your natural wake-sleep cycle.

DESTRESS. Find a way to manage stress and anxiety though meditation, prayer, yoga, nature walks, or simply listening to soft music to calm your mind, which is also good for your heart.

Blood Pressure: How Low Should You Go?

Millions of Americans take medication to combat hypertension—a silent killer that raises your risk for stroke and heart attack. If you're one of the more than seventy million American adults with high blood pressure, you've probably wondered how low you need to go. New research suggests that it might not be as low as previously thought. This means you might be able to take a lower dose of your medication or you might not need to pop a pill at all.

Until recently, most experts believed that everyone should be treated when their blood pressure hit 140/90 and that people with diabetes or chronic kidney disease should be treated when their level hit 130/90. Now, however, an increasing number of experts believe that 150/90 or lower for most people age sixty or older is acceptable. For those with diabetes or chronic kidney disease, a maximum of 140/90 is recommended.

The new higher numbers have been recommended by a panel of experts appointed by the National Heart, Lung, and Blood Institute (NHLBI) and by a number of heart doctors. The experts say it's a good idea to push down blood pressure toward the optimal level of 120/80 to prevent heart attacks and strokes. But they argue that this often requires high doses of multiple drugs, which increases the risk of side effects such as a nagging cough, frequent urination, dizziness, falls, and erectile dysfunction (ED).

A major NHLBI study is under way that might settle the argument for good, with the results expected in 2017. "No one likes to take medications that they don't need to take," says Dr. Lawrence Fine of the NHLBI. "Individual physicians and patients need to understand there's uncertainty. Given that and given their own preferences and views, they need to make a [treatment] decision that they're comfortable with."

If you do have high blood pressure, it's critical to make lifestyle changes before considering medication. Proven strategies include the following:

- Going on the low-fat Dietary Approaches to Stop Hypertension (DASH) diet reduces systolic blood pressure by 8–14 mmHg.
- Getting regular aerobic exercise at least thirty minutes per day most days of the week reduces systolic blood pressure by 4–9 mmHg.
- Losing weight. For every eleven pounds lost, systolic blood pressure declines by 2.5–10 mmHg.

- Reducing salt to no more than 2,300 mg per day reduces systolic blood pressure by 2–8 mmHg.
- Using natural remedies, such as beet juice and fruits and vegetables high in potassium (bananas, potatoes), has been shown to lower blood pressure.

Natural Ways to Lower Your Blood Pressure

Millions of Americans take blood pressure medications, including drugs known as angiotensin-converting enzyme (ACE) inhibitors, angiotensin-receptor blockers (ARBs), beta-blockers, alpha-blockers, calcium-channel blockers, central agonists, and diuretics.

Often it's a trial-and-error process to find one that works without triggering side effects that might include fatigue, breathing problems, heart palpitations, constipation, insomnia, joint pain, and ED, to name a few. But hypertension can be controlled by simple changes in lifestyle, diet, and exercise habits and by a variety of natural remedies. The following represent some of the most beneficial approaches:

EXERCISE. Walking one hour a day will reduce blood pressure naturally. Other forms of exercise—swimming, cycling, gardening, and even housework—can also be beneficial for the heart.

LOSE WEIGHT. Losing 10 percent of your body weight can effectively combat hypertension and even eliminate the need for medications and drugs to lower cholesterol.

REDUCE STRESS. Stress causes the body to release unhealthy hormones, like adrenaline and cortisol, known to raise blood pressure. Yoga, meditation, listening to quiet music, prayer, and other stress-reducing activities can help.

EAT HEALTHY. A good place to start is the Mediterranean diet, which limits sugars, refined carbohydrates, and saturated fat while going heavy on fruits, veggies, whole grains, and heart-healthy fats that combat hypertension.

GET ENOUGH SLEEP. Chronic insomnia and lack of sleep not only contribute to hypertension but can make the condition drug resistant. Aim for seven to nine hours every night.

In addition to these healthy lifestyle approaches, a number of dietary supplements have been shown reduce blood pressure in studies of heart patients and other research. Among them are the following:

MAGNESIUM. This essential mineral builds strong bones but also lowers blood pressure and can control irregular heartbeats (300–500 mg daily).

HAWTHORN TEA. This herbal remedy helps the heart function more efficiently and contains a beneficial flavonoid called proanthocyanidin, which causes the blood vessels to relax.

BEET JUICE. Beets are loaded with inorganic nitrate, which converts to nitric oxide in the body, which relaxes and dilates blood vessels. Many studies have found that one serving of beet juice daily lowers blood pressure. In one recent study published in the journal *Hypertension*, the systolic pressure of subjects who drank about 1 cup of beet juice a day fell eight points.

POMEGRANATE JUICE. A Scottish study found that when patients with hypertension drank about 16 ounces of pomegranate juice daily for four weeks, 90 percent experienced a significant drop in blood pressure. (Note: Be sure to check with your doctor, since pomegranate juice can react with some medications.)

TART CHERRY JUICE. British researchers found that hypertension sufferers who drank just 2 ounces of this bright-red juice a day averaged a 7 percent drop in blood pressure in a placebo-controlled study. They believe that the phenolic acids in the cherries were key in improving vascular flexibility and function.

WALNUTS. Replacing snack food with walnuts helped knock three points off the resting blood pressure of participants in a study at Penn State University. In another trial, adults who ate ½ cup of walnuts daily for four months also saw their blood pressure drop. The benefits are likely due to walnuts being rich in omega-3 fatty acids and magnesium, two nutrients that bolster blood vessel health.

FLAXSEED. In a six-month, double-blind, placebo-controlled study, systolic blood pressure dropped ten points in people who ate ¼ cup of ground flaxseed every day. Diastolic pressure went down by seven points. "In summary," say the researchers, "flaxseed induced one of the most potent antihypertensive effects achieved by dietary intervention."

YOGURT. Good-quality yogurt has two proven hypertension busters: calcium and probiotics. A calcium deficiency can contribute to high blood pressure, and a serving of yogurt has about one-third of the recommended daily allowance. Recent research shows that lowering blood pressure is just one of many health benefits of optimizing gut flora with the probiotics found in fermented food like yogurt. Just be sure to get yogurt that is low in sugar and fat and contains "live and active cultures" of good gut bacteria.

DARK CHOCOLATE. A popular choice, no doubt, but the key is in eating just one square a day. And it should be a type of chocolate that contains more than 50 percent cocoa. Do that, say researchers at Harvard University, and you can lower your blood pressure. And it works best for folks who already have hypertension. Apparently, the flavonoids in the sweet stuff dilate blood vessels.

NATURAL NUTRIENTS. A number of foods and supplements contain nutrients that naturally lower blood pressure, including phthalides (phytochemicals found in celery), melatonin, quercetin (an antioxidant flavonol found in apples, berries, and onions), magnesium, vitamin B6, and folate.

SUPPLEMENTS. You can also augment your diet with supplements. Studies show that CoQ10, omega-3 fatty acids, vitamin D, magnesium, and the amino acid acetyl-L-carnitine can all help you keep your blood pressure under control.

Miami-based cardiologist Dr. Michael Ozner, author of the best-selling book *The Complete Mediterranean Diet*, suggests that people with high blood pressure try natural methods before taking medication. But he adds that some people can't hit their target goals through natural alternatives alone.

"First, we try lifestyle intervention—get some exercise, learn relaxation techniques, and eat right. Nutrition plays a major role. The Mediterranean diet has been proven to lower blood pressure," Ozner notes. "The bottom line is, if you've tried lifestyle interventions and your blood pressure is still consistently higher than 140/90, then you need to be on medication. Hypertension is a major cardiovascular risk factor, not only for heart attack, but especially for stroke."

Blood Pressure: At a Glance

Blood pressure—a measure of the health of your arteries—is one of the four "vital signs" doctors use to assess your overall level of health, along with heart rate, body temperature, and respiration rate.

Your heart rate (measured by your pulse) is the number of times per minute that your heart beats, while your blood pressure indicates the force exerted on your arteries when your heart beats. If the blood flow is too forceful, the tissues that make up the walls of arteries risk stretching beyond their healthy limit.

Blood pressure levels normally rise and fall throughout the day. Being stressed or sick can temporarily elevate your blood pressure, which is measured in millimeters of mercury (mm/Hg) in a two-number series. Here is what the numbers mean:

- **Systolic pressure.** The first, or top, number measures the pressure in your blood vessels when your heart contracts, or pumps out blood.
- **Diastolic pressure.** The second, or bottom, number measures the pressure in your blood vessels when your heart rests, or relaxes between beats.

If your measurement reads 120 systolic and 80 diastolic, this is in the normal range and would be recorded as "120 over 80," or "120/80."

Federal health guidelines recommend maintaining blood pressure levels below 140/90 for Americans less than sixty years old. For those aged sixty and older, blood pressures of 150/90 are considered fine by US health officials.

Unfortunately, the aging process itself makes it more difficult to maintain your blood pressure in the normal range. Millions of Americans take high blood pressure medicine, and many others are at risk of developing hypertension.

"Nearly one out of every three American adults has blood pressure numbers that, while not yet in the high blood pressure range, are higher than normal," the CDC notes.

Salt: Is It Putting Your Heart at Risk?

For decades, cardiologists have warned their patients to cut back on salt to combat hypertension. But a number of recent studies have questioned the science that federal officials and doctors have used to establish national guidelines on salt.

Even if cutting salt lowers blood pressure, the effects are so small they're not likely to have much impact on overall cardiovascular risks, many experts say.

Your best bet is to not buy into the notion that one-size-fits-all guidelines to cut your salt intake will lower your blood pressure. Instead, talk to your doctor about the range of factors that might increase your risk for high blood pressure—including genetics, tobacco use, weight, activity level, diet, sleep habits, and stress management.

That discussion can form the foundation of a personalized program to help you stay healthy and keep your blood pressure in check. But if that discussion leads to a plan for you to reduce the amount of salt in your diet, it might not be as easy as putting down the salt shaker. That's because hidden sodium is in most of the processed foods that are part of the American diet.

Five classes of processed foods often contain high levels of salt: bread, cold cuts, sandwiches, poultry, and canned foods like soups and vegetables. For instance,

- A slice of white bread has 230 mg of salt; a plain bagel about 500.
- Two slices of bologna contain 578 mg.
- One ounce of salted potato chips has 180 mg of sodium; baked potato chips, 200 mg.
- A 6-ounce portion of ready-made rotisserie chicken has 468 mg of salt.
- A can of chicken noodle soup can have as much as 940 mg of sodium.

"Americans consume way too much salt," says Dr. Mark Creager, president of the American Heart Association (AHA) and director of the Dartmouth-Hitchcock Heart and Vascular Center in New Hampshire. He notes that eating foods high in sodium can lead to high blood pressure (hypertension), increasing the risk of congestive heart disease, stroke, and kidney failure.

The federal government's 2015–20 Dietary Guidelines for Americans recommends that adults consume less than 2,300 mg of sodium daily. But people with high blood pressure, middle-aged or older adults, and African Americans should consume less than 1,500 mg of sodium each day because of increased risks they face, doctors say.

A CDC study of the dietary habits of fifteen thousand Americans concluded that 98 percent of men and 80 percent of women consume too much salt.

More than three-quarters of people at greater risk of developing heart disease or stroke—individuals with high blood pressure or prehypertension, persons age fifty-one and over, and African Americans—exceed 2,300 mg of sodium daily, the CDC said.

Adults with hypertension consume less sodium than other adults and might be trying to follow their doctor's advice to reduce sodium in their diet. But 86 percent of adults with high blood pressure still consume too much salt, the study said.

While Americans have long known the risks of eating too much salt, little has changed in sodium consumption over the last decade, the study stated. And because more than three-quarters of sodium in the American diet comes from processed and restaurant food, people have little choice in lowering their daily consumption of salt.

So how do you reduce the amount of salt in your diet?

Be a savvy shopper. Be careful what you buy at the supermarket. Read labels for sodium content. In preparing meals at home, reduce the amount of foods from the food groups that are high in sodium.

Limit processed foods. Get meat from the butcher, go for fresh fish, and load up on fresh vegetables and fruits.

Check that restaurant menu. When eating in a restaurant, tell the server that you want a meal that is low in salt. Even if the menu contains few low-sodium items, the waiter or waitress can also ask the chef to prepare regular fare without salt.

Spice it up. When making meals at home, use herbs and spices or lemon and other citrus fruits as substitutes for salt, experts advise. Cook your own pastas, grains, and rice instead of using prepared options.

Eat it raw. Add more salads and a variety of raw vegetables to your meals. Be sure to use vinegar and oil or prepare your own dressings. Just two tablespoons of Italian dressing can contain 430 mg of sodium.

Avoid salty snacks. Instead of potato or corn chips, try healthier snacking alternatives, such as banana chips (1 once contains just 2 mg of sodium) or rice crackers (½ ounce has no sodium). Raw unsalted nuts like almonds, hazelnuts, pecans, and pistachios are also a good choice. Macadamia nuts, pine nuts, and walnuts are also low in sodium (1 ounce has 1 mg of sodium). And air-popped popcorn has little salt (2½ cups has 2 mg of sodium).

Fish Oil: Natural Medicine for a Strong Heart

Fish oil pills are among the most popular nutritional supplements sold in the United States, for good reason. A substantial body of medical research links omega-3 fatty acids to cardiovascular health and other benefits.

Cold-water fish and fish oil are rich sources of omega-3 fatty acids—known as docosahexaenoic acid (DHA) and eicosapentaenoic acid (EPA). They are unsaturated fats that play very important roles in the function of our bodies.

DHA and EPA are converted into hormone-like substances called prostaglandins that regulate cell activity and healthy cardiovascular function. DHA is a building block of tissue in the brain and retina of the eye that helps with forming neural transmitters that are important to mental health.

Many health experts advise older people to take fish oil pills containing DHA and EPA because our bodies produce less of these substances as we age. In fact, studies have suggested that lower levels of these fatty acids might be linked to reduced cognitive function and even contribute to such mental illnesses as Alzheimer's disease and dementia.

DHA and EPA also act as sources of energy, prevent skin from drying, and cushion tissues and organs. Some research has suggested that DHA's well-known anti-inflammatory properties might help combat cancer, diabetes, and other ills tied to inflammation.

Perhaps the most compelling evidence of fish oil's benefits comes from studies of people who follow the Mediterranean diet, which is rich in omega-3 fatty acids, fish, fruit, vegetables, and healthy fats, such as olive oil.

A landmark published in the *New England Journal of Medicine* found that the Mediterranean diet cut the risk of cardiovascular problems such as heart attack by 30 percent—even in people at high risk for them.

Experts recommend taking 2,000 mg of fish oil supplements daily. Major brands manufactured in the United States or imported from Scandinavian countries are the most reliable. Two other nutrients, vitamin E and CoQ10, are known to boost heart health.

You can also get omega-3s straight from the source. Eating cold-water fish—like salmon, trout, and sardines—three times a week will supply you with the omega-3 fatty acids you need.

The latest research also shows that high doses of omega-3 fatty acids not only help prevent cardiovascular problems but might protect against further damage in patients who've already suffered a heart attack. About 735,000 Americans suffer a heart attack each year, according to the CDC.

In many ways, the new research is just catching up with what cardiologists and alternative medicine practitioners alike have known for a long time.

Magnesium: The Rodney Dangerfield of Nutrients

Magnesium is the Rodney Dangerfield of natural nutrients. It's been shown to combat heart disease as well as stroke, diabetes, and even depression. But chances are, you aren't getting enough of it and might not even know about it.

"It affects every organ, tissue, and cell in the body," says Dr. Carolyn Dean, author of *The Magnesium Miracle* and a Hawaii-based holistic medicine physician. "Magnesium deficiency is killing people, and it's a simple solution to many of our chronic diseases."

Federal studies show that the average American diet fails to meet the FDA's recommended daily allowance of magnesium—of 400–420 mg per day for men;

310–20 mg for women. One reason for this is that public health officials and the mainstream medical establishment aren't doing enough to raise awareness of magnesium's many benefits.

Magnesium is involved in more than three hundred metabolic reactions but is particularly beneficial for the heart. It is found in the body's muscles, bones, blood, and tissues. It's involved in regulating everything from blood pressure to heart activity, energy production, nervous system function, metabolism, cell growth, bone density, fat and protein synthesis, muscle strength, and metabolism.

Sources of dietary magnesium include supplements, fruits, green leafy vegetables such as spinach, whole grains, dairy products such as yogurt, fish, wheat germ, brown rice, beans, tofu, soybeans, and a variety of nuts.

Because magnesium is inexpensive and readily available, many health experts are calling it a medical marvel—even though most people have never heard about its many benefits and doctors are often unable to tell if their patients are at risk of magnesium deficiency.

Commercial agricultural processes have depleted the levels of the mineral in soil and in a variety of crops over the past sixty years. "A hundred years ago, we were getting 500 mg in our daily diet. Today we are lucky to get 200 mg, which is about half the very low RDA [recommended daily amount]," Dean says. "Most people think that their doctors would have warned them about this problem. But doctors are as ignorant as the public."

A US Department of Agriculture study, published in the *Journal of the American College of Nutrition*, found a decline in the overall levels of key nutrients—protein, calcium, phosphorus, iron, riboflavin, and ascorbic acid—in forty-three crops between 1950 and 1999. "Perhaps more worrisome would be declines in nutrients we could not study because they were not reported in 1950—magnesium, zinc, vitamin B6, vitamin E, and dietary fiber, not to mention phytochemicals," notes lead researcher Dr. Donald Davis, a biochemist at the University of Texas at Austin. In addition, current diagnostic tests don't provide an accurate indication of whether a patient has magnesium deficiency.

Symptoms include muscle cramps, twitching, heart palpitations, migraines, insomnia, angina, irregular heartbeat, asthma, anxiety, gastrointestinal problems, fatigue, poor concentration, depression, and numbness of hands or feet.

Numerous studies have found that adding magnesium to the diet can provide a variety of health benefits, according to the National Institutes of Health (NIH). Here are some of the areas in which magnesium is most beneficial:

Heart disease. Researchers have found that magnesium can help prevent cardiovascular disease. There is also evidence that low levels of the mineral raise the risk of abnormal heart rhythms and complications after a heart attack, as well as angina, sudden cardiac death, and congestive heart failure. Studies have found that magnesium supplements help in the recovery of heart attack patients.

Blood pressure. Smoking, lack of exercise, and a diet high in salt are all well-known contributing factors to hypertension. But studies show that magnesium deficiency can also lead to high blood pressure. Magnesium relaxes the muscles that control blood vessels, allowing blood to flow more freely and reducing blood pressure. In addition, it helps equalize the levels of potassium and sodium in the blood, which also lowers blood pressure. In a study published in 2012 in the *European Journal of Clinical Nutrition*, researchers from England reviewed twenty-two clinical trials involving 1,173 people and found that magnesium supplementation resulted in a significant reduction in blood pressure.

Stroke. A study of Finnish male smokers aged fifty to sixty-nine found that those who consumed the most magnesium had a 15 percent lower risk of ischemic stroke over a fourteen-year follow-up period.

Diabetes. Magnesium is essential for regulating insulin and the metabolism of carbohydrates. As a result, bolstering the body's magnesium might prevent diabetes, studies show. Researchers in China analyzed thirteen studies involving 536,318 people and found that those who consumed the highest amounts of magnesium had the lowest risk of diabetes.

Osteoporosis. Studies show that magnesium deficiency is a risk factor for postmenopausal osteoporosis. This is probably because magnesium deficiency alters calcium metabolism and the hormones that regulate it.

In addition, dozens of other studies have linked magnesium to a host of mental health benefits—in treating migraines, tension headaches, insomnia, depression, panic attacks, stress, and anxiety.

"Magnesium supplements support the production of serotonin in the brain and gut and assist in the proper functioning of the adrenal glands," Dean says. "Therefore, magnesium reduces the severity of such attacks and also helps in reducing the rate of recurrence."

Some research has also found that it can help prevent and treat preeclampsia, eclampsia, premenstrual syndrome (PMS), dysmenorrhea, kidney stones, fibromyalgia, blood clots, tooth decay, insomnia, and muscle and nerve problems.

Federal Magnesium Guidelines

Federal health officials recommend the following daily levels of magnesium:

- **Children 1–3 years old:** 80 mg/day
- **Children 4–8:** 130 mg/day
- **Children 9–13:** 240 mg/day
- **Teens 14–18:** 410 mg/day (boys); 360 mg/day (girls)
- **Adults 19–30:** 400 mg/day (men); 310 mg/day (women)
- **Adults 31+:** 420 mg/day (men); 320 mg/day (women)

Resveratrol Supplements Ranked: Which Are Best Bets?

Resveratrol, a natural antioxidant found in wine and grapes, has been widely hailed for its potential to boost heart health and longevity. But which resveratrol supplements are the best, most effective, and budget-friendly?

A new review published by ConsumerLab.com—a leading provider of consumer information and independent evaluations of products that affect health and nutrition—aims to answer those questions by ranking the best available supplements on the market.

The organization's Resveratrol Supplements Review rates nineteen products evaluated by the group. Among the findings are the following:

- All but one product contained the listed amount of resveratrol.
- Nearly all had consistently high quality.
- Supplement costs varied wildly, with some providing 100 mg of resveratrol for $0.10 or less and others fetching as much as $1.50 for that dosage.

Based on the organization's research findings, the review's authors identified three products as "Top Picks":

1. **ShopRite resveratrol** provides 100 mg of resveratrol per softgel for $0.10. Although this product was not the cheapest product overall, it ranked number one because it's an easy-to-take, single-ingredient product. "It is often best to stick with single-ingredient supplements so you can judge the effects and potential side effects of an ingredient," the authors stated.

2. **BulkSupplements.com resveratrol** is a loose-product powder that provides 100 mg of resveratrol for $0.09. Although this is also a single-ingredient product, the authors ranked it number two because it must be stored in a cool, dry, and dark place, and each dose must be carefully measured.

3. **Trunature Resveratrol Plus (Costco)** provides 100 mg of resveratrol for $0.06. It ranked number three because it also contains a modest amount of green tea extract (25 mg of epigallocatechin gallate [EGCG], about the same amount found in 1 cup of tea).

Other products on ConsumerLab's "approved" list included Country Life Resveratrol Plus, Doctor's Best Trans-Resveratrol 100, Dr. Whitaker Triveratrol Gold, Finest Nutrition Resveratrol (Walgreens), Life Extension Optimized Resveratrol, Longevinex, Pure Encapsulations Resveratrol VESIsorb, Puritan's Pride Resveratrol, Puritan's Pride Resveratrol 250 mg Plus Red Wine, Resvinatrol Complete, ResVitále Resveratrol, Solgar Resveratrol, Spring Valley Resveratrol (Walmart), Vitacost Trans-Resveratrol, Vitamin Shoppe Reservie Trans-Resveratrol, Vitamin World Youth Guard Resveratrol, and Vitamin World Youth Guard Resveratrol 250 mg Plus Red Wine.

ConsumerLab's researchers noted that resveratrol is a plant chemical found in red grape skins, grape seeds, purple grape juice, and red wine. Some researchers believe that high consumption of grape products might be partly responsible for the "French paradox"—the low rate of heart disease among the French, despite an extremely high intake of rich, fatty foods.

More than $40 million of resveratrol-containing supplements are purchased in the United States each year, according to *Nutrition Business Journal*. Although grape products are the most significant dietary source of resveratrol, most supplements contain resveratrol extracted from the Japanese knotweed plant.

Resveratrol supplements have been popular since 2006, when studies in animals showed "life-extending" and "endurance-enhancing" effects, among other potential benefits.

Although such dramatic effects have not been demonstrated in people, other potential uses are being explored relating to age-related macular degeneration (AMD), cardiovascular health, diabetes, and memory.

In releasing its findings, ConsumerLab called for more research into the health benefits of resveratrol. They also summarized recent clinical evidence for resveratrol as well as potential side effects and drug interactions.

Common OTC Drugs Raise Heart Risks

A wide range of medications, over-the-counter (OTC) drugs, and even herbal products can interact negatively with heart medications, according to a new AHA report. Among them are heartburn medications, painkillers, and allergy remedies.

"Since many of the drugs heart failure patients are taking are prescribed for conditions such as cancer, neurological conditions, or infections, it is crucial but difficult for health care providers to reconcile whether a medication is interacting with heart failure drugs or making heart failure worse," says Robert L. Page II, who coauthored the new AHA report published in the advocacy organization's journal, *Circulation*.

Page says the report underscores the need for patients to talk to their doctors about all prescription and OTC medications they're taking, as well as nutritional supplements and herbs. The AHA has compiled a comprehensive guide to prescription medications, OTC drugs, and complementary and alternative medicine products that can worsen heart failure. Among them are the following:

Painkillers. Nonsteroidal anti-inflammatory drugs (NSAIDs), including commonly used painkillers such as ibuprofen, can trigger or worsen heart failure by causing sodium and fluid retention and making diuretic medications less effective.

Heartburn medications. OTC medications that treat acid reflux often contain significant amounts of sodium, which can boost blood pressure, and are usually restricted in patients with heart failure and those on low-salt diets.

Cold and allergy remedies. Certain OTC medications that knock down allergy and cold symptoms (including antihistamines and decongestants) might cause increases in heart rate or blood pressure that could exacerbate some cardiac conditions. They might also contain sodium.

Supplements. Commonly used nutritional supplements and alternative medicines are generally safer than prescription medications, according the FDA's risk-assessment reports. But some can cause or worsen heart failure when taken with cardiovascular medications. Among them are products containing ephedra, St. John's Wort, ginseng, hawthorn, danshen, and green tea.

According to the AHA, such medications and remedies can cause problems by

- being toxic to heart muscle cells or changing how the heart muscle contracts,

- interacting with medications used to treat heart failure so that some of their benefits are lost, or
- containing more sodium than advised for patients with heart failure.

Heart failure is the leading cause of hospitalization for seniors, and the average heart failure patient takes an average of seven prescription medications per day, according to the AHA.

How Canine Companions Help Your Heart

Chalk up another reason dogs are man's—and woman's—best friend. New research shows that canine companionship has a number of heart-healthy benefits.

In fact, the health benefits of dog ownership, detailed in the latest edition of the Harvard Heart Letter, are tied to not only increased levels of exercise from daily walks but also lower levels of daily stress.

"Research shows that people who have a dog are far more likely to get the recommended 150 minutes of moderate physical activity each week," says Dr. Elizabeth Frates, assistant professor at Harvard Medical School and an editor of the new report entitled, "Get Healthy, Get a Dog."

The findings echo those of a second recent study, conducted by the AHA, that found that dog owners are more active physically, are more likely to stick to daily walking routines, and have greater heart-healthy "social support" than people without pets.

"Over the last decade or so, there have been periodic reports on the association between pet ownership and cardiovascular risk," notes Dr. Glenn N. Levine, a cardiologist with the Michael E. DeBakey Veterans Administration Medical Center in Houston, who led the new AHA study examining the influence of pets on heart health.

Most of those studies focused on dogs and heart disease, he explains. According to the study, "dog owners who walk their dogs are more likely to achieve the recommended level of physical activity than dog owners who do not walk their dogs."

According to the Humane Society of the United States, Americans own about 78.2 million dogs and 86.4 million cats. Nearly half of American households include dogs, which are the "ultimate exercise partners," according to the Harvard researchers. "Unlike a human walking buddy, a dog will never choose to grab a cup of coffee instead of going for a brisk walk, no matter how miserable the weather," they noted.

Among the findings of recent research on the benefits of dog ownership are the following:

- Having a dog encourages physical activity, particularly among seniors and others who traditionally get less exercise.
- Walking a dog can lessen the embarrassment some people might feel about their physical appearance and level of fitness.
- Pets can help you stick with a healthy new habit or behavior, such as taking a daily walk.
- A pet's companionship can enhance a person's sense of well-being and social connectedness by providing opportunities to meet and interact with other dog or cat owners. This is especially beneficial to older people or others who might feel socially isolated.
- Dog owners have lower blood pressure than nonowners. In fact, just petting a dog has been shown to reduce a person's blood pressure and heart rate.

Studies have also shown that people with dogs are less likely to experience dangerous spikes in blood pressure and heart rate when mentally stressed. Researchers attribute this to a reduction in levels of the stress hormone cortisol.

If you don't have a dog because your landlord or work schedule doesn't allow it, the Harvard researchers suggested offering to take a neighbor's dog out for a daily jog or volunteering for such services at a local animal shelter.

Chocolate: A Valentine for Your Heart

Good news for chocolate lovers: the cocoa-derived candy—once portrayed as a dietary villain—is now touted for its health benefits, especially those that are heart-related. But there are a few catches. First, you can't eat too much of it—moderation is key. And second, and you have to choose the right type of chocolate. Dark is better than milk chocolate.

The health benefits of chocolate are so significant that researchers have launched a new initiative—dubbed the Cocoa Supplement and Multivitamin Outcomes Study (COSMOS)—that aims to determine the effects of cocoa and multivitamin supplements on heart disease and cancer.

The research project is being spearheaded by the Brigham Children & Women's Hospital, the Fred Hutchinson Cancer Research Center, and the Women's Health Initiative, which is the influential group that transformed how hormone therapy is used to treat postmenopausal women.

The study will determine whether concentrated cocoa extract can reduce the risk of developing heart disease and stroke and whether commonly used multivitamins can reduce the risk of cancer, particularly in older women.

The idea that the cocoa bean has medicinal properties dates back centuries, particularly in Mexico and Spain, where it has long been used in healing practices. Chocolate, particularly the dark type, contains flavanols that have antioxidant-like properties that protect the body from the effects of aging. High concentrations of flavanols are found in cocoa, tea, wine, and certain types of fruits and vegetables.

Chocolate has also been found to boost nitric oxide levels in the blood, which can widen coronary arteries and increase blood flow. Although people have consumed chocolate as a healing agent since ancient times, modern food manufacturers have added sugar and dairy products to chocolate—turning it into a high-calorie, less-healthy confection.

Many studies tout the following health benefits of chocolate:

Combat heart disease. A recent study in the United Kingdom, published in *Heart*, found that middle aged and older adults who eat up to 3.5 ounces of chocolate a day (that's more than two standard Hershey bars) have lower rates of heart disease than those who spurn chocolate.

Lower cholesterol. Cacao—made by cold-pressing unroasted cocoa beans—contains plant sterols, which also occur naturally in small amounts of other cholesterol-lowering foods, such as certain grains, legumes, nuts, and seeds.

Lower blood pressure. More than twenty studies, analyzed by the *Cochrane Library*, found that chocolate reduced blood pressure by at least a few points, which they attributed to the flavanols.

Prevent stroke. Canadian scientists conducted a study involving nearly fifty thousand people and found that chocolate eaters were 22 percent less likely to suffer a stroke.

Prevent memory decline. A Harvard Medical School study found that participants who drank 2 cups of specially prepared cocoa a day did better on learning and memory tests.

Boost your sex drive. Maybe there's a reason chocolates are a gift of choice for Valentine's Day? In fact, eating chocolate can lead to higher levels of desire, arousal, and sexual satisfaction because it contains a compound called phenylethylamine (PEA), which releases the same mood-altering endorphins that occur during sex, according to an Italian study reported in the *Journal of Sexual Medicine*.

Why Sugar, Not Fat, Is Public Health Enemy No. 1

Big Sugar has been as hazardous to public health as Big Tobacco. That's the upshot of recent revelations that the sugar industry has funded scientific research since the mid-1960s, casting doubt on sugar's role in heart disease and claiming that fat was the biggest risk factor.

So say a growing number of health experts, citing new scientific research that shows that sugar consumption by the average American—about 20 teaspoons daily—is driving the nation's obesity crisis and high rates of cardiovascular disease, diabetes, and a host of mental health problems.

"This news definitively shows how the sugar industry [Big Sugar] is comparable to Big Tobacco in the singularity of its goal—keeping us addicted to their product, irrespective of the health consequences," says Dr. Susan Peirce Thompson, PhD, one of the nation's leading brain and cognitive scientists.

Thompson is CEO of Bright Line Eating Solutions, which specializes in sharing the psychology and neurology of sustainable weight loss and helping people achieve it. She says the misinformation spread by the sugar industry pushed federal health recommendations to limit fat intake for decades, despite the fact that "the real culprit in a myriad of health problems, including obesity, is sugar."

She adds that sugar changes brain chemistry in ways that are comparable to nicotine and addictive drugs, resulting in more cravings for sweets. "What is so dangerous about sugar is that it doesn't just impact us based on what we consume of it today; it rewires our brains to ensure that we will consume more of it tomorrow," says Thompson. "The intensity of the sugar our brains are processing on a daily basis is hijacking our dopamine reward system exactly the same way as drugs and is highly addictive."

Thompson is one of many health experts who believe most Americans need to cut back on sweets and desserts. It's also important to cut high-carb processed foods—many of which are labeled "nonfat" or "low-fat" but contain more sugar and carbs than full-fat foods to compensate.

In addition, consumers need to recognize that many products contain hidden sugar—including salad dressings, tomato sauce, protein bars, crackers, and baked goods. Americans consume nearly twice as much added sugar each day (88 grams) as the World Health Organization (WHO) recommends (52 grams)—no more than 10 percent of a person's diet.

Switching to diet sodas and sugar-free foods containing artificial sweeteners is not the answer, experts say. In fact, doing so might do more harm than good and actually increase weight gain, according to research by the University of Texas Health Science Center.

The latest revelations about the dangers of sugar emerged in late 2016, when the *Journal of the American Medical Association* published papers revealing that in 1965, the sugar industry paid scientists from Harvard University to downplay links between sugar and heart disease and focus instead on fat.

In an accompanying editorial, New York University professor of nutrition Marion Nestle noted that the Harvard research shaped health advice and polices targeting fat—not sugar—for decades to come. That, in turn, increased sugar levels in many packaged and processed food products. At the same time, federal dietary guidelines encouraged Americans eat lower-fat products that, in many cases, were higher in sugar and carbs.

Since 1965, the nation's collective waistline has been expanding, with nearly one-third of Americans now considered obese and another third overweight, according to the CDC. Obesity-related health care costs now top $150 billion year, by some estimates.

Thompson says research shows that sugar damages the brain and changes the way the body processes hormones like insulin and leptin, the chemical that tells us that we're full and need to move. "The sugar in our diet is elevating insulin levels far beyond [what] our bodies were intended to [handle]," she states, noting that high levels of insulin block the brain's ability to recognize leptin. "Research on overweight kids has shown that their average insulin levels rise 45 percent between grade school and high school, creating a surge in type 2 diabetes."

Over time, a steady diet of sugar also results in brain chemistry changes that actually lead to more sugar cravings. By contrast, fat is not addictive and doesn't change the brain in such negative ways. Fat is also filling and can make healthy foods more palatable. "If you put butter and salt on broccoli, people will eat just a bit more broccoli," Thompson points out.

The take-home message?

Americans need to limit sugar—as well as low-fat, high-carb processed foods—and eat more healthy fats (from nuts, fish, olive oil, dairy products, and even certain cuts of meat).

Thompson says there is another lesson here: health advice and information can come with strings attached, so it's important to consider the sources—and financial ties—of the experts providing it. "As I sit here, I can't help but wonder what would have happened if those [Harvard] scientists hadn't been bought off—could we have started this conversation fifty years ago?" she muses. "Could we have saved millions of people from a demoralizing food addiction they don't understand?

"We now know what we're doing when we put a cigarette in our mouth and light up. But too many of us still think that a pack-a-day cookie habit is harmless. It isn't. They knew it in 1965—and now we know it too."

Five Fatty Foods That Are Good for You

For decades, health experts have advised cutting back on dietary fat and choosing low-fat and fat-free foods—such as margarine over butter and skim milk over whole—to lose weight, combat heart disease, and boost overall health. Since the 1970s, nutritionists have suggested that the best way to avoid *being* fat was to simply avoid *eating* fat.

But it turns out that's not entirely true. In fact, the latest nutritional studies show that fat is not the great dietary evil we've been led to believe it is. What's more, new research indicates that not all fats are created equal; some are even good for us. And the real culprits in the nation's ever-expanding waistline are sugary, high-carb, processed foods—many of which carry reduced-fat labels.

Dr. Richard Stein, a cardiologist with New York University Langone Medical Center, explains that there are certain fats that we should avoid, of course—such as artery-clogging trans fats in baked goods and those in deep-fried foods. But it's also true that some fatty foods are essential to our health, such as the staples of the heart-healthy Mediterranean diet, including olive oil, nuts, and fish.

"Clearly, fats like in fish oil and in vegetable fats and nuts are fats that are not thought to promote atherosclerosis or heart disease; in fact, they are felt to be protective in some regard," says Stein.

He also notes that even the kind of saturated fat that's in dairy products like butter, poultry, and red meat isn't as big a problem as once believed in terms of cardiovascular risks. "Fats that are saturated fats—in animal fats [and] in whole milk—were traditionally thought to be a bad fat," he says. "[But] we're beginning to understand that area between good fats and bad fats is becoming very blurred, and small amounts of appropriate fats from milk [and] small amounts of appropriate fats from meat and from fowl are absolutely part of a heart-healthy diet."

Yet at the same time, many of the low-fat foods that have been pushed as healthy alternatives to fatty foods are being consumed in ever-larger amounts and contributing to the nation's obesity crisis, with nearly two out of three Americans now considered clinically obese or overweight, according to the CDC.

By taking fat out of our diets, "we've actually increased calories, and America has gotten very fat on a low-fat diet," Stein says. "And the incidence of heart disease has not gone down, and the precursors of heart disease, like diabetes and high blood pressure, have actually gone up."

Meanwhile, Americans are consuming more total calories—about five hundred more per day, on average—than two decades ago and getting too little exercise to burn off those extra calories. While the changing view of dietary fat might be confusing to many Americans, Stein suggests what we need to be doing is focusing more on the foods we should be eating and less on the foods we should avoid.

"I think now what is going to replace the good-fats-bad-fats concept [is] not what you *don't* eat but what you *do* eat. And what you should be eating is a lot of fruits and vegetables, a lot of nuts, [and] more whole grain than processed grain," he says. "Chewing a toasted piece of white bread will get more sugar into your bloodstream quicker than will actually [eating] a teaspoon of sugar."

Stein identifies five healthy fats that do not pose significant health risks for most people when consumed in moderation, and some are even essential to our health:

Fish. Polyunsaturated fats, or "good" omega-3 fatty acids—such those found in fatty fish like salmon and fish oil supplements—are healthy nutrients that have been shown in many studies to lower the risk of heart disease, boost brain function, ease arthritis symptoms, and help prevent dementia.

Nuts. Natural fatty acids in tree nuts have been shown to reduce the risk of coronary heart disease and the risk of developing type 2 diabetes. A recent Canadian study published in the journal *Nutrition, Metabolism & Cardiovascular Diseases* by researchers with the University of Toronto and St. Michael's Hospital found that incorporating about 2 ounces of tree nuts—almonds, Brazil nuts, cashews, hazelnuts, pecans, pine nuts, pistachios, macadamias, walnuts, and peanuts—into the diets of people with diabetes helped boost their heart health.

Dairy products. Moderate amounts of saturated fat in butter, milk, and cheese don't clog arteries and might even be beneficial in moderate amounts. Scientists once believed that saturated fat raised the level of dangerous cholesterol in the blood. But the latest research shows there are two different kinds of cholesterol particles: small and dense (the kind linked to heart disease) and large and fluffy (which don't pose a risk). Saturated fat in dairy foods and other animal products raise the level of larger particles that are not harmful, but refined carbohydrates boost the level of smaller, more dangerous cholesterol particles.

Vegetable oils. Olive oil and other vegetable-based fats—such as canola and palm oils—are loaded with alpha-linolenic acid, a type of omega-3 fatty acid also found in walnuts and avocados. Recent research by the University of Toronto found that switching to a diet low in simple sugars and high in healthy fatty oils can help people with type 2 diabetes control their blood sugar and lower their heart disease risks.

Beef, poultry, and pork. All animal fats were once demonized as unhealthy, but the latest research shows that, in moderate amounts, certain cuts of beef, poultry, and pork are healthy sources of high-quality protein and nutrients, despite their fat content. Like dairy products, they also contain types of fats that won't significantly raise your heart risks but will leave you feeling full longer than carbs (and less likely to chow down on unhealthy snacks). And if you think chicken or pork are always a healthier alternative to beef, consider this fact: almost half of the fat in beef is oleic acid, the same heart-healthy fat found in olive oil, and it also contains important nutrients such as iron, zinc, and B vitamins. And new research out of Penn State has found that, contrary to popular belief, eating lean beef daily can actually reduce heart disease risks by lowering blood pressure.

Dr. Joel Fuhrman, author of six *New York Times* best-selling books on health and nutrition, argues that a healthy diet is as important to heart health as exercise, if not more so. In fact, Fuhrman's latest book, *The End of Heart Disease: The Eat to Live Plan to Prevent and Reverse Heart Disease*, maintains that dietary changes could prevent more than 95 percent of heart-disease related deaths—"and that is a conservative estimate," he says. "People think that meds make them OK," he says. "But their risk continues to get worse. My contention is that if people had informed consent, and if they understood the risks of meds and surgery, millions would embrace diet change."

His new book is based on evidence from extensive studies that show that a diet rich in nutrients—which he calls a "nutritarian diet"—can decrease heart disease. Fuhrman's book is also supported by his recent groundbreaking study, published in *The Journal of Lifestyle Medicine*. "There is a preponderance of evidence supporting a nutritarian diet," he says.

His three-step plan involves these strategies:

1. Get rid of high-glycemic foods like white bread and ingredients like sugar and refined carbohydrates that boost blood sugar and increase the risk of diabetes, heart disease, and other chronic health conditions.

2. Eat a diet rich in natural foods like vegetables. "The full rainbow of veggies—the full spectrum—is full of phytochemicals that benefit the heart," he says.
3. Limit animal products, including meat, pork, fish, eggs, and chicken. "Americans eat twenty-one servings a week of animal products when three servings would be much better," he says. Significantly reducing the intake of animal products would reverse heart disease.

Food Is Medicine

Fuhrman argues that we should think of the food we eat as medicine. "Diet is not just preventive, but therapeutic," he explains. "After a short period of time—it doesn't take years—you will see benefits."

One major obstacle to eating a healthier diet is the fact that that sugar affects dopamine and brain chemistry, boosting cravings for unhealthy foods. "People want the ice cream and cake. It's possible for motivated people to make change, but you have to change your taste buds, which takes three to six months," Fuhrman notes.

Although some people won't adopt a nutritarian diet, he feels that it is the obligation of doctors to give them this information. Fuhrman—a board-certified family physician and research director of the Nutritional Research Foundation—recommends the following tips for adopting a nutritarian diet:

- Make one meal a day a salad.
- Change the types of fats you use. Make your own salad dressings, for instance, by blending nuts and seeds, roasted garlic, and balsamic vinegar.
- Make a big pot of vegetable bean soup and put it in five containers for the week ahead.
- Try healthy desserts like a cake made of pineapple, banana, carrots, and beets.

L-Arginine: Surprising Safeguard for Heart and Blood Vessel Safety

Everyone knows that Viagra was the first federally approved treatment for ED. But few people realize that Viagra (sildenafil) was originally tested as a treatment for cardiovascular problems—including angina pectoris, which is associated with coronary heart disease.

In fact, the first men enrolled in those early Viagra clinical studies did not want to give back their unfinished bottles of the little blue pills after the heart research was completed—for reasons that gave scientists their first clues about the *other* beneficial effects of the wonder drug.

But the truth is that the same mechanism that makes Viagra such a dynamo in treating ED also safeguards the heart and blood vessels. That culprit is nitric oxide (NO), a signaling molecule for the cardiovascular system. And you don't need Viagra—or other drugs—to benefit from it. In fact, the amino acid L-arginine regulates the production of NO in the body and is readily available in supplement form.

The 1998 Nobel Prize for Physiology or Medicine was awarded to three medical doctors—Robert F. Furchgott, Louis J. Ignarro, and Ferid Murad—who discovered the role of NO in heart health. That groundbreaking research provided a deep understanding of the nutrient's heart-healthy benefits and opened the door to many medical uses of L-arginine, including the following:

- heart protection
- blood pressure control
- memory-boosting effects
- sexual enhancement
- growth hormone release
- increased immune function

Dr. Valentin Fuster, former president of the AHA and head of cardiology at Mount Sinai Hospital in Manhattan, called the findings of Furchgott, Ignarro, and Murad "the most important [discovery] in the history of cardiovascular medicine."

NO: How It Works

NO is a gas that transmits important signals in our bodies by penetrating membranes and regulating the function of cells. In 1980, Furchgott, a New York pharmacologist, discovered that certain drugs had varying effects on blood vessels—sometimes causing them to contract and at other times causing them to dilate. He speculated that the integrity of the blood vessel's surface cells (the endothelium) was a factor and conducted experiments that showed blood vessel dilation occurs because of a then unknown signaling molecule, produced by the endothelial cells, that makes vascular smooth muscle cells dilate.

Independently, Murad found that NO relaxes smooth muscle cells and that the gas could regulate important cellular functions, including blood vessels. And several years later, Ignarro performed a series of experiments confirming the work of both Furchgott and Murad.

The idea that NO—an air pollutant, formed when nitrogen burns—could have beneficial effects on the human cardiovascular system was a surprise to many scientists but ultimately led to the Nobel Prize for the three doctors.

How Is NO Produced?

L-arginine is the only known way NO is produced in the body. As arginine circulates in the blood, it triggers a reaction in which an atom of the amino acid combines with an oxygen molecule to form NO and the amino acid L-citrulline.

Arginine supplements can boost this process, which not only protects the heart but also enhances the immune system, sexual function, and memory. Studies have shown the following effects:

- In the cardiovascular system, NO signals the nervous system to combat infections, regulates blood pressure, and controls blood flow to different organs and helps prevent clots.
- In the immune system, NO is produced in white blood cells to attack and destroy bacterial and viral pathogens.
- In the brain, where NO is formed in nerve cells, it activates neurons involved in many functions, including behavior and the digestive system.
- NO is also believed to be involved in long-term memory formation as well as our ability to identify different scents.

A recent analysis of eleven separate randomized, double-blind, placebo-controlled trials published in the *American Heart Journal* concluded that oral arginine supplementation influences both systolic and diastolic blood pressure, suggesting that arginine supports overall heart and immune system function.

Do You Have a Heart Attack Gene?

Many of us know someone who did all the right things to prevent coronary artery disease, the most common cause of cardiovascular death. He didn't smoke. He ate a healthy diet, got regular exercise, and maintained an ideal body weight. He also had optimal levels of cholesterol, blood pressure, and blood sugar. Yet he dropped dead of a heart attack or stroke, possibly at a tragically young age.

How could such a thing happen?

An increasing number of experts believe the culprit is something that few people ever check: their genes. "About 40 percent of coronary artery disease risk is actually based in the genes," says Dr. Bradley Bale, a nationally recognized cardiovascular specialist and coauthor of the book *Beat the Heart Attack Gene: The Revolutionary Plan to Prevent Heart Disease, Stroke, and Diabetes*.

According to Bale, more than half of Americans carry one or more gene defects that can dramatically increase their risk of a heart attack or stroke. Some variants can even increase the risk as much as heavy smoking.

All in the Family

It's long been known that coronary artery disease runs in families. If one or both of your parents had an unusually early heart attack or stroke (before age fifty for men and before age sixty for women), it doubles or even triples your risk of suffering the same fate.

Only in recent years, however, have researchers identified the inherited gene variants that increase the risk of coronary artery disease. Thanks to the decoding of the human genome, at least 174 gene variants have been associated with heart attacks, strokes, and other cardiovascular conditions.

Of these, the following are the four most powerful predictors of risk:

1. 9P21 (often called the "heart attack gene")
2. variants of the apolipoprotein E (Apo E) gene
3. defects of the K1F6 gene
4. mutations of the interleukin-1 (IL-1) genes

Because of rapidly advancing technology, the cost of testing has decreased from thousands of dollars to as little as $100 per gene. Such tests must be ordered by a doctor and might not be covered by insurance.

Knowing Your Risks

There are many advantages to knowing your genetic status. First is being aware of your true risk profile. According to the AHA, up to 70 percent of patients who undergo genetic testing might be reclassified as having a higher risk for a heart attack or stroke than their standard risk factors would suggest.

"As we understand more about the variants that are associated with coronary artery disease or cholesterol levels, we'll be able to build genetic prediction models that may distinguish people who should be treated earlier or treated more aggressively," says Dr. Donna Arnett, a former president of the AHA. "The potential value [of genetic testing] cannot be overstated. But we need more time to develop the evidence base."

In short, knowledge is power. If you learn that you carry one or more risky genetic variants, you can take steps to reduce your risk of a heart attack or stroke that go beyond the usual lifestyle recommendations—eating a better diet, ramping up your exercise program, and losing weight if necessary—and medical recommendations to take certain drugs. Genetic testing has advanced to a state where it can help your doctor practice the kind of personalized care that is promising to revolutionize twenty-first-century medicine.

If you have a doctor who is up to date on genetic research, he or she can recommend a diet and medical regimen that's optimized to fit your unique genetic profile. "Right now, the guidelines are driven by huge studies, which average populations. So people are being treated as if they're the average," explains Bale. "But everybody is unique. You can get much better results if you manage their issues based on their biological uniqueness, which is determined by their genes."

Fearsome Foursome Heart Genes

Here's what you need to know about the four most serious genetic threats to your cardiovascular health:

9P21. The 9P21 gene predicts cardiovascular events independently of established risk factors such as obesity, diabetes, and high blood pressure. It's also as dangerous to your health as cigarette smoking. About 25 percent of Caucasians and Asians carry two copies of the gene (one from each parent), which means that they are homozygous for 9P21. Compared to noncarriers of 9P21, those with two copies have a 102 percent increased risk for developing early heart disease or having a heart attack and a 74 percent increased risk for developing an abdominal aortic aneurysm, which is fatal in up to 90 percent of cases.

Among diabetics with poorly controlled blood sugar, those who test positive for 9P21 have a far greater risk of coronary artery disease and death compared to those who are noncarriers.

Apo E. The Apo E gene has three variants—E2, E3, and E4—and affects how you metabolize nutrients. If you're one of the 25 percent of Americans who have an Apo E 3/4 or 4/4 genotype, you have a high risk of developing coronary artery disease and should limit dietary fat to 20 percent or less of your daily calories. You also should avoid alcohol because it increases levels of LDL cholesterol while decreasing levels of HDL cholesterol.

But if you're one of the 64 percent of Americans who have an Apo E 2/4 or 3/3 genotype (intermediate risk), or 11 percent of Americans who have an Apo E

2/2 or 2/3 genotype (low risk), you might benefit from a 25 percent fat Mediterranean diet or even a 35 percent fat diet from healthy sources such oily fish and olive oil. You also can safely consume a moderate amount of alcohol because it decreases levels of LDL cholesterol while increasing levels of HDL cholesterol.

K1F6. The K1F6 gene makes a protein that transports nutrients within cells. If you're one of the 40 percent of Americans who carry a particular variant of this gene, you have a significantly increased risk of heart attack, stroke, and death compared to the 60 percent of people who don't.

Even more alarmingly, you might still have an increased risk of such adverse outcomes if you take atorvastatin (Lipitor) or pravastatin (Pravastatin). That's because the "bad" variant of K1F6 is associated with a 40 percent chance that these drugs won't provide any real cardiovascular protection even if they reduce your cholesterol to normal levels. If you have this variant, you might need a different statin, such as lovastatin (Mevacor).

IL-1. The IL-1 genotype regulates the immune system's inflammatory response. If you carry the IL-1 A or IL-1 B gene, you react to any assault on your body with increased inflammation, which is the most important driver of coronary artery disease.

Of the two, IL-1 B is the worst because it places you at the same risk of having a heart attack as being a lifetime cigarette smoker. IL-1 B also increases your risk of developing periodontal disease, an often-overlooked risk factor for coronary artery disease (CAD).

If you test positive for IL-1, it's a good idea to get screened for the several types of oral bacteria that can promote hardening of the arteries. If these bacteria are found in your mouth, you'll probably need to brush and floss twice a day, use an antibacterial mouthwash, and schedule more frequent dental exams.

Attention, Diabetics

If you have type 2 diabetes, you also should consider being tested for variants of the haptoglobin (HG) gene, which also increases your risk of cardiovascular disease as much as smoking. If you have the HG 2/2 genotype, you have a five-fold increased risk of heart attack and stroke. But recent research suggests that you can mitigate that risk by taking 400 IU of vitamin E daily, which improves the function of HDL cholesterol.

On the other hand, if you're a type 2 diabetic with the HG 1/2 genotype, vitamin E will actually *impair* HDL function. So this is one those cases where uninformed self-treatment with supplements can be hazardous, says Bale.

New Blood Test for Heart Disease Genes

Practically every day brings fresh evidence confirming the connection between genes and cardiovascular disease. In 2016, researchers developed what many cardiovascular experts are calling a "breakthrough" in the diagnosis of inherited heart conditions—a simple blood test that detects all known genes associated with cardiovascular disorders.

The TruSight Cardio Sequencing Kit, devised by researchers from the United Kingdom and Singapore, can identify all 174 genes linked to 17 inherited heart conditions. The advance, reported in the *Journal of Cardiovascular Translational Research*, will allow doctors to rapidly and accurately diagnose such inherited conditions as structural heart disease, aortic valve disease, long and short QT syndrome, Noonan syndrome, familial atrial fibrillation, and most cardiomyopathies.

Peter Weissberg, medical director of the United Kingdom's British Heart Foundation, which helped fund the group's research, calls the test a milestone in heart care. "As research advances and technology develops, we are identifying more and more genetic mutations that cause these conditions. In this rapidly evolving field of research, the aim is to achieve ever-greater diagnostic accuracy at ever-reducing cost," he says. "This research represents an important step along this path. It means that a single test may be able to identify the causative gene mutation in someone with an inherited heart condition, thereby allowing their relatives to be easily tested for the same gene."

Inherited heart conditions caused by gene mutations are common causes of cardiovascular disease. In the United States, about one hundred thousand people die from sudden cardiac arrest each year as a result of inherited heart conditions.

Genetic testing has enabled early diagnosis of inherited heart conditions and allowed patients to take steps to lower their risk of sudden death from such disorders. But existing genetic tests can only flag a small numbers of genes, which means that they often overlook gene mutations that could be keys for diagnosing an inherited heart condition.

By contrast, the new TruSight test—developed by Dr. James Ware of the National Heart and Lung Institute at the MRC Clinical Sciences Centre at Imperial College London and colleagues—analyzes the DNA in patients' blood samples to identify, with 100 percent accuracy, all genes tied to inherited heart conditions.

"Without a genetic test, we often have to keep the whole family under regular surveillance for many years, because some of these conditions may not develop until later in life. This is hugely costly for both the families and the health system," noted Ware. "By contrast, when a genetic test reveals the precise genetic abnormality causing the condition in one member of the family, it becomes simple to test other family members.

"Those who do not carry the faulty gene copy can be reassured and spared countless hospital visits. This new comprehensive test is increasing the number of families who benefit from genetic testing."

Other Heart Problems and How to Treat Them

In addition to CAD, which is the leading cause of heart-related deaths, a variety of other heart problems claim thousands of US lives every year.

Angina. Technically not a disease, angina is chest pain, discomfort, or pressure caused when your heart muscle doesn't get enough oxygen-rich blood. Symptoms can also be felt in the shoulders, arms, neck, jaw, and back and might even feel like indigestion in some cases.

Congestive heart failure (CHF). CHF occurs when your heart muscle doesn't pump blood as well as it should because of certain conditions, such as narrowed arteries (e.g., CAD) or high blood pressure. These gradually leave your heart too weak or stiff to fill and pump blood efficiently. Symptoms include shortness of breath upon exertion, ankle swelling, and circulatory problems.

Heart valve disease. Valve problems occur if one or more of them don't work well, because of either birth defects or issues that develop later in life. The heart has four valves: the tricuspid, pulmonary, mitral, and aortic valves. All have tissue flaps that open and close with each heartbeat. The flaps make sure blood flows in the right direction through your heart's four chambers. Heart valves can have three kinds of problems:

1. Regurgitation, or backflow, occurs if a valve doesn't close tightly and blood leaks back into the heart rather than flowing forward through the heart or into an artery. The most common cause of this is prolapse, usually of the mitral valve, when the flaps bulge back into an upper heart chamber during a heartbeat.
2. Stenosis occurs if the flaps of a valve thicken, stiffen, or fuse together, which can prevent it from fully opening. As a result, not enough blood flows through the valve.

3. Atresia occurs if a heart valve lacks an opening for blood to pass through.

Abnormal heart rhythms (arrhythmias). Cardiac arrhythmia occurs when electrical impulses in the heart don't work properly, which can cause feelings of heart racing, pain or a fluttering in the chest, fainting, or dizziness. As a result, the heart might beat too fast (tachycardia), too slowly (bradycardia), too early (premature contraction), or irregularly (fibrillation). Many heart arrhythmias are harmless, but if they are particularly abnormal or result from a weak or damaged heart, they can cause serious and even potentially fatal symptoms. Arrhythmias are different from heart palpitations (which are usually not dangerous), which make it feel like your heart has skipped a beat or that your pulse is racing, pounding, or fluttering.

If you experience any of these heart symptoms, you should consult a doctor. A variety of treatments, from medications to surgery, can address and correct serious problems. But you should also ask your doctor about natural remedies and lifestyle modifications that can boost your heart health.

Many scientific studies have shown that several key natural treatments can improve heart muscle efficiency and ease symptoms. Among them are the following:

- **Ribose.** This sugar-like nutrient produced by the body can improve energy production in the body and the heart muscle. It is typically used to improve athletic performance and the ability to exercise by boosting muscle energy. But published research has shown it can help combat abnormal heart rhythms, CAD, and improve symptoms of chronic fatigue syndrome (CFS) and fibromyalgia.
- **CoQ10.** This nutrient, sold as a dietary supplement, is particularly important for those taking cholesterol-lowering statins, which can cause CoQ10 deficiency, research shows. The nutrient is critical for energy production and heart health. Your cells use it to produce energy your body needs for cell growth and maintenance. It is also a potent antioxidant, which protects the body from damage caused by harmful molecules.
- **Magnesium.** This nutrient is involved in more than three hundred bodily functions and is crucial to nerve function, muscle contraction, blood coagulation, energy production, nutrient metabolism, and bone

and cell formation. Taken as supplement, it can increase heart muscle strength and combat abnormal heart rhythms, studies have found.

- **Acetyl-L-carnitine.** This amino acid (a building block for proteins) is naturally produced in the body and helps produce energy. It is important for heart and brain function, muscle movement, and many other body processes. It is used to treat a variety of mental disorders, including Alzheimer's disease, age-related memory loss, and late-life depression, as well as to boost circulation in the brain, treat cataracts, ease nerve pain due to diabetes, and improve symptoms of "male menopause" (low testosterone levels due to aging).

Chelation: Alternative Heart Treatment
Leaping into the Mainstream

Pioneers in cardiovascular medicine are few and far between. Some examples include Chicago surgeon Dr. Daniel Hale Williams, who performed the first open-heart operation; Dr. Michael DeBakey, a forerunner in bypass surgery; and Paul Winchell, who invented the artificial heart.

Now add to that list of medical visionaries Dr. Gervasio Lamas, a Harvard University–trained Miami doctor, whose research on a promising alternative therapy for heart disease is being hailed as a revolution in the treatment of the nation's number-one killer—an advance on par with the work of Williams, DeBakey, and Winchell.

Lamas, chief cardiologist with the Columbia University Division of Cardiology at Mount Sinai, is the nation's leading expert on chelation therapy, an alternative technique for heart patients that has long been dismissed by mainstream medical doctors. However, as a result of Lamas's research, the treatment has taken a giant step toward becoming a first-line cardiovascular therapy, thanks in part to a boost from the NIH.

The federal health agency's National Center for Complementary and Integrative Health (NCCIH) recently awarded a $37 million grant to the Mount Sinai Medical Center of Florida, the Duke Clinical Research Institute, and other leading medical institutions to conduct a comprehensive study of chelation as a standard treatment for cardiovascular disease.

The NIH grant, announced in September 2016, will allow Lamas and his colleagues to conduct a follow-up study of promising preliminary research suggesting that chelation therapy—combined with high-dose vitamins—might be as beneficial as the use of conventional medication and treatments (or more so) in preventing heart attacks.

The study, known as the "Trial to Assess Chelation Therapy 2" (TACT2), will involve 1,200 patients and will examine the use of intravenous chelation treatments in combination with oral vitamins in diabetic patients with a prior heart attack. The goal is to determine if chelation can prevent recurrent heart episodes, such as heart attacks, stroke, death, and others, by removing toxins from the blood.

"If TACT2 is positive, it will forever change the way we treat heart attack patients and view toxic metals in the environment," says Lamas, noting that chelation therapy cleanses the body of environmental pollutants that might be implicated in heart disease. "Therefore, with NIH support and in collaboration with the Duke Clinical Research Institute, Columbia University, New York University, Mount Sinai [NYC], and hundreds of physicians and nurses throughout the United States and Canada, we are moving forward with TACT2."

Early Findings Promising

The $37 million grant follows preliminary research Lamas spearheaded that showed the therapy provided a huge health boost to heart attack survivors. That study, published in the *American Heart Journal*, found that the combination treatment cut the death risk for some patients by half and is particularly beneficial to those with diabetes. If follow-up studies confirm the benefits, chelation would rival the benefits of statin drugs and other conventional treatments prescribed for tens of millions of Americans.

Lamas, once a skeptic himself about chelation's benefits, says the results came as a complete surprise to the researchers, who expected the study to prove the alternative therapy was a sham treatment. The NIH's support for new research could catapult the therapeutic approach into the mainstream, he adds.

"I think this a huge step forward," Lamas says. "When we started this research—in 2002, when we received our initial grant award, and in 2003, when we enrolled our first patient—we expected this would be a negative study that would be debunking chelation and this would prove it doesn't work. But in fact, we didn't find that . . . it was a complete turnaround from what we expected."

Lamas petitioned the FDA and NIH after his preliminary findings to support the new follow-up study and take chelation therapy to the next level. "It was such spectacular results—and it isn't just me that looked that his and said, 'Wow, this is dynamite.' But it is also hard-headed scientists at the NIH, my colleagues at Duke, and many other topic academic institutions that have looked that this and said, 'Wait a minute, this has such potential that we can't let this go,'" he notes.

Lamas's initial study involved 1,708 heart patients at 134 clinics in the United States and Canada, including such prestigious facilities as Johns Hopkins and the Mayo Clinic. All the patients were heart attack survivors—fifty and older, a third of them diabetics—who were taking heart medication.

The study participants were divided into four groups. The first received chelation injections (known as "infusions") plus high-dose oral multivitamins; the second was given chelation with a placebo (in place of vitamins); the third received placebo infusions (in place of chelation) with high-dose multivitamins; and the fourth were administered placebo infusions with oral placebo.

For seven years, the researchers tracked the participants to see which patients experienced a second heart attack, stroke, bypass surgery, other cardiovascular events, or died. The results showed that those who received chelation therapy plus vitamin supplements had a 26 percent lower risk of heart complications compared with those given placebos. In diabetic patients, the combination therapy was associated with a 49 percent lower risk of heart complications. Chelation (with or without vitamins) was also found to cut the risk of death among diabetics by 50 percent over the course of the study.

"There is nothing like this for diabetes care," Lamas explains. "There just isn't."

Getting the FDA on Board

In follow-up meetings with the FDA, Lamas presented his findings and pressed for a federal review of chelation therapy as an approved treatment for heart patients, alongside other conventional therapies such as the use of cholesterol-lowering statins, aspirin, and other heart drugs.

Chelation has long been approved by the FDA to rid the body of lead by using a synthetic amino acid (ethylenediaminetetraacetic acid) that binds to toxic metals and minerals in the bloodstream, allowing a patient to excrete them.

Some experts believe heavy metal contamination causes or contributes to heart disease and that chelation rids the body of deposits that can lead to atherosclerosis, which causes coronary arteries to narrow, leading to heart attacks. But it is not currently approved for other medical applications.

With the NIH's blessing and support, Lamas is now beginning the next leg of research (TACT2), which focuses on patients who received the greatest benefits from chelation—those with a prior heart attack and diabetes. The researchers also hope to delve more deeply into how chelation benefits heart patients.

He expects to enroll 1,200 patients in the United States and Canada over the next year, including more women and minorities than were included in the initial study. The patients will be treated and tracked for five years. "Unless we can show a consistent effect across the two TACT trials and establish a similar mechanism to deliver the treatment safely, it will be difficult for chelation to enter the mainstream of other cardiovascular therapies," Lamas says.

But he is convinced the therapy offers great promise to heart patients. Patients like Eduardo Angeles, who enrolled in Lamas's study after suffering a sudden heart attack and believes the treatment is keeping him healthy.

"Dr. Lamas said I benefited from the trial 100 percent, and I started feeling a change after joining the study. Now my risk of having a second [heart attack] is very low," says Angeles, sixty, who also has diabetes. "So I feel like it helped me, but in my mind, I was also doing something for somebody else. I feel like I have made a little contribution to science."

Changing Minds about Chelation

Lamas says he hopes such success stories from his continuing research will convince other cardiologists to embrace chelation, but he acknowledges the treatment still faces deep skepticism in conventional medical circles.

"Although not approved by the [FDA] for treating heart disease, chelation therapy has been used for nearly sixty years and has generally been believed by conventional medical practitioners and cardiologists to be without value, though TACT suggested otherwise," he notes. "A definitive answer on chelation therapy that will be embraced by the cardiology community will require this additional research."

Dr. Josephine P. Briggs, director of the NCCIH, notes that Lamas's research is targeting a particularly vulnerable group of Americans. "A subgroup analysis of the original trial results suggests major benefit in diabetics with cardiovascular disease," Briggs says. "The disease burden in this group of patients is devastating, so a replication of these findings is of some urgency."

Dr. Eugene Braunwald, a professor of medicine at Harvard Medical School, adds that the results of Lamas's first study "were both surprising and intriguing" and that there is a great need for new treatments for heart disease. "I am very pleased that TACT2 is building on these findings to determine if they can be replicated in diabetic patients who have experienced a [heart attack]—a particularly high-risk group of patients in need of effective therapy," he says.

Dr. David M. Nathan, director of the Diabetes Center at Massachusetts General Hospital and a professor of medicine at Harvard Medical School, explains that the nation is facing a growing epidemic of Americans with both heart disease and diabetes—one that requires urgent attention. "The excess heart disease that continues to accompany diabetes is a major public health problem with enormous human and economic costs," he says. "If the original findings in the TACT study are replicated in TACT2, we will have a new and powerful weapon to ameliorate heart disease in diabetes."

Lamas notes that scientific advances are often the result of research that challenges conventional thinking and earlier study findings. "When you do research and you get the findings that you expect, they are always less interesting than when you do research and you get findings you don't expect," he explains. "That's where you learn—that's where you have to be able to go to the next step, where you can really help patients."

He believes chelation could become a vital way for Americans to undo the cardiovascular damage many studies have linked to environmental pollutants and chemicals.

In addition, he hopes his research will encourage traditional doctors to spend more time exploring the potential benefits of other legitimate and promising alternative medical practices and less time dismissing them as junk science.

"I told many patients that chelation was junk, but once I took a closer look at what we found, I had to believe it [is beneficial]," he acknowledges. "I absolutely think that what one of the lessons of the chelation trial is that we have to look and see what the alternative medicine practitioners are doing. Now, some of the stuff that they do doesn't work, but there may be other gems that we as conventional scientists and doctors have not yet arrived at—they've leaped ahead—and so there may be other gems . . . out there in complementary and alternative medicine. I'd bet on it."

Q&A: Chelation Primer

Q: What is chelation therapy?

A: The word *chelation* comes from the Greek word "to claw." It was first used during World War I as an antidote against arsenic-based chemical weapons and to treat sailors suffering from lead poisoning from paints used on navy vessels. Now it is an FDA-approved method to treat lead and other toxic metal poisoning, and alternative doctors use it to treat heart disease, Parkinson's, Alzheimer's, cancer, vision problems, and autism.

Q: How does it work?

A: The therapy uses a synthetic amino acid (ethylenediaminetetraacetic acid), which binds to toxic metals and minerals in the bloodstream, allowing a patient to excrete them. Some experts believe heavy metal contamination causes or contributes to heart disease and that chelation rids the body of deposits that can lead to atherosclerosis, which causes coronary arteries to narrow, leading to heart attacks.

Q: How are heart patients treated?
A: For heart disease, chelation is done intravenously over a three-and-a-half hour session. Two or three infusions are administered weekly, and a course of therapy can include twenty to thirty sessions or more.

Q: How common is the procedure?
A: More than 110,000 Americans undergo the treatment each year, according to the National Center for Health Statistics. Its popularity has skyrocketed over the last decade, even though it is time-consuming and expensive—$5,000 is the average cost—and it is not covered by insurance.

Heart Disease: By the Numbers

Heart disease is the leading cause of death for American men and women. According to the CDC,

- About 610,000 people die of heart disease in the United States every year—that's one in every four deaths.
- While the disease is slightly more common in men, women are also far more likely to die from cardiovascular problems than any other disease. In fact, about five times as many women die from heart disease than breast cancer annually.
- Coronary heart disease is the most common type of heart disease, killing more 370,000 people annually.
- Every year, about 735,000 Americans suffer a heart attack. Of these, 525,000 are a first heart attack and 210,000 occur in those who have already had a heart attack.

HEPATITIS C

One of the biggest health threats facing baby boomers is something most know little to nothing about—namely, hepatitis C.

Three-quarters of all hepatitis C cases in the United States are among those born between 1945 and 1964, according to the US Centers for Disease Control and Prevention (CDC). What's more, 75 percent of those who have this disease don't know it because typically, there are no symptoms.

Although baby boomers are five times more likely to have been exposed to the hepatitis C virus, most fail to get tested. Yet hepatitis C is the leading cause of liver cancer and the primary reason patients eventually require a liver transplant.

"Hepatitis C is . . . actually the leading cause of all chronic liver disease in the United States," says Dr. Ilan S. Weisberg, director of hepatology at Lenox Hill Hospital in New York City. "We have a big important mission right now to try to identify all the patients with hepatitis C so we can prevent [cancer] and cure them."

Up to 30 percent of all people with hepatitis C will develop cirrhosis of the liver, which can take twenty to thirty years to develop. During that period, the infection is completely asymptomatic, but once cirrhosis takes hold, the odds that a patient will develop liver cancer increase.

A simple blood test can detect antibodies that indicate someone has been exposed to the virus, which can be spread through blood transfusions, IVs, tattoos, and sexual activity. The CDC and the US Preventive Services Task Force (USPSTF) recommend that all Americans born between 1945 and 1965 have the simple test, which is designed to detect and prevent illness before the virus wreaks havoc. The latest treatment takes about twelve weeks and has a cure rate of up to 95 percent.

Investigators at the University of Michigan have also recently developed an easy way to help primary-care physicians ensure that a hepatitis C virus (HCV) screening is part of the checkup routine by using electronic medical record alerts. These alerts, programmed to appear if a patient is within the at-risk age group, remind doctors to issue the test and provide educational materials about the virus.

Implemented in fall 2015 in primary-care clinics throughout the university health system, the strategy contributed to an eightfold boost in screening in the first six months alone. "A large part of the success was figuring out how to take the logistical work away, which involves more than looking at a patient's date of birth," says Dr. Monica Konerman, a hepatologist at the University of Michigan who treats patients facing the prospect of hepatitis damaging their liver.

Why Infection Risks Are High

According to the CDC, many boomers were probably infected during the 1970s and 1980s, before screening tests for donated blood and organs became available in 1992. The screening checks for the HCV antibody. If detected, a confirmation test for the virus's RNA (genetic material) is recommended to confirm chronic infection, and antiviral medication can eliminate it.

"The availability of direct-acting antiviral agents has been a game changer," says Konerman. "Previously, many providers thought screening had low utility—[that] the treatment was terrible and didn't work well. Today, short courses of all oral treatments are highly effective and can prevent progressive liver disease."

New Drugs Are Costly Game Changers

The makers of two high-priced hepatitis C drugs are embroiled in a price war for the revolutionary treatments.

Gilead Sciences Inc. set off a heated debate about drug costs after it priced its new drug Sovaldi at $84,000 per treatment, or $1,000 per pill. That drug has since been followed by a combination pill that is more expensive: Harvoni, which can cure a majority of patients who take it, has a retail price of $94,500. But Gilead is now facing competition from AbbVie Inc.'s new Viekira Pak, which is priced about $10,000 lower at $83,319.

Top Natural Supplements for Treatment

Since ancient times, natural supplements have been used for hepatitis C treatment. However, you should be aware that anything you eat or drink or apply on your skin goes through your liver. As a result, you need to be sure that any supplement you take is completely safe and check with your physician before using natural supplements for hepatitis.

That said, a number of herbal supplements have been found to be beneficial to the liver:

MILK THISTLE. This herb contains a chemical called silymarin, which is known for its medicinal properties. It has been used as a natural supplement in the treatment of jaundice and some liver diseases. It helps prevent oxidation damage to liver cells and promotes growth while also reducing inflammation and pain.

LICORICE. This supplement contains a chemical, glycyrrhizin, that has some beneficial effects in the treatment of hepatitis C—namely, it has been shown to prevent the occurrence of liver cancer in chronic hepatitis C patients.

OTHER NATURAL SUPPLEMENTS. Thymus extract, ginseng, schisandra, and sophora roots are also used in hepatitis C treatment. But laboratory studies have not proven the health benefits of these supplements.

You should also be aware that research suggests natural supplements that should be avoided are kava, vitamin A, beta-carotene, and iron, since they can get deposited in the liver and cause complications.

High doses of essential fatty acids can cause fatty liver and should be avoided. Some of these natural supplements contain contaminants like arsenic, cadmium, mercury, thallium, and lead. These are all toxic substances that can cause harm to the body.

Pregnant or nursing women, liver cirrhosis patients, patients with serious comorbidities, infants, and organ transplant recipients should stay away from natural or dietary supplements for hepatitis C treatment unless advised otherwise by a qualified physician. Some supplements have bleeding risk, and some do not go well with anesthesia.

The dosage of the natural supplements in the treatment of hepatitis C is important. High doses might cause side effects like nausea, vomiting, headache, and fever and can worsen the liver condition.

IMMUNE SYSTEM DISORDERS

Modern conventional medicine tends to focus on therapies that treat diseases after they develop—through drugs, surgery, and radiation. As a result, the US health care system could be more accurately described as a *sick* care or *disease* care system.

Alternative medicine practitioners, on the other hand, aim to prevent diseases from developing or keep them in check by boosting the body's own natural defenses. Increasingly, even conventional medicine is embracing the idea of harnessing the power of the body's natural defenses to fight cancer and other diseases through the emerging field of immunotherapy.

But what both sides of the conventional-alternative medicine divide agree on is that the immune system is our greatest ally when it comes to combatting disease and living a long and healthy life. Yet many of us don't take even the simple steps that researchers have found can keep the immune system in tip-top shape—that is, until something goes wrong. And then, in many cases, it's too late.

Here's a primer on what you can do to boost your own immune defense.

Ounce of Prevention versus Pound of Cure

Think of your immune system as your own personal biological army—a well-trained corps of defenders that guard against foreign invaders to keep you safe. When the army's soldiers are well-nourished and in good shape, they can generally prevent illness or at least minimize its effect.

Your immune system constantly seeks out and destroys foreign invaders like influenza, staphylococcus, and salmonella. It also guards against defective and damaged cells that give rise to chronic disease. But when it doesn't get the nutrients it needs or becomes otherwise compromised, it loses its ability to combat ailments. That opens the door for invading bacteria, viruses, and other pathogens. A weakened immune system also allows aberrant cells to wreak havoc on your body like little homegrown terrorists.

Sometimes stressed immune system soldiers go haywire and overreact, attacking healthy tissue and organs. "They fight things that aren't really a threat," says Dr. Elson Haas, a family physician and author of the book *Ultimate Immunity*. "It's like worrying too much about something that will never happen. When you get a hyperactive immune system, it causes autoimmune diseases and allergy problems."

An overwhelming number of studies have found that taking steps to boost your immune system—through diet, exercise, supplements, and adopting healthy lifestyle habits—can stave off everything from the common cold to chronic diseases like heart disease, diabetes, and cancer. A healthy immune system can also improve the functioning of your brain and digestive organs.

The immune system is made up of special cells, proteins, tissues, and organs that defend us against germs and microorganisms every day. The special cells, called lymphocytes and leukocytes, are like tiny soldiers and are located in various parts of the body—including the lymphatic system, which includes the lymph nodes, the bone marrow, the thymus, and the spleen.

In recent years, scientists have learned that a large portion of our body's immunity—upward of 80 percent—is actually located in the gut. This makes sense because the gastrointestinal (GI) tract is the entry point for most invading organisms and toxins that come from the foods we eat.

But what is only now becoming clear to medical scientists are the vital connections among the immune system, healthy gut bacteria, and the brain. In a recent scientific discovery, researchers found that a previously unknown set of blood vessels directly link the immune system to the brain, influencing everything from body weight to various disease risks. They called this the "missing link" in determining how immunity might play a key role in protecting us from such neurological diseases as autism, multiple sclerosis, and even Alzheimer's disease.

Some of the most significant and effective cancer treatments have come from the emerging knowledge of the immune system as well. This latest understanding of the link between immunity and cancer has given birth to the exciting new field of cutting-edge cancer therapy known as immunotherapy.

Unlike surgery, radiation, and chemotherapy—which aim to cut out, burn away, or poison tumors—immunotherapy causes few side effects and increases (rather than suppresses) the body's own natural defenses against cancer.

Maintaining a well-functioning immune system has become increasingly import-ant because Americans are living longer than ever before, and our natural defense mechanisms tend to decline dramatically with age.

Expanding Lifespan Increases Immune System Risks

Centuries ago, when the human lifespan was less than forty years, a declining immune system was not a problem. But now, people are outliving their immune system's nat-ural lifespan, sometimes by forty or even fifty years.

Fortunately, there are a number of natural ways to bolster your immune system, including exercising regularly (at least 150 minutes a week) and eating a healthy diet rich in nutrient-dense fruits, vegetables, lean protein, and whole grains.

In fact, to a large degree, your immune soldiers are only as good as your diet, says Dr. Joel Fuhrman, a family physician and author of the book *Super Immunity*. "They are our defenders, and we rely on them to keep us healthy," he says. "But the conventional American diet weakens these defenders, and that's led to an explosion of cancer, autoimmune diseases, and other problems . . . asthma, allergies, autism, lupus . . . you name it."

Fuhrman, who also hosts the PBS program *Eat to Live*, has developed an eating plan he call his "G-BOMBS diet," which emphasizes the following nutrient-rich foods to boost your immunity.

GREENS. Leafy greens and cruciferous vegetables have a wide array of nutrients to support the immune army with vitamins, minerals, and antioxidants. Among other benefits, they stimulate the production of isothiocyanates (ITCs), which have proven anticancer powers.

BEANS. The most nutrient-dense carbohydrate, beans and other legumes contain a lot of fiber and resistant starch, slowing digestion and optimizing nutrient absorption. They are also fermented by gut flora, creating fatty acids that feed the immune system.

ONIONS. The allium family of vegetables, which includes onions, leeks, garlic, chives, shallots, and scallions, has immune-boosting organosulfur compounds and flavonoid antioxidants. To reap the full nutritional benefits, eat them raw.

MUSHROOMS. These edible fungi have been used therapeutically for centuries. Their beta-glucans help modulate the immune system. Shiitake, reishi, and maitake are known to be particularly effective, but even the common button mushroom has a host of beneficial compounds. Unlike most other produce, cooking helps unleash their full potential.

BERRIES. The vibrant colors of these sweet treats means that they are loaded with antioxidants, including flavonoids and vitamins, and that is great fuel for the soldiers of the immune army.

SEEDS. Flax, chia, hemp, sunflower, sesame, and their nutty cousins—almonds, pecans, pistachios, and so on—are rich in a broad spectrum of micronutrients, including healthy fats, minerals, and antioxidants. As a bonus, their fats help the body process nutrients from vegetables.

OTHERS. Other immune-boosting foods include oysters, green tea, citrus fruit, watermelon, wheat germ, sweet potato, and the spices turmeric, cinnamon, and clove.

In addition to adding foods to your diet that boost your immune system, it's important to know that some foods can lower your defenses or cause negative reactions. Among them are processed, high-glycemic foods loaded with sugar and simple carbs.

Food allergies and sensitivities can wreak havoc on your immune system and make you sick. The list of common causes of food allergies typically includes gluten, dairy, soy, eggs, corn, pork, beef, chicken, lentils, coffee, citrus fruits, and nuts. The best way to tell if you're having problems with a particular food group is to try a so-called elimination diet, which involves not eating several foods or food groups for a few weeks and then reintroducing them into your diet one at a time to gauge the effects.

Healthy Gut Bacteria: Keys to Healthy Defenses

Because the digestive tract is your immune system's central command, it's important to maintain a healthy balance of good versus bad bacteria through diet and lifestyle modifications. Research shows that five hundred or so species of beneficial bacteria live in the gut, where they help process food, produce immune molecules, and battle bad bacteria.

"There is a conversation between our immune system and our resident bacteria," says pathologist June Round, senior author of a University of Utah study about the relationship between the immune system and gut flora. "The microbes can send signals that tell our immune system how to develop, and in turn, our immune system can shape what types of microbes live on our body."

While a G-BOMBS diet fosters the growth of beneficial bacteria, the usual suspects—sugars, simple carbs, and processed foods—feed harmful bacteria. And when things like toxins, antibiotics, and stress wipe out good bacteria, the bad guys rush in. Illness typically follows, often in the form of irritable bowel syndrome (IBS).

The best defense is a good offense. That includes a healthy diet, which you can reinforce by eating fermented food like yogurt, kimchi, tempeh, sauerkraut, natto, and kefir or taking probiotic supplements that contain live active cultures.

Don't Neglect Your Sleep

Getting a good night's sleep is also critical to a healthy, functioning immune system. In fact, a recent survey of health experts found that many believe the single best way to strengthen the immune system is to get plenty of sleep.

Among those experts is Michael Asaly, founder of Practical Sleep Solutions in Irvine, California. "Sleep is one of the most important things we do in our lives, and not just any sleep—quality sleep," Asaly says. "Sleep refreshes everything to keep us alive and vibrant."

A lack of shut-eye has the opposite effect. Sleep deprivation stimulates proinflammatory cytokines, an immune overreaction. The same holds true if you disrupt the sleep-wake circadian rhythm. That's one reason it's common for travelers who cross time zones to catch viruses.

Salas notes that poor sleep is linked to many chronic diseases, including diabetes, heart disease, obesity, and even dementia. A recent British study, for instance, tied lack of sleep to diabetes and heart disease and a 12 percent increase in death. People who sleep less than six hours nightly—and that's more than one in three Americans between forty and ninety years of age—are more likely to die prematurely than people who sleep for six to eight hours.

Dr. Craig Title, an obesity expert from New York City, notes that sleep deprivation disrupts the balance between the crucial hormones leptin and ghrelin, which regulate the appetite. "When you are sleep deprived, there is an increase in ghrelin, a hormone that signals the brain you are hungry, and a decrease in leptin, [which] tells your brain you are full," he explains. "Therefore, you tend to eat more. So what we see is more fat storage and decreased insulin sensitivity, which can lead to obesity, diabetes, and heart disease."

Lack of sleep also triggers your body's stress response, says Title, which leads to increased cortisol levels that also cause fat storage and organ damage.

Dr. Helen Emsellem of the Center for Sleep Disorders in Chevy Chase, Maryland, explains that sleep is restorative for both body and mind. "There is a natural purpose for sleep that if disrupted can wreak havoc with your health," she says. "Numerous studies have shown that too little sleep increases blood pressure, which can lead to heart disease and stroke."

Here are your best bets for getting a good night's sleep:

- **Keep a consistent bedtime.** Try to go to bed and wake up at approximately the same time every day. Make going to bed a pleasant ritual, perhaps by taking a lavender-scented bath or reading an inspirational passage.

- **Keep electronics out of the bedroom.** Avoid having a TV or computer in the bedroom or using an e-reader thirty minutes before you turn in. Prayer and meditation can also help you sleep more peacefully.
- **Avoid a nightcap.** It's a myth that alcohol can help you sleep better. In fact, it can upset your sleep cycle so that you might awaken in the middle of the night. Too much daytime caffeine can have a similar effect. Try drinking chamomile tea in the evening to help you sleep soundly.
- **Exercise.** Daily exercise has been proven to help you get a good night's sleep. Even a thirty-minute walk in the fresh air is beneficial for good zzz's.
- **Check your medications.** Often, medicine like beta-blockers can impact your sleep. Ask your health care provider for the best time to take your meds.
- **Avoid sleeping pills.** Taking an occasional sleeping pill is fine, but relying on medical sleep aids (such as sedatives) regularly can actually make it harder to get sleep over time.

If you have trouble sleeping, Emsellem recommends keeping a sleep log and taking care of issues—such as snoring or sleep apnea—that can disrupt your sleep pattern. "Make sure you also get a metabolic testing to rule out medical issues that may be causing your sleeplessness," she says.

Banish Stress

Stress is another enemy of your immune system. It triggers the release of cortisol and other hormones that suppress your natural defenses, which is why you've got to learn how to relax.

"It is not possible to not have stress," notes psychologist Rob Pennington, author of the book *The Upside of the Down Times: How to Turn Your Worst Experiences into Your Best Opportunities*. "But we can learn how to recognize it quicker and move through it faster. And that makes all the difference."

Stress-busting practices include yoga, deep breathing techniques, Tai Chi, meditation, exercise, prayer, hot baths, nature walks, or simply listening to music you enjoy to calm the mind.

Laughter: The Best Medicine

The cliché is true: laughter really is the best medicine for enhancing your immune system. In addition to relieving tension, a good laugh increases the flow of feel-good endorphins in the brain as well as lymphatic fluid—producing more lymphocytes, antibodies, and other soldiers in the immune army.

"When you get medical treatment, a clinician is not necessarily going to tell you to take two aspirins and watch Laurel and Hardy," says Lee Berk, an associate professor of pathology and anatomy at California's Loma Linda School of Medicine. "But the reality is, there's a real science to this, and it's as real as taking a drug."

Vaccines and Vitamins: What You Need to Know

Vaccines are controversial in some alternative medicine circles. There is no doubt that inoculations have an impressive track record in preventing polio, smallpox, rubella, diphtheria, whooping cough, the flu, and other diseases that strike children and adults.

They are considered to be safe, effective, and necessary by the vast majority of mainstream physicians as well as the US Centers for Disease Control and Prevention (CDC), but some natural health proponents fear that vaccinations might have some insidious side effects.

Jean Sniffin, a community health nurse for Century Health Systems, speaks for the majority of health care professionals in saying, "Although good nutrition, exercise, [and] knowing your family health history, [as well as] physical, social, emotional, and spiritual health are all important to keep your immune system strong, being up to date with all your adult vaccines tops the list."

But many studies have also found that key vitamins, minerals, and natural supplements can also keep the immune system in optimal shape.

ANTIOXIDANT VITAMINS (A, C, E). Aging is one of the greatest causes of damage to the immune system. A by-product of normal metabolism is called oxidation, and like rust on a car, this process damages the cells of the immune system as we age. But antioxidants—such as vitamins A, C, and E—combat this process and can even reverse the effects of age on our immune systems. In addition, vitamin C is essential for good immune health. Along with vitamin E, both mitigate damage caused by oxidation, a recent study published in the journal *Toxicology* noted.

VITAMIN D. This essential vitamin has been known to boost immunity since before the advent of antibiotics, when it was used to treat tuberculosis. More recently, vitamin D has been shown to fight autoimmune disorders. Yet researchers find that three-quarters of Americans suffer from vitamin D deficiency.

VITAMIN E. Known for its antioxidant powers, vitamin E has also emerged as a superstar in boosting the immune system and neutralizing the damaging effects of common environmental contaminants, especially in the elderly. A study published in the *Journal of Experimental Medicine* found that adding vitamin E to foods protected immune cells from such environmental stresses as UV radiation, air pollution, and tobacco smoke.

ZINC. Four in ten Americans are deficient in zinc, which helps the immune system guard against the development of many chronic diseases (as well as the flu and common cold), according to a study published in *Molecular Nutrition & Food Research*. Also, since the body cannot store this essential element, daily supplementation is usually needed.

ASTRAGALUS. An herb used in Chinese medicine for thousands of years, astragalus not only helps regulate the immune system but also functions as an antioxidant and reduces inflammation, a 2014 study in the journal *Phytotherapy Research* found.

MAITAKE MUSHROOM. The maitake mushroom has long been used in botanical folk medicine and is prized for its immune-boosting and antioxidant powers, which were documented in the scientific journal *Annals of Translational Medicine*.

OLIVE LEAF EXTRACT. Multiple studies have shown that the bioactive components of olive leaves can help optimize the body's natural defense system, protect it from environmental stress, and even reduce inflammation.

BETA-GLUCAN. Derived from baker's yeast, beta-glucan strengthens the key immune function of neutrophils, which comprise 40 to 75 percent of white blood cells and are an essential part of the immune system. It is also considered a potential probiotic that could benefit the gut microbiome, which plays a key role in the immune system. Beta-glucan is also believed to have cholesterol-lowering and cancer-fighting properties.

KIDNEY STONES

In findings that sound more like a Walt Disney World promotion than a medical science discovery, researchers have found that roller coaster riding might help pass kidney stones. The findings are just the latest addition to a long list of ways to pass—and prevent—the painful condition that strikes millions of Americans.

David D. Wartinger—the lead author of the 2016 study published in *The Journal of the American Osteopathic Association*—says he became interested in roller coaster riding as a therapy when a series of patients reported passing kidney stones after riding the Big Thunder Mountain Railroad roller coaster at Walt Disney World in Orlando, Florida.

Previous research reports have also identified cases of patients who passed kidney stones after riding a roller coaster or bungee jumping, he said. Wartinger was especially intrigued by a patient who spontaneously passed a stone after each of three consecutive rides on the Orlando roller coaster. So he and coauthor Marc A. Mitchell decided to perform an experiment using 3D printing to create a clear silicone anatomical model of the patient's kidney.

They filled the model with urine and three kidney stones of differing sizes. With the permission of Walt Disney World, they placed the sealed model in a backpack and took twenty two-and-a-half-minute rides on the roller coaster, which makes sharp twists and turns and reaches speeds up to thirty-five miles per hour.

The researchers found that the coaster ride not only helped the stones to pass, but sitting in the back was associated with a nearly quadrupled passage rate (about 64 percent) compared with sitting in the front (nearly 17 percent). "Preliminary study findings support the anecdotal evidence that a ride on a moderate-intensity roller coaster could benefit some patients with small kidney stones," Wartinger says.

"Passing a kidney stone before it reaches an obstructive size can prevent surgeries and emergency room visits. Roller coaster riding after treatments like lithotripsy and before planned pregnancies might prevent stone enlargement and the complications of ureteral obstruction."

A Common, Painful Affliction

Kidney stones are one of the nation's most common urinary tract disorders. Each year, they account for more than one million visits to doctors and more than three hundred thousand trips to emergency rooms. The annual cost of treating kidney stones is estimated at $2.1 billion.

The most common types of kidney stones—which range in size from a grain of sand to a golf ball—contain calcium. They're more likely to occur in people who are overweight or obese, non-Hispanic whites, and men. In the United States, an estimated 11 percent of men and 6 percent of women will develop a kidney stone during his or her lifetime. Kidney stones are associated with risk factors such as

- a family history of stones,
- recurrent urinary tract infections, and
- a condition affecting levels of calcium, phosphorus, and oxalate, substances in urine that foster kidney stone formation.

Because kidney stones are strongly associated with an insufficient fluid intake, one of the best ways to prevent them is to drink two to three liters of fluid per day. Although experts say plain water is best, beverages such as orange juice and lemonade also might be effective.

Other ways to prevent kidney stones include limiting intakes of the following:

- sodium
- animal protein
- calcium
- oxalate (concentrated in tea, rhubarb, leeks, spinach, beets, Swiss chard, almonds, cashews, peanuts, wheat germ, and quinoa)

Although small kidney stones often cause no symptoms and pass on their own with little or no discomfort, the following are symptoms of problematic kidney stones:

- pain during urination
- blood in urine
- sharp and persisting pain in the back or lower abdomen

- fever and chills
- vomiting

If you have a large kidney stone or a blockage of your urinary tract, treatment options include surgical removal or procedures to break it into small pieces:

- shockwave lithotripsy
- ureteroscopy
- percutaneous nephrolithotomy

Wartinger and colleagues said kidney stone sufferers should talk to their doctors before considering roller-coaster ride therapy. Factors such as the size and location of the kidney stone—as well as medical history—might influence how well a kidney stone responds to the ride's force of gravity.

But the authors are hopeful that further research might establish roller-coaster ride therapy as an effective alternative to oftentimes painful medical treatments. "The osteopathic philosophy of medicine emphasizes prevention and the body's natural ability to heal," Wartinger says. "What could be more osteopathic than finding a relatively low-cost, noninvasive treatment that could prevent suffering for hundreds of thousands of patients?"

MENOPAUSE AND ANDROPAUSE

When Hollywood starlet Suzanne Somers hit her midthirties, she started feeling lousy and didn't know why. The popular actress and best-selling author went from doctor to doctor without getting any relief for the unexplained mood swings, weight gain, and serious PMS that plagued her.

Eventually, she realized she was suffering from the classic symptoms of perimenopause. In her book *I'm Too Young for This!*, Somers chronicles her journey through the challenging rite of passage for women and offers advice to help them cope—before, during, and after menopause.

The *Three's Company* star notes that many women turn to synthetic hormone replacement therapy (HRT) to ease menopausal symptoms. But those treatments carry increased risks for breast cancer and other problems in some women. However, many natural remedies can ease perimenopause without these risks. The first step is recognizing the symptoms of the condition, which she likens to a medical version of the supporting cast of Disney's *Snow White*.

"I call it the Seven Dwarves: Itchy, Bitchy, Sleepy, Sweaty, Bloated, Forgetful, and All Dried Up," says Somers cheerfully. "What I try to teach in this book is that those dwarves I just mentioned are symptoms."

Symptoms Common in Women—and Men

Many women—and some men—experience at least a few of the symptoms of menopause caused by age-related hormonal changes (in men, the condition is sometimes called andropause). But they might fail to recognize that they are tied to hormone deficiencies that promote the aging process and should be addressed early.

That's especially important for those experiencing the first signs of perimenopause—the stage in a woman's life just before she enters menopause—which can occur as early as the thirties or forties, as hormone levels begin declining. Hot flashes, mood swings, sleeping problems, and vaginal dryness are common. Perimenopause ends once a woman goes a full year without a menstrual period, after which she has reached menopause.

There are two types of hormones—considered major and minor—that regulate key bodily functions. Major hormones include insulin and cortisol as well as thyroid and adrenal hormones. Minor hormones include testosterone, estrogen, progesterone, and dehydroepiandrosterone (DHEA).

The good news, antiaging experts say, is that bioidentical hormone therapy can counteract the effects of aging on your health. Blood tests can turn up hormone deficiencies that can be addressed with therapy to boost your overall health and well-being by keeping weight down and energy levels and libido up.

Bioidentical hormones differ from conventional therapeutic hormones in that they are derived from plant products that have the exact same chemical structure of human hormones, unlike synthetic drugs.

"I'm in my sixties. I sleep eight hours every night without drugs," Somers says. "I have a sex drive, which is one of things [you lose] when you lose your minor hormones, your sex hormones. . . . So when you get everything balanced again, you get your sex drive back, your hair gets thick and more lustrous. Older women get stringy hair; I'm not getting stringy hair because my hormones are replaced, [and my nails are] strong."

Somers notes that advances in medical technology are allowing Americans to live longer but not necessarily better. She says she was driven to become a health advocate by a single question: "What if we could make aging aspirational?"

"I realized for the last twenty years that I have been restoring what I have lost in the aging process with natural bioidentical hormones . . . so technology is great, technology has figured out how to extend life—we're all going to live 90, 100, the futurists say 110, 120," she says. "But nobody has thought about quality of life in that second half. And so what I write about is quality of life."

HRT: Other Ways to Combat Menopausal Symptoms

Conventional HRT involves a combination of estrogen and progestin and has been shown to reduce menopausal symptoms as well as those linked to hormone-blocking medications like the breast cancer drug Tamoxifen.

Doctors used to routinely prescribe HRT to relieve symptoms and also because research suggested it could potentially lower the risk of heart disease. But in 2002, a large US study called the Women's Health Initiative found that women using estrogen and progestin had a slightly higher risk of breast cancer, heart attack, and blood clots. As a result, many women stopped using HRT after those results were released.

Because many women do not want to take hormones—whether they are bioidentical or synthetic—or cannot take them for medical reasons, the European Menopause and Andropause Society (EMAS) recently commissioned a multinational team that analyzed past studies on treatments ranging from exercise to antidepressants and behavioral therapy.

The researchers reviewed studies that assessed a wide range of alternatives—including clinical trials—and smaller or observational studies covering lifestyle modifications, diet and food supplements, prescription medications, and behavioral and alternative/complementary therapies. Lead study researcher Gesthimani Mintziori of the Aristotle University of Thessaloniki, Greece, said the group drafted the position paper on hormone alternatives because it could be confusing for women to figure out what works best for them.

The results were decidedly mixed, they reported in the journal *Maturitas*. But there was some evidence that certain alternative approaches can help. Based on the new review and other scientific reports, research has demonstrated that the following natural remedies might offer at least some relief:

EXERCISE. Not all studies have found that working out relieves hot flashes, but the consensus of many researchers is that it is worth trying. Some studies have shown that it can reduce the frequency and intensity of such symptoms. In addition, exercise improves overall quality of life and can offset the increase in heart disease risk women face after menopause.

SOY, PHYTOESTROGEN SUPPLEMENTS. The evidence for supplements or a diet rich in phytoestrogens is mixed. But some research has found that women might benefit by trying phytoestrogens, compounds derived from plants that are similar in structure to estrogen and are found in a variety of foods, especially soy. Many alternative health practitioners tout them as safe alternatives to standard HRT to ease menopausal symptoms such as hot flashes or to protect against bone loss.

Dr. Ivonne Rietjens, PhD, of Wageningen University in the Netherlands and her colleagues analyzed previously published studies and concluded that phytoestrogens can ease menopausal symptoms in addition to lowering risks of cardiovascular disease, obesity, metabolic syndrome and type 2 diabetes, brain function disorders, and various types of cancer. But there is a caveat: phytoestrogens are endocrine disruptors, which means they have the potential to cause negative health effects, including infertility and increased risks of cancer in estrogen-sensitive organs, such as the breast and uterus.

RELAXATION. A study published in the *International Journal of Clinical and Experimental Hypnosis* found that hypnosis relaxation therapy decreased hot flashes and lowered levels of the stress hormone cortisol. In another study, women who suffered severe hot flashes also benefited from relaxation therapy. After three months of treatment, their cortisol levels had dropped significantly, and their hot flashes had decreased from at least seven a day to only two.

ACUPUNCTURE. A study published in the journal *Menopause* found that women who underwent acupuncture experienced a notable decrease in the number and severity of menopausal symptoms after twelve weeks compared to women who received a placebo treatment.

HERBAL REMEDIES. The Indian ashwagandha root has been found to reduce cortisol levels, which can increase the risk for hot flashes, according to a study published in the *Indian Journal of Psychological Medicine*. In addition, a supplement called phosphatidylserine was found to lower cortisol levels in as little as ten days.

Testosterone Therapy: What Men Need to Know

Testosterone therapy has been hailed as a medicinal fountain of youth for many men over fifty, with a growing body of research showing that low-T treatments can significantly boost a man's energy, memory, and libido.

But in recent years, conflicting studies about potential downsides of hormone therapy have prompted the US Food and Drug Administration (FDA) to investigate the risks and benefits of testosterone. That review was prompted by studies suggesting that the popular treatments might lead to heart problems in some men who take hormone supplements.

So what do men need to know about the pros and cons of low-T treatments?

Dr. David Samadi, a leading men's health authority, says men who opt for low-T therapy can take comfort in the many studies that show it is safe and healthy for men. Samadi says the warnings on testosterone therapy are "overblown" and that men—whose levels of testosterone naturally fall as they age—don't need to worry, just so long as they work closely with a doctor who can be sure they are getting appropriate amounts.

"Almost every time you turn on the TV or radio, all you hear is all these ads about . . . how this testosterone therapy is going to add more to your life," says Samadi, chairman of urology and chief of robotic surgery at Lenox Hill Hospital in New York City. "And we all have seen the picture[s] of the older man who really looks muscular, and we all want to be like him. . . . But we want to be sure that people are very careful about this."

He believes some of the warnings about testosterone therapy are "completely exaggerated" but adds that treatments must be tailored to the unique needs of individual patients, because having too much of the hormone can be as risky to some men as having too little.

"We see that patients come in that are very tired, they have a loss of libido," he explains, "they have no interest in any kind of socializing in with other people, they become like a real couch potato, they just want to play with that remote control and not do anything else. . . . And that's the low-T we see; those are the symptoms of it."

But Samadi notes that you can get too much of a good thing when it comes to hormone therapy. "If you take too much testosterone, that doesn't make it any better. You add the risk of clotting. You add the risk of heart attack and stroke and many other things," he says. "So too much testosterone is not necessarily the right answer. That's why [the] FDA is getting involved; they want to make sure that people are aware of this."

In addition, some men—particularly those at risk for prostate cancer or those with enlarged prostates—are not good candidates for low-T therapy, which can make things worse.

The key, Samadi says, is for men to work closely with a doctor who knows the risks and benefits of hormone therapy and can determine, through blood testing, the appropriate treatment options. An experienced doctor can also help men determine which formulations of low-T therapy—including injections, patches, or gels—are best. "So it's a little tricky," he says, adding, "Testosterone is not the answer for every man out there. We have to select them carefully, and then it will do the trick."

Samadi also notes that there are other ways to boost testosterone naturally—through a healthy diet, exercise, and managing stress levels. Belly fat, for instance, can lead to low-T, which might be why increasing activity levels keeps hormone levels up. Depression and thyroid problems can also affect hormone levels.

"So guess what? Try to lose weight. And that's one of the cures for metabolic syndrome; [it can] lower your blood pressure, lower your cholesterol. So . . . losing some of that weight automatically will shift up your testosterone.

"The knee-jerk reaction of someone coming in and just get[ting] a shot and leav[ing], thinking that it's going to take care of everything. . . . It's really bad medicine."

Wellness expert Dr. Erika Schwartz also notes that both male and female hormones are critical to men's health in midlife and beyond. Making sure all men have adequate levels tailored to their individual needs—by supplementing them with natural bioidentical hormones—can stave off obesity-related conditions and boost their overall health.

"Men, just like women, need hormones as they get older, as long as the testosterone you're giving them is bioidentical," she says. She adds that there is no one-size-fits-all prescription for hormone replacement therapy for men. Some might benefit from a small dose; others might need more.

"There is such variation in levels of testosterone that men need, so they are gradually coming to idea that we are not all the same—what a shocking idea!" she says. "As men get over the age of forty, they start to have symptoms of weight gain, loss of muscle, loss of libido. Now, some men with those complaints will have higher levels of testosterone and some will have lower levels."

"Low-T" is typically diagnosed in men with hormone levels under 200 or 300 ng/dl of blood. But Schwartz says treatment needs to also take into account a patient's symptoms and particular physiology. Current medical practices don't call for testing hormone levels in men when they are younger to establish a baseline for comparison—something she advocates doing for men's health—so doctors can't say whether a man with a level of 200 or 300 is necessarily deficient.

"Because everybody is different and we don't have baseline testosterone levels when men are eighteen, you should treat people based on clinical symptoms, in addition to [considering] blood test levels," she says. "You have to tailor a treatment program to individuals, and it always has to use bioidentical hormones—not synthetic hormones or drugs like Arimidex."

But even healthy individuals experience declines in hormones as they get older. "With aging, you will still need hormones," she adds. "So rather than waiting for a disease and then treating a disease with a drug, if we actually treat people with hormones that they're losing as they age and change their diet, exercise, and lifestyles, then we'll have a population of healthy people—and we won't be spending our money on developing new ways of treating disease with drugs."

OBESITY

Cut the fat, lose the weight.

For decades, that advice has been the mantra of health and nutrition experts who urged cutting back on dietary fat to shed pounds and combat obesity. The consensus view was that the best way to avoid *being* fat was to simply avoid *eating* fat.

But as it turns out, it's not that simple. Despite embracing that advice—with many Americans choosing margarine over butter, skim milk over whole, nonfat yogurt over full—the nation's collective waistline has continued to expand since the 1960s. Today, nearly two-thirds of Americans are clinically obese or overweight, according to the US Centers for Disease Control and Prevention (CDC).

Dr. Mark Hyman is one of a growing number of nutritional specialists who believe that's not merely a coincidence. In fact, he says, the low-fat food movement has fueled the nation's obesity crisis. The reason being, low-fat foods are often loaded with empty calories, additives, sugar, and unhealthy carbohydrates that boost weight gain and aren't very nutritious.

Hyman, the author of *Eat Fat, Get Thin*, challenges the orthodoxy of conventional nutritional advice and offers a simple message: add more *healthy* fats to your diet, which have been proven to help people shed pounds and boost their overall health.

"Healthy fats are crucial for our brain, our hormones, our skin, [and] our gut flora, and often when people limit healthy fats, they replace those fats with processed carbohydrates," Hyman says. "This is what our government recommended when the Food Pyramid came out in 1992, and it led to one of the biggest health epidemics of all time."

Obesity Undermines US Health Care System

By virtually any measure, the US health care system is among the best in the world—offering a wide variety of patient choices, the latest treatments for a wide range of life-threatening conditions, a qualified cadre of doctors and health care workers, high standards for care, and top-notch hospitals, clinics, and medical facilities.

As a result, Americans' average life expectancy is greater than it's ever been and continues to grow every year. Yet despite the fact that we are living longer than ever, obesity-related health problems and chronic conditions are rising every year. The primary reasons for this are unhealthy lifestyles, bad diets, lack of exercise, and other disease-causing habits.

A recent report card on the nation's wellness by the not-for-profit United Health Foundation (UHF) underscores what might be called the "American longevity paradox."

On the one hand, the America's Health Rankings report indicates that an American born today can expect to live to celebrate his or her seventy-ninth birthday, on average—with US life expectancy growing by about two years since 2000. On the other hand, the UHF report also found that older Americans are more likely to be obese or overweight and suffer from diabetes, cancer, or cardiovascular disease than merely a decade ago.

In addition, the United States spends more on health care per capita than any other wealthy nation, yet trails other affluent countries when it comes to life expectancy—ranking thirty-fourth (tied with Costa Rica, Nauru, and Qatar), according to the UHF report. Citizens of Western European countries, Japan, Australia, Singapore, Canada, and New Zealand all have a longer life expectancy than those from the United States. Inhabitants of nineteen different countries have a life expectancy that is at least three years longer than the average American's.

Several factors account for this reality, including the high cost of health care in the United States, insurance gaps, and lack of access to timely, effective health care among many Americans. But another critical factor is the epidemic of obesity in the United States, with poor dietary habits and inadequate exercise contributing to many costly health conditions.

In fact, obesity-related health care spending adds up to nearly $147 billion every year, by some estimates. Other key findings of the UHF report include the following:

- Nearly one in three Americans is clinically obese, which is defined as being at least thirty pounds overweight. That's nearly seventy million people. One reason for this might be that one in four people do not engage in any structured physical activity of any kind.

- The incidence of diabetes has grown to nearly one in ten Americans, about 30 percent of the population has high blood pressure, and cardiovascular diseases remain the nation's leading cause of death.
- Mississippi and Louisiana are the unhealthiest states largely because of high rates of obesity, diabetes, inactivity, tobacco use, and low infant birth weight. Vermont is the healthiest state, partly due to a low rate of infectious diseases and a high rate of health insurance.

The report is based on an examination of twenty-four measures of health—including tobacco and alcohol abuse, infectious diseases, and cancer and heart disease rates—from the files of the CDC, American Medical Association (AMA), US Census Bureau, and the Federal Bureau of Investigation (FBI).

"The good news is, we're living longer; the bad news is, while we're living longer, we're living sicker," notes Dr. Reed Tuckson, chief of medical affairs for UHF. "But it doesn't have to be this way. These are largely preventable illnesses.

"The point we're making is what's underneath the chronic disease rates, of course, are the risk factors that lead to them. Number one on that list would be obesity, with 28 percent of the US population obese now and 26 percent of the population exhibiting sedentary lifestyles."

The UHF's findings were echoed by other studies in recent months that have reached similar conclusions about the impact of obesity-related health problems:

- The AMA reported that cardiovascular causes still account for one in every three deaths in the United States, even though the death rate has fallen by a third since 1999.
- The CDC has found only 3 percent of all Americans without cardiovascular problems meet the key criteria for heart health—maintaining an ideal weight, normalizing blood pressure, getting regular exercise, and eating a healthy diet.
- Washington University researchers noted that great strides have been taken in fighting killer diseases around the world, but many nations face rising financial costs tied to chronic diseases. The fifty-nation Global Burden of Disease study found that malnutrition has dropped as a cause of death, but the effects of overeating are taking its place, with thirteen million deaths due to stroke and heart disease—tied to eating and drinking too much, smoking, and inactivity.
- The nonpartisan Commonwealth Fund found that the United States leads fifteen other high-income nations—including Germany, France, and the United Kingdom—when it comes to the death rate from such preventable

diseases as cancer, diabetes, infections, and heart disease before age seventy-five. Despite the fact that the US health care system accounts for nearly one-fifth of the US economy, we still trail the European Union when it comes to preventing deaths. The study, published in the journal *Health Policy*, found that the preventable mortality rate in the United States is ninety-six per one hundred thousand people—nearly twice the rate as in France. "We spend far more than any of the comparison countries [up to twice as much]," noted Cathy Schoen, Commonwealth Fund senior vice president, "yet are improving less rapidly."

Tuckson believes the new alarms health experts are sounding should prompt aggressive campaigns—comparable to antismoking and polio-eradication initiatives—to change Americans' behaviors as we grow older.

Without a change, the already stressed US health care system won't be able to handle the growing number of seniors who will need care in coming decades, with doctor shortages already emerging in many regions.

His prescription for America is simple: most people need to move more, eat less, and take more active steps to take better care of themselves. "It doesn't need to be more complicated than that," he says. "Just get up and move. Get on a bicycle, walk, garden . . . just do something. Because what we're learning is that if you can just go from no activity at all to just a little bit of activity, that will significantly help you in terms of longevity."

Combatting Obesity: A Doctor's Perspective

As director of the Cleveland Clinic's Center for Functional Medicine, Dr. Mark Hyman has watched health and food trends come and go over the years. He has also learned, the hard way perhaps, what works and what doesn't when it comes to weight loss.

A former vegetarian, Hyman once limited his intake of dietary fat and loaded up on whole grains, wheat bread, beans, pasta, and fruits and vegetables—following a diet in line with the federal government's dietary guidelines.

Despite following those recommendations, and getting regular exercise, he found himself gaining weight. So he began examining the latest nutritional research and found that many studies have concluded that healthy fats—those contained in olive oil, fatty fish, nuts, and certain vegetables like avocados—boost weight loss.

As a result, he started eating *more* fat—not less—and found that he lost weight. He then began urging his patients to follow suit and found that many lost weight and improved their cholesterol levels. Some even reversed their type 2 diabetes.

One of his patients became a very public example of the benefits of a healthy-fat diet: former president Bill Clinton—a friend of Hyman's—lost a significant amount of weight (thirty pounds since he left the White House, by his account) after giving up his low-fat vegan diet and following the doctor's advice to eat more healthy fats.

In an interview, Hyman took aim at the confusing dietary advice out there and the disconnect between conventional nutritional guidelines and the scientific research on diet. An excerpt from the interview follows:

Q: Do you believe the federal dietary guidelines on fat have fueled the nation's obesity crisis?

A: Yes, 100 percent. We were told to replace fats with carbs and sugars. Not only that, we were told to eat six to eleven servings of rice, bread, cereal, and pasta every day! This has made us fatter and sicker than ever.

Our government, the media, and many doctors and nutritionists can't let this low-fat recommendation go, despite the flawed research and the scientific evidence proving that healthy fats are the way to go.

Q: You argue that, essentially, not all fats are created equal—that is, some are actually good for you. How so?

A: Fat is a complicated topic that inspires a lot of debate among experts. We can't say that all fat is good or bad. Sugar is sugar is sugar. There are 257 names for sugar, and with a few exceptions, they're pretty much all the same. But fat is not fat is not fat.

You have trans fats, which are evil; stay away from those! You have omega-3 fats that come from foods like wild fatty fish. These are what I like to call the happy fats. They make your brain happy, they regulate cholesterol, protect your heart, and so much more.

Q: What types of fat should you include in your diet?

A: Some of my favorite fats include organic, unrefined, cold-pressed coconut oil and organic, unrefined, cold-pressed extra virgin olive oil; nuts and seeds; wild fatty fish; grass-fed meats; and avocados. These are healthy fats.

Q: What's your take on the latest US Dietary Guidelines, which for the first time remove their long-standing restrictions on dietary fat?

A: The most powerful recommendation is to avoid or limit added sugars. Fat and cholesterol have also been exonerated with no restrictions on total fat or cholesterol in the diet after thirty-five years of previous guidelines advising a low-fat and low-cholesterol diet.

The other key focus is whole, nutrient-dense foods and healthy dietary patterns, which moves away from the confusion in past guidelines by highlighting whole foods, not just ingredients.

But the recommendations do not go far enough in addressing the need to reduce refined carbohydrates and processed meat. They also sidestepped and did not include the environmental impact and sustainability issues caused by factory farming of animal products that were a main focus of the 2015 US Dietary Guidelines Advisory Committee, on whose recommendations these guidelines are based.

TYPE OF FAT	GOOD	BAD
Animal fats	Grass-fed, organic, sustainably raised lamb, beef, bison, venison; organic chicken, duck, and turkey; omega-3, pasture-raised eggs; organic, free-range, pasture-raised lard	Feedlot animal meats, nonorganic poultry
Fish and seafood	Wild fatty fish (sardines, mackerel, herring, black cod, salmon); shellfish (clams, oysters, mussels, shrimp, scallops, crab); calamari or octopus	Tuna, catfish, king mackerel, Chilean sea bass, swordfish (fish high in mercury and unsustainable fish)
Dairy and dairy substitutes	Grass-fed butter, ghee, nut, and seed milks (almond, cashew, hemp, hazelnut)	Milk, yogurt, cheese, cream, regular butter, soy milk
Nuts and seeds	Nuts (almonds, macadamia, walnuts, pecans, Brazil nuts); seeds (hemp, chia, pumpkin, sesame, flax); nuts and seed butters (without added sugars or bad oils)	Peanuts
Oils	Coconut butter; organic, virgin, cold-pressed, unrefined coconut oil; organic, extra virgin, cold-pressed olive oil; medium-chain triglyceride (MCT) oil; organic flaxseed oil; organic, expeller-pressed, refined avocado oil; walnut, pumpkin seed, pistachio, hemp oils	Safflower, soybean, sunflower, corn, cottonseed oils; hydrogenated or partially hydrogenated oils; margarine, shortening
Whole food fats	Avocado, olive, cacao butter, dark chocolate	

Green Diet Plan: Best Way to Lose Weight

Fad diets. Extreme exercise plans. Diet pills. Complicated calorie-cutting methods. Americans spend millions every year on costly, unproven weight-loss strategies. But in fact, the key to shedding pounds is far less complex; all you have to do is start eating "green."

So says Dr. Charles T. Nguyen, coauthor of *The Thinsulin Program: The Breakthrough Solution to Help You Lose Weight and Stay Thin*. Nguyen argues that the number-one culprit in weight gain and obesity is your insulin level. High levels of the hormone cause the body to store fat, whereas low insulin levels cause it to burn fat.

So how can you keep your insulin levels low?

"If you eat green, leafy vegetables, the pancreas doesn't need to produce insulin, so the insulin levels are lowered because there's no fat, no carbs, in these foods," Nguyen says. To help dieters follow his plan, he's come up with a tri-color dining scheme modeled after traffic lights.

Green-light foods. Vegetables like asparagus, bok choy, spinach, kale, and arugula are prime examples of "green-light foods," which lower a person's insulin levels and boost weight loss. Proteins are also good choices, especially those found in meats and egg whites.

Yellow-light foods. Eating only greens would make for a pretty boring diet, so Nguyen suggests adding a few "yellow-light foods," which are fine in moderation but can raise insulin levels in excess. These foods include nuts and fruits (apples, oranges, grapes, and berries).

Red-light foods. Avoid or limit your consumption of sweets and starchy vegetables—like potatoes, carrots, and beets—because these "red-light foods" will spike insulin levels and cause your body to pile on the pounds. "Any type of grain will raise the insulin levels, causing weight gain," Nguyen adds, "regardless of how 'healthy' they may be."

Nguyen also advises against extreme low-calorie diets, which he says are doomed to fail. "In order to beat this cycle of obesity, to really change it, we have to reject this idea of dieting," he says. "People looking to lose weight should look at it as a journey. In this way, people want to lose the weight and understand that there will be little bumps in the road but that they're still getting where they want to go."

Are "Natural" Sugars Really That Bad for You?

Americans' overconsumption of sugar has been linked to a variety of chronic health problems, including heart disease, cancer, diabetes, and Alzheimer's disease. But does the kind of sugar you consume make any difference in the risk it poses? The answer, it turns out, is not as straightforward as you might think, expert say.

On the one hand, the latest research shows that all sugars are basically the same, whether they come from fruit, honey, maple syrup, candy, or the sugar bowl. But on the other hand, nutritionists note that eating naturally sweet foods—such as fruit—is a better option than loading up on processed cakes, cookies, pastries, bread, and pasta.

"There's some truth in saying 'sugar is sugar,'" notes Joy Dubost, a registered dietician based in Washington, DC. "The body can't tell the difference between natural sugar and added sugar and processes it all the same way."

Still, there's a big difference in how the sugar is packaged. For example, a large apple has the same amount of sugar as six Oreo cookies. But it's much healthier to eat the apple. Fruit fiber, in particular, has a beneficial effect because it changes the pace at which the sugars are processed. Fiber is also satiating, so you feel fuller when you consume a piece of fruit as opposed to sugary junk food or drinks.

"Fiber slows down the digestion of carbohydrates, so it has a buffer effect on blood sugar rise," explains Carol Sherman, a registered dietitian based in Boca Raton, Florida. "That's why you don't get the same blood sugar spike from an apple that you would get from a soft drink."

Caveman Diet: Intermittent Fasting Drives Weight Loss

Fasting, even occasionally, has been linked to a host of health benefits, including lowered blood pressure, weight loss, better insulin sensitivity, and improved mental sharpness.

While fasting for long periods of time not only is difficult but might be bad for your health, occasionally forgoing food for a day or so—known as intermittent fasting—can be a great way to lose weight and boost your overall health, experts say.

"It's only in periods where you don't have food that your body goes into a sort of repair mode," says Dr. Michael Mosley, a British physician and author of the best-selling book *The FastDiet: Lose Weight, Stay Healthy, and Live Longer with the Simple Secret of Intermittent Fasting*. "Some of the proteins get denatured. New ones get created. Your mitochondria cells originate. There's a lot of fundamental biochemistry, which completely validates this argument."

If you'd like to give intermittent fasting a try, here are some key variations on the idea promoted by health researchers:

Leangains diet. Promoted by Swedish nutritionist Martin Berkhan, this plan requires that you fast sixteen hours a day but eat three meals during the other eight.

Warrior diet. Eat just one meal a day. In a study published in the *Journal of Clinical Nutrition*, researchers found that people who ate one meal a day lost more weight and built more lean muscle tissue over time than those who ate three.

Alternate-day fasting. This is just what it sounds like. You eat pretty much all you want, but only every other day.

This One Simple Trick Helps You Lose Weight

Here's a weight-loss trick so simple, it probably didn't need a scientific study to discover it: simply use a smaller plate.

In what is probably the most obvious scientific finding ever reached, an analysis published in the *Journal of the Association for Consumer Research* found that smaller plates reduce the amount of food a person eats. For the review, researchers examined fifty-six previous studies and found that overall, smaller plates can cut consumption under specific conditions. The following factors were evaluated in the analysis:

- **Type of food consumed:** Snack foods, popcorn, ice cream, breakfast cereal, rice, vegetables, fruit, and so on
- **Type of plate:** Bowls versus plates; serving platter versus plate from which the food is consumed
- **Portion size:** Fixed amount of food served; amount varied in line with the plate size; self-served portions
- **Setting:** Consumers invited to a food laboratory; unaware consumers in natural settings such as a buffet

In general, the studies showed that using plates that are half the normal size prompted volunteers to eat an average of 30 percent less food. The researchers found that small plates worked best if people served their own food. They also found that smaller plates were more effective if consumers weren't aware their actions were being monitored.

Overall, the research shows that simply switching to smaller plates can curb overeating among individuals who serve themselves, either at the dinner table or at a buffet. "Just changing to smaller plates at home can help reduce how much you serve yourself and how much you eat," says coresearcher Natalina Zlatevska of Bond University, Australia.

Another study found that the size of a dinner table might also influence how much we eat. This new study, published in the *Journal of the Association for Consumer Research*, found that people ate less when food was served in smaller portions and placed on a large table and ate most when large portions were served on a small table.

For the study, the researchers divided four large round pizza pies of the same size into regular-sized slices (eighths) or smaller slices (sixteenths). They then placed two pies on small tables that were just a little bigger than a pizza pie. And they placed the other two pies on large tables that were much bigger than a pizza pie.

They then asked 219 university students to one of the four tables and invited them to take as much pizza as they would like to eat. Those at small tables took about twice as many slices as people at large tables. In other words, people who saw a pizza pie with smaller slices took about the same number as those who saw one with regular slices when served on a large table. This meant they ate a lot less pizza overall.

"To eat less food," lead researcher Brennan Davis recommends, "serve food in small portions and on large tables."

Other simple tricks to help you drop extra weight include the following:

Weigh yourself daily. A study published in the Public Library of Science journal *PLOS ONE* found that the more dieters weighed themselves, the more weight they tended to lose. Those who went more than a week without weighing themselves gained the most weight over the course of the study.

Chew food thoroughly. A recent study revealed that people who were at an ideal weight chewed their food almost forty times before swallowing, while those who were overweight chewed fewer than ten times before swallowing.

Drink before eating. Studies show that people who drink a lot of water while dieting lose more weight than people who don't. In fact, one study found that people who drink a glass of water before each meal tend to eat less. "Water makes your stomach feel fuller, suppressing your hunger as well as your overall caloric intake," says nutritionist Elizabeth DeRobertis.

Flavonoid-Rich Foods: Natural Way to Lose Weight

Health researchers have long known that people who eat lots of fruits and vegetables are less likely to gain weight as they age. But they haven't pinpointed exactly which ones are best for weight control. Until now.

A new large-scale observational study suggests that the key to minimizing middle-aged spread is to increase your intake of flavonoids, which are naturally occurring bioactive compounds found in some but not all fruits and vegetables.

For the study, researchers analyzed data on diet, weight, and other lifestyle factors from 124,086 American adults who were tracked for up to twenty-four years. The data came from three ongoing studies:

1. **The Health Professionals Follow-Up Study.** This study began in 1986 and enrolled male health professionals ages forty to seventy-five.
2. **The Nurses' Health Study.** This began in 1976 and enrolled female nurses ages thirty to fifty-five.
3. **The Nurses' Health Study 2.** This began in 1989 and enrolled younger female nurses ages twenty-five to forty-two.

"Most of the study participants were actually gaining weight over time—about one pound per year," says lead researcher Dr. Monica Bertoia, PhD, of the Harvard T. H. Chan School of Public Health in Boston.

But Bertoia and her colleagues found that participants with a flavonoid-rich diet gained significantly less weight over time. The results were most noticeable in those with high intakes of three flavonoid subclasses:

1. **Anthocyanins**, the main sources of which were blueberries, strawberries, apples, and red wine.
2. **Flavonoid polymers**, the main sources of which were tea, apples, and strawberries.
3. **Flavonols**, the main sources of which were tea, apples, and onions.

Other flavonoid-rich foods and beverages included beer, celery, grapefruit, oranges and orange juice, pears, peppers, prunes, and tomato juice. "We can get flavonoids from juices such as citrus juices," Bertoia says. "But whole fruits are better sources than juice because a lot of flavonoids are found in the pulpy parts of the fruit."

Flavonoids had a relatively modest effect on reducing weight gain, particularly as we age. Over a four-year period, for example, each 10-mg increase in daily anthocyanins intake was associated with only 0.2 fewer pounds gained. "They were not associated with big changes in weight," explains Bertoia.

In theory, however, increased flavonoid intake could make a big difference. For example, if you eat ½ cup of blueberries per day—which contains 120 mg of anthocyanins—it's possible that you could reduce your weight gain by 2.4 pounds over four years.

"Preventing even small amounts of weight gain or losing even small amounts of weight can have an important impact on your personal health," says Bertoia.

Research shows that even modest changes can significantly reduce your risk of developing high blood pressure, diabetes, heart disease, and several different kinds of cancer.

Bertoia's colleagues are now conducting follow-up research to see if one or two daily servings of blueberries have significant effects on body weight, blood pressure, cholesterol, and other measures of metabolic health. To maintain a constant level of flavonoids, which can vary in fresh fruit, the researchers are giving participants either freeze-dried blueberries or an inactive placebo.

Another of Bertoia's colleagues is looking at the association between alcohol consumption and weight change over time. "It'll be interesting to see if people who increase their alcohol intake either increase their weight, stay the same, or even lose weight," says Bertoia.

The new Harvard study, which was published in the *British Medical Journal* (*BMJ*), builds on previous small-scale research suggesting that the flavonoids in green tea can help control weight. Experts currently recommend that Americans consume 2 cups of fruit and 2½ cups of vegetables daily. Most Americans consume far less—namely, about 1 cup of fruit and less than 2 cups of vegetables daily.

Bertoia's first-of-its-kind study not only supports these current recommendations; it also suggests a more discerning approach to diet. "Our overall conclusion is that if you're choosing to eat more fruits and vegetables, it's best to consider choosing higher-flavonoid sources," she says.

Fiber and Probiotics: Nature's Weight-Loss Solution

You are what you eat, as the saying goes. That's a big reason obesity has reached epic proportions in the United States—the typical American diet is loaded with unhealthy processed foods that are fueling the nation's ever-expanding waistline.

It's not that we're not trying to stay fit. In fact, Americans spend $20 billion a year on diet pills, weight-loss books, and bariatric surgery, according to industry estimates. But health experts suggest that there are better, more natural ways to lose weight and boost your health at the same time—and you only have to go as far as your refrigerator or kitchen pantry to find what they are.

They keys are dietary fiber—from fruits, vegetables, and whole grains—and probiotics, which are naturally occurring beneficial bacteria in yogurt, sauerkraut, aged cheeses, and other healthy foods.

Many studies show that a diet rich in fiber, probiotics, and other nutrients can help you shed pounds and cut your risk for diabetes, heart disease, cancer, and other chronic health conditions. Yet most Americans don't get enough of these natural health boosters in their diets or through supplements to make a difference.

Fiber: Digestive Aid and Health Booster

Fiber—also called "roughage"—is the indigestible part of plant foods that absorb water and ease bowel movements as it moves through our digestive systems.

There are two broad types of fiber, soluble and insoluble:

1. **Soluble fiber** dissolves in water and is fermented by bacteria in the digestive tract, becoming gelatinous.
2. **Insoluble fiber** does not dissolve in water and does not change as it moves through the digestive tract.

Both types of fiber are present in fruits, vegetables, legumes, and whole grains. Dairy products, white bread, and other starches are low in fiber. Most foods that are high in fiber are also rich in health-boosting vitamins and other essential nutrients.

Foods packed with insoluble fiber include dark-green leafy ones, root vegetable skins, fruit skins, whole-wheat products, wheat bran, corn bran, nuts, and seeds. Foods rich in soluble fiber include kidney beans, pinto beans, brussels sprouts, broccoli, spinach, zucchini, apples, oranges, grapefruit, grapes, prunes, oatmeal, and whole-wheat bread.

Two Key Types of Fiber

Two types of fiber have been a key focus of nutritional research:

Fibersol-2 (maltodextrin) is a soluble corn fiber that acts as a low-calorie bulking agent containing 90 percent dietary fiber.

Inulins are a group of naturally occurring polysaccharides produced by many plants but most often extracted from chicory. Inulins are part of a class of dietary fibers known as fructans and are present in more than thirty-six thousand species of plants, including wheat, onion, bananas, garlic, asparagus, sunchoke, and chicory.

Eating at least five servings of fruit and vegetables each day, as well as some servings of whole-grain products, will generally provide sufficient fiber levels. But for some Americans, a fiber supplement can fill in the gaps.

Probiotics: "Good Bacteria"

Most people associate diseases and health problems with the word *bacteria*. But in fact, not all bacteria in your body are "bad." In fact, some "good bacteria" boost your health, and eliminating them could actually be dangerous to your well-being.

The average person's intestinal tract contains about one hundred trillion bacteria, weighting about two to three pounds. Some bacteria not only help digest your food, but emerging research shows they play an important metabolic role that impacts your overall health—including weight levels and your risk for obesity, heart disease, and other conditions.

Numerous studies have linked significant benefits to introducing more "good" bacteria called probiotics into your diet. Consuming probiotics, in foods and supplements, can help balance your digestive system and boost your immune system, which is more affected by the digestive system than many people realize.

In fact, about 70–80 percent of your immune system is controlled by the bacteria and cells in your digestive system. As a result, when your friendly bacteria become imbalanced or decreased in your gut, your immune system can become compromised, making you more vulnerable to illness.

Some probiotics are more effective than others. Many experts recommend eating foods with good bacteria, including fermented dairy products such as kefir and organic unsweetened yogurt, fermented teas such as kombucha, and cultured vegetables like sauerkraut and the spicy Asian dish kimchi.

But you can also take supplements containing prebiotics as well as probiotics. Prebiotics, such as fiber and inulin, contain nondigestible food matter that nourishes and promotes the growth of good bacteria. By taking prebiotics, you are setting the stage for probiotics to flourish.

To choose an effective probiotic, follow these methods:

- Use a formula with multiple strains of researched and clinically documented probiotic bacteria.
- Use a formula with high quality controls to make sure strains remain alive and effective through the manufacturing process.
- Use a formula that has been tested to see that it is resistant to stomach acids and enzymes in the digestive tract.
- Choose products with important strains of probiotics, including *Bifidobacterium bifidum, Bifidobacterium longum, Lactobacillus acidophilus, Lactobacillus casei, Lactobacillus rhamnosus,* or *Lactobacillus sporogenes.*

Metabolism: Key to Weight Loss

Remember when as a teenager you could eat whatever you wanted and still not gain weight? Then the years rolled by, and those stubborn pounds piled on, despite dieting and exercise. Now an internationally known weight-loss expert and bariatric surgeon has come up with an easy-to-follow weight-loss plan that can turn back the clock in only six weeks and help you get the metabolism of a teenager.

In his new book *The Appetite Solution: Lose Weight Effortlessly and Never Be Hungry Again,* Dr. Joseph Colella details how to boost your metabolism and permanently reduce your cravings for foods that pack on the pounds. In it, he offers scientific evidence on why we are becoming an obese nation and how we can permanently and effortlessly lose weight once and for all.

"It's really simple," he says. "There's nothing magical or complicated about my lifestyle plan. We're plagued with obesity and other chronic diseases not only because we've become a sedentary nation but because we are consuming far too many simple sugars. They're in just about everything we eat, from processed foods to condiments like ketchup."

Step 1: Cut the Sugar

By eliminating simple sugars almost entirely from our diet and adding clean, power-packed protein, we combat hunger and support muscle repair, both of which lead to permanent weight-loss success.

"Simple sugars not only add pounds but . . . trigger food cravings, so you [end] up eating more of them," explains Colella. "Simple sugars are saboteurs because they are so easy to digest. They don't have to travel through the intestines to deliver glucose to your body. They go right into the bloodstream, and for the first few moments, you feel great! You've received an IV shot of sugar!"

The bad news is that a few hours later, after the pancreas pumps insulin into the body to drive the sugar into your body's cells, you "crash." "Of course, you then crave another sugar hit, so the vicious cycle goes on," says Colella. "Whole foods, especially protein and complex carbohydrates, must travel through the intestines to be digested and deliver sugar to the body at a much slower rate, so your metabolism stabilizes."

Step 2: Eat Regular Meals

Another factor that contributes to sugar cravings and weight gain is missing meals regularly. "Nothing spins [you] faster into a sugar cycle than missing meals," says Colella.

Other factors include sleep deprivation, stress, medications, depression, anxiety, and heartburn. "All these factors make us want to dive into that bowl of comforting mashed potatoes and other starchy foods," he says.

Amazingly, the current fad of drinking smoothies and fresh juices is also a potential health hazard, according to Colella. "Fruit and veggie juices without their fibrous pulp are pure sugar," he says. "Sure, you feel great after drinking a blended beverage, but that's the same sugar high you'd get from eating a candy bar."

Step 3: Build Muscle

The three-phase program of *The Appetite Solution* promises to wean you off the sweet stuff while building fat-burning muscle. There's plenty to eat with more than two thousand calories a day consisting of 30–40 percent protein, 30–40 percent complex carbohydrates, and 30–40 percent fat at every meal. As phases progress, you drop the amount of simple sugar intake to a total of 5 grams per meal and 20 grams daily.

Exercise is critical and added in the second phase. "You only need fifteen minutes daily, and it can be done in the comfort of your home," says Colella. "It's important to work on the big muscle groups—the thighs, quadriceps, glutes, and chest. For example, doing a few sets of pushups and squats will achieve this goal."

By the sixth week, the body's metabolism has been transformed, and the weight comes off naturally and will stay off if you read labels and avoid simple sugars.

Here's a handy chart to identify sources of simple sugars and better alternatives.

SIMPLE SUGARS	COMPLEX CARBS
White potato	Sweet potato
White rice	Brown rice
Corn	Beans
Cow's milk	Almond milk
Juices, sauces	Whole fruits and vegetables
Processed foods	Whole fruits, grains, vegetables, and legumes

OSTEOPOROSIS

Loss of bone density—known as "osteopenia" when mild and "osteoporosis" when severe—has become increasingly common in the United States as the nation grows older and ever more sedentary.

About 10 million older Americans have osteoporosis, which leads to an estimated 1.5 million bone and hip fractures every year—bone breaks that can be life threatening.

Several medications, such as Fosamax and calcitonin, are typically prescribed to strengthen bones, but they can cause serious side effects. But a handful of simple, safe, and cheaper natural remedies have been proven to treat osteoporosis.

Supplements and food products containing calcium are the most popular nondrug option for increasing bone density—along with estrogen and exercise, which can build bone strength. Studies show that taking 1,000 mg a day of calcium can help. But calcium isn't the only option. Here's what you need to know about the best bets for keeping your bones strong as you grow older.

STRONTIUM. When most people think of strontium, they tend to think of strontium-90, the dangerous radioactive compound released during nuclear testing. But in fact, low-dose levels of strontium are highly effective at improving bone density.

A recent study of strontium in the treatment of 353 osteoporosis patients showed a 15 percent increase in spine bone mineral density (BMD) over two years in patients using 680 mg of strontium a day. A second placebo-controlled study that involved 1,649 osteoporotic women found that new fractures decreased by 49 percent in the first year of treatment. In addition, BMD in the lumbar spine increased by an average of 14.4 percent after three years.

SOY. Many people drink milk for calcium to build strong bones. But research suggests that soy protein might a better option. A recent study available online in the *FASEB Journal*, published by the Federation of American Societies for Experimental Biology, found that early dietary nutrition heavy in soy protein isolate can protect against serious bone loss during adulthood.

The study, led by Dr. Jin-Ran Chen, a researcher with the Skeletal Development Laboratory at Arkansas Children's Nutrition Center at the University of Arkansas for Medical Sciences in Little Rock, involved rats fed a soy protein isolate diet for thirty days (from postnatal day twenty-four to fifty-five) and then switched to a regular standard diet until six months of age.

The rats were engineered to mimic postmenopausal bone loss in women to determine the amount of bone loss. The researchers found that the soy helped combat bone density loss in the animals more than a standard diet.

HORMONES. US researchers have found that a natural hormone called parathyroid hormone (PTH) can stimulate the reconstitution of bone cells called osteocytes. The study, published by Massachusetts General Hospital (MGH) researchers in the journal *Nature*, notes that PTH is secreted by the small glands at either side of the thyroid and plays a key role in regulating calcium distribution. Its main role is to stimulate the release of calcium from bones, which is then absorbed in the kidneys to increase blood calcium levels.

PTH therapy is generally used to stimulate bone formation in women who have already suffered at least two vertebral fractures. The MGH researchers found that daily PTH injections—from prefilled pens, similar to the insulin pens used for treating diabetes—were able to stop the action of certain enzymes (SIK2) that block bone formation.

In turn, this might reduce the risk of vertebral and peripheral fractures. Fractures can occur in any bone in the body, but the vertebrae, the neck of the femur, and the wrist are the most commonly damaged bones.

VITAMIN AND MINERAL SUPPLEMENTS. A healthy, nutrient-rich diet—free of refined foods—is a must when it comes to building strong bones. But it's also important to be sure you're getting enough vitamins and minerals. Magnesium, boron, calcium, copper, manganese, and strontium are all minerals that strengthen bones. Vitamins C, D, K2, B1, B2, B3, B6, and B12 are also needed for optimal bone health.

LIFESTYLE FACTORS. While drug treatments are the most common ways to combat osteoporosis, a number of lifestyle modifications can be crucial in preventing the condition:

- Safe sun exposure is recommended to boost vitamin D production, which helps the body naturally absorb calcium.
- Exercise is important for maintaining and increasing bone density.
- Cigarette smoke, alcohol (two glasses per day maximum), and caffeine (coffee, cola, energy drinks) should be limited.
- Avoid unnecessary use of heartburn medicines and acid blockers (proton pump inhibitors like Prilosec), which reduce your ability to absorb calcium and other nutrients, setting the stage for osteoporosis.

"Don't forget the basics," notes Dr. Jacob Teitelbaum. "Walk more—one half to one hour a day. If your problem is severe enough that you have osteoporosis, I would use bisphosphonate medications (like Fosamax) with . . . natural therapies at least until you have improved from osteoporosis to osteopenia."

PARASITIC INFECTIONS

Imagine that you have a stress fracture, but your doctor dismisses it as muscle strain and prescribes a painkiller. This absurd situation is not likely to occur in real life, but similar misdiagnoses happen all the time when it comes to parasitic infections.

Often, people who complain to their doctors of low energy, moodiness, stubborn weight gain, bloating, or digestive discomfort are told they might have irritable bowel syndrome (IBS) or chronic fatigue syndrome (CFS).

But if, after treatment, those conditions don't improve, it could be signs of a parasitic infection, says certified nutrition consultant Mary Vance, author of *Vitality for Life*. "I see a very common pattern where my clients have been to numerous—sometimes up to eight or nine—gastrointestinal doctors, and they are told, 'We can't find anything wrong with you,' after extensive testing," says Vance. "They are typically given a diagnosis of IBS, which is a diagnosis of exclusion, given when nothing else obvious is present."

Neglected Parasitic Infections Prevalent in United States

Parasites draw their nourishment from a host and vary greatly in size. Some are microscopic (blood parasites), while others are visible (worms). Parasites harm the host that they live on . . . or in. Often, their symptoms masquerade as other illnesses.

An example is *Babesiosis*, a tick-borne parasitic illness that infects red blood cells and can be mistaken for Lyme disease. A common misconception is that human parasites thrive primarily in underdeveloped countries, but in this increasingly globalized culture, infections are present in the United States. In fact, the US Centers for Disease Control and Prevention (CDC) has classified several parasites as neglected parasitic infections (NPIs) because little attention has been devoted to their surveillance, prevention, and treatment.

In other words, you might not know you have them, and your doctor might not know to test for them. Symptoms range from extreme fatigue to acute gut pain. Once diagnosed, patients can be treated with either traditional antibiotics or natural treatments.

How We Are Infected

Hand-to-mouth contact after touching infected surfaces can transmit pinworms, hookworms, or roundworms, and the parasite trichinosis can be transmitted by undercooked meat. But one of the main culprits is simply poor gut health. One of the biggest causes of gut problems is stomach acid that is too alkaline.

"We are all equipped with a very acidic stomach. If your digestion is working properly and you have good levels of probiotic bacteria and a strong immune system, you will fight off parasites and pathogens," Vance says. "This is rarely the case, however, due to diet and stress, which raise the pH of the stomach, making it too alkaline to kill pathogens."

How to Identify Parasitic Infections

The symptoms of parasitic infection can be subtle, and not all doctors are trained to look for them. If you have gut symptoms that persist after being treated for a condition assumed to be IBS, you should ask your doctor for a DNA-based, pathogen/parasitic stool test to detect gut parasites.

Hookworms can cause rash and abdominal pain and can eventually lead to anemia if the infection persists. Roundworms travel through the body and cause a myriad of symptoms—such as abdominal pain, wheezing, poor appetite—and can even travel to the eye. Both parasites can be detected through basic blood tests. If parasites are found, your doctor can prescribe a straightforward regimen of antiparasitic medications and antibiotics.

Prevention: The Best Medicine

Practicing good hygiene is the start of prevention. Wearing gloves and washing your hands when gardening is a proactive measure to avoid exposure to some parasites in the first place. But maintaining strong gut health can also equip your body to naturally fight off exposure. Here's how:

- Include fermented foods and probiotic foods in your diet, such as sauerkraut and yogurt.

- Eat foods rich in omega-3 fatty acids, such as salmon, and/or take fish oil supplements.
- Eat plenty of anti-inflammatory foods, such as blueberries, and vegetables from the cruciferous family, like broccoli.
- Address daily stress levels.
- Get eight hours of sleep.
- Do not pop medications like candy.

Is Yeast Ruining Your Health?

Do you suffer from sinusitis, IBS, CFS, depression, fibromyalgia, or an inability to lose weight? If you've been treated but your symptoms persist and your doctor shrugs his or her shoulders, don't be discouraged.

You could be a victim of candida.

Candida is an overgrowth of the yeast *Candida albicans*, and it is the culprit behind yeast infections commonly found in women and thrush in babies. But that same overgrowth could be lurking in your digestive system and wreaking havoc on your health. Since the symptoms masquerade as other diseases, it can be tricky to catch.

What Is Candida?

Candida is normally harmless and thrives alongside other bacteria in the digestive tract, mouth, and other areas of the body. The problem starts when there's simply too much of it. If there is an overgrowth, candida can lead to significant health problems in men, women, and children.

Your digestive tract is home to trillions of bacteria—about two to three pounds' worth—outnumbering human cells ten to one. About 90 percent are "good bacteria" that help digest food and are involved in many bodily functions; about 10 percent are "bad" bacteria that can cause disease. It's important to maintain a healthy balance of bacteria for the immune system to function properly and keep candida and other potentially harmful pathogens in check, experts note.

Candida generally manifests as sore throats and yeast infections in adults. One serious consequence of candida is leaky gut syndrome, which occurs when an overpopulation of candida causes the intestinal wall to become permeable. This allows partially digested proteins and other toxins to be absorbed in the body, which causes inflammation and can release candida into the bloodstream as well.

Once Candida is free to travel to other parts of the body, it can set off a number of symptoms that mimic other diseases, such as joint pain commonly associated with fibromyalgia. According to the CDC, candida is one of the most common causes of bloodstream infections in hospitalized patients.

What Causes Candida Overgrowth

Candida is a product of modern life, and a number of factors encourage it to overmultiply, even in people with normal immune systems:

- poor diet
- refined foods
- lack of sleep
- overprescribed antibiotics or medications
- daily stress levels

When and How to Seek Help

If you think you might have a candida overgrowth, your medical professional can conduct a comprehensive stool test to detect candida yeast or a blood test to detect candida antibodies. If the test is positive, there are many healthy lifestyle changes you can make to restore your body's natural balance:

- **Eliminate sugar.** Candida is a yeast and is nourished by sugar. Switching to a low-carbohydrate diet is essential for starving out the candida overgrowth. Avoid sugars, carbohydrates, alcohol, and fermented foods. Your medical professional or nutrition consultant can provide a more comprehensive list of foods to avoid.
- **Eat antifungal foods.** In addition to eliminating candida-enabling foods from your diet, you can also introduce herbs and foods that combat candida. Herbs include garlic, oregano, and cloves. Foods include onions, rutabaga, and seaweed. Coconut oil is also recommended as a strong fungal fighter, as it contains caprylic acid. Caprylic acid, which can also be taken in supplement form, is a powerful antifungal.
- **Consume probiotic foods or supplements.** Your medical professional might prescribe an antibiotic instead of advising you to rely on diet alone to combat candida. As a consequence, you might lose essential healthy gut flora in the process. Be sure to load up on probiotics, such as probiotic yogurt or supplements, to maintain a healthy balance.

Since treatments for other diseases with symptoms similar to candida can make the overgrowth worse, it is important to rule candida out. If you are treated with steroids for suspected IBS, the steroids can stimulate the growth of candida.

Heavy antibiotics given to treat chronic sinus infections can kill the "good" gut bacteria that normally balance the candida out, making the imbalance even worse and causing infections to recur.

Symptoms of Candida Overgrowth

If you are frequently experiencing one or more of the following problems, you could be suffering from a candida overgrowth:

- bloating or difficulty losing weight
- digestive discomfort, such as diarrhea, constipation, and indigestion
- irresistible craving for sweets, carbohydrates, or alcohol
- constant fatigue
- mood disorders, mood swings, or anxiety
- brain fog, difficulty focusing, or poor memory
- persistent seasonal allergies, ear infections, or frequent cases of the cold or flu
- chronic joint ache

PROSTATE PROBLEMS

For most men, prostate health isn't exactly a topic of polite conversation. In fact, prostate problems have been described as a "silent epidemic," in part because many men are reluctant to discuss them—even with their doctors. Although breast cancer awareness has been a rallying point for women's health advocates, the same can't be said of prostate health. Yet prostate problems—from cancer to infections to enlargement of the gland—are among men's most common health concerns.

In addition to the hundreds of thousands of men diagnosed with prostate cancer each year, millions more suffer infections (prostatitis) and enlarged prostate (benign prostatic hyperplasia [BPH]). In fact, prostate cancer is the second most common type of the disease among American men (after skin cancer), with federal statistics showing that nearly 200,000 new cases are diagnosed each year, with more than 32,050 deaths.

Conventional treatments range from antibiotics and other drugs to surgery, radiation, hormone therapy, and chemo, all of which carry the risk of side effects. But a handful of natural remedies have shown progress in warding off infections, treating BPH, combatting cancer, and boosting overall prostate health. Here's a primer.

Common Prostate Problems and Remedies

BPH. For most men, the prostate—a walnut-sized gland that sits below the bladder and produces fluid for semen—slowly grows bigger with age. In fact, more than half of men over age sixty have BPH. The condition typically puts pressure on the bladder, slowing the flow of urine through the urethral canal, causing pain and increasing a sense of urgency that typically requires men to wake up multiple times during the night to urinate.

Doctors typically diagnose BPH by checking the patient's prostate gland with a digital rectal examination. Severe cases can be treated with medications such as alpha-blockers (Cardura and Hytrin), which temporarily relieve the symptoms. But they do not treat the underlying cause of BPH or stop the progressive enlargement of the gland.

Doctors might also perform surgery to open up the urethra in a procedure called a transurethral resection of prostate (TURP). But certain key supplements—including saw palmetto—are better alternatives for many men, research suggests.

Made from a palm (*Serenoa repens*) that grows in the southern coastal regions of the United States, the active ingredient in saw palmetto (taken from the berries of the plant) has long been used by American Indians for healing and has caught on in the United States and around the world.

One reason for its growing popularity is that multiple scientific studies have shown that saw palmetto can ease symptoms of BPH—reducing the need to urinate in the night and improving urinary flow and painful urination. In fact, one analysis of multiple studies concluded that the benefits of saw palmetto are comparable to finasteride (Proscar), a drug for enlarged prostate, and also boosts the quality of life for men with BPH.

Other studies of saw palmetto's health benefits have been less conclusive but suggest it might also be effective against baldness, chronic pelvic pain, chronic nonbacterial prostatitis, and urinary problems due to prostate conditions.

PROSTATITIS. An inflammatory condition often caused by an infection, prostatitis can cause painful and difficult urination as well as discomfort in the abdomen, groin, penis, testicles, rectum, or lower back.

About 15 percent of prostatitis cases are caused by acute bacterial infection of the prostate gland, which can be associated with fever, chills, nausea, vomiting, and poor appetite. It can also be caused by an infection of the bladder, sometimes brought on by trauma from activities such as biking or horseback riding.

In many cases, doctors prescribe tetracycline antibiotics (minocycline or doxycycline) or quinolones (Cipro or Levaquin) to clear the infection and treat symptoms. But such medications carry well-known side effects—nausea, diarrhea, vomiting, headaches, and tendon damage—and are often ineffective.

Better options include eating a healthy diet, avoiding certain foods and dehydration, getting regular sexual activity and exercise, and adding nutritional supplements—including saw palmetto—that boost prostate health, studies show.

PROSTATE CANCER. One in six men who live to celebrate their eighty-fifth birthdays will develop prostate cancer, according to the National Cancer Institute (NCI). The risk grows with age, with some estimates suggesting that nearly three out of every four men age eighty and older have it.

But statistics also show just one in thirty-five men diagnosed with prostate cancer actually die from it because tumors are usually very slow-growing and never progress to the point that they spread beyond the gland and become life-threatening. The problem is that doctors can't readily tell which cancers are slow-growing and which are aggressive.

Typically, after age fifty, men are advised to get a yearly rectal exam and prostate-specific antigen (PSA) test, which assesses the level of the enzyme secreted by the gland. If a doctor's manual rectal exam is abnormal or the PSA level is elevated, men are typically referred to an urologist for a further work-up, which can include a biopsy to confirm or rule out the presence of cancer.

But PSA testing is imperfect, and elevated PSA might simply indicate the presence of an infection or BPH and not necessarily cancer. What's more, conventional prostate cancer treatment—surgery, radiation, hormone therapy, and chemo—is not always successful.

That's why routine PSA screening is controversial among some doctors, with most recommending a detailed discussion of the pros and cons of testing based on a man's particular risks. However, there is no controversy about how prevention—by maintaining prostate health—is the best approach when it comes to reducing risks. That approach includes lowering inflammation and maintaining the right balance of hormones.

Scientific studies have shown that saw palmetto lowers the levels of several sex hormones tied to cancer and overall prostate health, including estrogen. The primary culprits in elevated estrogen levels are obesity, eating a diet of refined foods that have estrogen-like hormones added to the animal feed, and exposure to pesticides and other toxins that have estrogen-like effects in the body.

Maintaining a healthy diet and weight level, getting regular exercise, eating nutritious foods and, in some cases, taking supplements like saw palmetto can help. In addition to saw palmetto, the following supplements have been shown to boost prostate health:

- **Beta sitosterol.** This plant-derived nutrient is shown to promote prostate and urinary tract health by lowering levels of the 5-alpha reductase enzyme to reduce dihydrotestosterone (DHT).
- **Pomegranate extract.** Biologically active compounds in pomegranate juice, known as ellagitannins, contain powerful antioxidants that lower inflammation and support healthy cells in the prostate and urinary tract.

- **Pumpkin seed.** Protective compounds called phytoesterols in pumpkin seeds promote proper prostate size and function and contain chemicals that reduce the transformation of testosterone into DHT.
- **Pygeum africanum.** The bark of the African plum tree has been used in healing for thousands of years to promote both proper inflammatory response and overall prostate health by easing urinary hesitancy and urinary frequency, particularly at night.
- **Boswellia extract.** Derived from the sap of the boswellia tree, boswellia is a potent herb that reduces inflammation.
- **Stinging nettle root powder.** This compound is widely used in Europe to treat prostate swelling and contains numerous biologically active chemicals that promote proper inflammatory response and inhibit the production of DHT.
- **Lycopene.** A powerful antioxidant found in tomatoes, lycopene is known to combat prostate cancer as well as heart disease by combatting inflammation.
- **Others.** Studies have also suggested that several other supplements might boost prostate health, including flower pollen, selenium, zinc, copper, and vitamins D3 and E.

Prostate Cancer: By the Numbers

One in six. That's how many men will be diagnosed with prostate cancer—most of them over the age of sixty-five. In fact, after lung cancer, prostate cancer is the most common cause of cancer death in American men. The American Cancer Society (ACS) estimates that in the United States, about 220,800 new cases of prostate cancer will be diagnosed this year and about 27,540 men will die from the disease.

The good news is that nearly three million men in the United States are living with prostate cancer today, but only about one in thirty-eight will die from it. Those survival figures are due, in large part, to new conventional cancer treatments but also to natural alternatives that scientific research has proven to be effective in staving off prostate cancer death. But many non-traditional therapies—including supplements, herbal remedies, and healthy lifestyle habits—have also been shown to be effective against other noncancer prostate ailments.

Allspice: Natural Treatment for Prostate Cancer

Prostate cancer can be a killer, but a flavorful spice typically used in pumpkin pie might help disarm it. A promising study suggests that allspice zaps cancer cells by starving them of their main fuel—male hormones called androgens.

"Allspice may reduce your chances of getting cancer or, if you already have it, prevent it from becoming more serious," says Dr. Bal Lokeshwar, a professor of medicine and surgery at Georgia Regents University Cancer Center.

In one experiment, the researchers exposed prostate cancer cells to an allspice extract. Within days, the extract stopped the progression of cancer growth and ultimately began killing the cancer cells. In another experiment, the researchers injected three groups of mice with human prostate cancer cells, causing tumor growth. One group was given allspice extract to drink every day, a second group was injected with the extract three times a week, and the third group was given nothing.

After six weeks, tumors were 62 percent smaller in the group that drank the extract and 58 percent smaller in the mice injected with the extract compared to the mice that didn't receive the allspice. The researchers discovered that ericifolin, a compound in allspice, blocks the production of androgen receptors in cancer cells. That's key because prostate cancer can't survive without androgen receptors promoting its growth.

"We're trying to determine if people can delay or stop cancer growth by taking allspice in sufficient quantity," Lokeshwar says. "But the devil is in the details. Human cancer is more complex than single cancer cells, and human beings are . . . unique creature[s] much different from rodents."

Men would have to eat about 2 teaspoons of powered allspice a day to equate to what the mice ingested. However, some people already seem to be benefitting since 2013, when Lokeshwar's research was published in the medical journal *Carcinogenesis*. "Since the study, I have received letters from people who say that after eating allspice, their cancer went away," he notes. "Of course, that's not reliable evidence. But it is encouraging."

And prostate cancer might be just the beginning. In a 2015 study, researchers including Lokeshwar found that allspice also showed promise in battling breast cancer, particularly when coupled with mainstream therapies. "Allspice has the medical potential for cancer prevention and treatment, not necessarily on its own, but in combination with other treatments," he says.

Native to Central America and the Caribbean, allspice comes from the berries of a small evergreen tree. Its name is testament to its unique quality of tasting like a combination of cinnamon, nutmeg, ginger, and clove, with peppery undertones. Along with pumpkin pie, it's used in a variety of dishes and cuisines, including Jamaican jerk sauce, curry, chutney, and pickling.

A nutrient-packed natural anti-inflammatory, allspice is also used as a home remedy for digestive issues, arthritis, muscle aches, menstrual cramps, and other ailments. "I've always been interested in dietary cancer prevention," says

Lokeshwar. "Spices are ideal subjects for study because they have a history of therapeutic uses. They also have a long shelf life, retaining their anticancer nutrients a long time."

Unlike some other natural cancer fighters, allspice is hearty enough to stand up to cooking. "Garlic, chili peppers, and turmeric all have compounds that seem to fight cancer," explains Lokeshwar, "but cooking destroys the effective compounds. That doesn't seem to be the case with allspice, which we extracted by boiling."

Lokeshwar plans to continue his research, striving to unlock the full potential of allspice as a cancer therapy. "Allspice is a fascinating spice." he says. "It has multiple aromas and flavors and is used in many ways. I myself use it in cooking. It makes something like rice pilaf taste very good, and you can add it to sweets. Now we're finding that it could also be a general cancer-fighting agent."

SEXUAL PROBLEMS

Aging takes a toll on many aspects of our lives and health, and one of its most distressing side effects is a flagging love life.

At least one in three middle-aged men experience erectile dysfunction (ED) at one time or another, by some estimates. Many men with ED have problems with blood flow to the penis. Viagra, Cialis, and other ED medications address such underlying conditions and are among the top-selling drugs in the United States. These phosphodiesterase type 5 (PDE5) inhibitors increase the amount of nitric oxide in the body.

But blood flow isn't the only factor in ED and other sexual problems. Stress, heart disease, clogged blood vessels, diabetes, and obesity can all contribute to ED. So can decreasing testosterone, levels of which begin dropping in men after the age of thirty at about 1 percent each year.

In addition to changes in sexual function, low levels of testosterone also cause insomnia, reduced muscle strength and smaller muscles, depression, and an inability to concentrate. Testosterone medications might seem to be the answer, but they come with risks.

Prescription testosterone can contribute to sleep apnea, acne, reduced sperm production, and prostate enlargement and slow production of the body's own testosterone. It can also spur the spread of prostate cancer. Fortunately, there are supplements that can boost the production of testosterone and help you cope with some of the most common causes of ED to give your love life a boost.

Here's a look at some of the most popular and promising nondrug options:

DEHYDROEPIANDROSTERONE (DHEA). This hormone, which is produced by the adrenal glands, is broken down by the body into a hormone called androstenedione, which is then changed into testosterone and estrogen. By age sixty, a man possesses only one-third of the level he had as a young man. Lab tests can determine if you are deficient in this critical hormone and supplements can boost it.

L-CARNITINE. A recent study published in the journal *Urology* found that elderly men who regularly used this natural substance saw their ED significantly improve—without the complications common to drugs or testosterone therapy.

The study was a randomized, double-blind, placebo-controlled trial of 150 older men who complained of decreased libido and impotence. All were diagnosed with very low levels of testosterone. The men receiving L-carnitine supplements used two types of L-carnitine taken together (propionyl-L-carnitine and acetyl-L-carnitine). After six months, those taking L-carnitine showed improvements in testosterone that were significantly greater than those taking only testosterone medication.

VITAMIN D. Although it's called a vitamin, vitamin D is actually a hormone. A majority of Americans are deficient, especially seniors. A three-year study of older men published in *Hormone and Metabolic Research* found that men who had higher levels of vitamin D also had higher levels of free testosterone. Another study found that men with low testosterone who were given a vitamin D supplement (3,332 IU) every day for a year experienced a 20 percent rise in free testosterone.

L-ARGININE. This amino acid fights ED by making nitric oxide, which relaxes smooth muscles around blood vessels and dilates vessels—letting more oxygen-rich blood flow to the penis, which allows for an erection. One study published in the *Journal of Sex & Marital Therapy* found that when 1,700 mg of L-arginine was combined with 40 mg of pycnogenol (a form of pine bark that is also a nitric oxide booster), the success rate for improving ED was 80 percent.

HORNY GOAT WEED. This colorfully named herbal remedy contains an ingredient called icariin, which several studies have found increases testosterone levels. Similar to ED drugs, icariin inhibits the PDE5 enzyme to increase testosterone levels. It also allows the smooth muscles of the penis to relax and boosts blood flow in the pelvic area by increasing the production of nitric oxide. Some experts suggest using a horny goat weed extract with 10 percent icariin.

GINGKO BILOBA. Used in Chinese herbal medicine for almost five thousand years, ginkgo biloba is believed to fight ED by increasing blood flow. Studies have shown that it is most effective in improving sexual function in elderly men and women who take antidepressants. Gingko was shown to be 76 percent effective in men and was even more effective—an astounding 91 percent—in women.

Top Foods to Prevent ED

Viagra, healthy lifestyle changes, and supplements aren't the only ways to combat ED and other sexual problems. Specific berries and other fruits and vegetables can prevent these issues, and you don't have to eat enormous amounts of them.

"The benefits for reducing risk of ED can be found by including a few portions of fruits people already eat," says Aedin Cassidy, a nutrition professor at the University of East Anglia in the United Kingdom and lead researcher of the first study to identify the top foods that fight ED. The study, a collaboration between Harvard University and British scientists, analyzed the diets and sexual health of more than fifty thousand American men between 1986 and 2008. The findings were published in *The American Journal of Clinical Nutrition*.

"Total fruit was associated with a reduction in risk, but in particular, citrus fruits and berries—including blackberries, strawberries, blackcurrants, blueberries, grapes, and cherries—were associated with the greatest reduction in risk," Cassidy says. These are all rich sources of flavonoids, a category of nutrients found in plant foods.

The Underlying Mechanism

Viagra works by increasing blood flow to the penis. Flavonoids have a similar effect, although they work in a more subtle way. "Exactly how flavonoids cause these [health benefits] is not fully known, but we know from clinical trials that some flavonoids can improve blood pressure, make our arteries more flexible, and help open blood vessels, resulting in improved blood flow," says Cassidy. They also give fruits and vegetables some of their vibrant colors.

In nature, there are six types of flavonoids, and any one fruit or vegetable contains different combinations and amounts of these. The study analyzed foods with all the types and found that two, in particular, are especially beneficial for erectile function:

1. **Anthocyanins** are found in red, blue, and purple fruits and vegetables, such as blackberries, strawberries, blackcurrants, blueberries, red and purple grapes, cherries, cranberries, eggplants, radishes, and red wine.
2. **Flavanones** are found in citrus fruits, such as oranges and grapefruit.

More Ways to Avoid ED

Other studies have found better sexual and overall health among men who follow a Mediterranean diet, one that is rich in plant foods—including plenty of fresh fruits and vegetables—whole grains, and fat from olive oil rather than other types of vegetable oils or dairy fats. Such a diet includes small amounts of fish or meat but is dominated by fresh foods from plants.

Exercise also plays an important role in the health of blood vessels and sexual function. The greatest benefits come from eating the high-flavonoid foods and getting regular exercise. "As well as improving sexual health for middle-aged men, there is another important benefit linked to heart health," says Cassidy. "ED is often an early barometer of poor vascular function and offers a critical opportunity to intervene and prevent cardiovascular disease, heart attack, and even death."

What to Eat

The Harvard-UK study found that the richest sources of ED-fighting nutrients are blueberries and strawberries. Other top sources are citrus fruits, blackberries, blackcurrants, grapes, and cherries. Eating four or more portions of these per week reduced the risk for ED by 19 percent. Other fruits, such as apples and pears, and red wine, were also beneficial.

One portion consists of the following:

- 1 cup of berries
- 1 medium orange or grapefruit
- 1 medium apple or pear
- 5-ounce glass of red wine

Here are the best ways to eat these portions:

- Have a bowl of berries for dessert or as a snack.
- Add berries to cereal or a smoothie at breakfast.
- Eat an orange as a snack.
- Instead of potatoes for a side dish, have grilled eggplant seasoned with olive oil and herbs.

Here's a shopping tip: Berries can be pricey. When they are in season, shop at farmers markets or buy directly from farms. At other times of year, buy frozen berries. Spread them out on a flat surface so they aren't touching each other and allow them to thaw at room temperature. You can also use a low setting in the microwave for a few minutes.

SLEEP DISORDERS

More than forty million Americans are chronically sleep deprived, according to the US Centers for Disease Control and Prevention (CDC). That's one reason Americans spend some $2 billion a year on sleeping pills. But sleep medications are often ineffective, can be addictive over time—making it even harder to get to sleep naturally—and can cause serious side effects.

The latest research has even linked prescription and over-the-counter (OTC) sleeping aids to Alzheimer's disease. A recent study by the University of Washington School of Pharmacy found that the sleeping medication Nytol and antiallergy pills Benadryl and Piriton have "anticholinergic" blocking effects on the nervous system that significantly boost the odds of developing dementia.

In addition, new research published in the *British Medical Journal* (*BMJ*) noted an increased risk of cancer and death in people who regularly take sleeping pills. Dr. Erika Schwartz, a leading advocate of disease prevention and wellness, says too many Americans simply reach for the medicine cabinet when they can't get a good night's sleep.

Conventional physicians often encourage the trend by readily writing prescriptions before recommending proven drug-free alternatives, including healthy lifestyle changes, natural compounds, and supplements that can all be safer alternatives. In fact, doctors write nearly sixty million prescriptions for sleeping pills in the United States each year, in addition to antidepressants and medications for anxiety, irritability, psychosis, and other mental health conditions that can interrupt sleep.

"Research consistently demonstrates that taking sleeping pills is not a healthy way to get those much-needed seven to eight hours of sleep a night. In fact, the more sleeping pills people take, the more likely they are to become addicted and the less likely they are to get a good night's sleep," Schwartz notes. "Also, the more sleeping medications taken, the more likely the occurrence of dangerous side effects—including problems with mental acuity, harmful interactions with other drugs, and even death. There also are many studies that fail to make those connections, but physicians have always scared patients into fearing addiction to sleeping pills rather than raise the issue of dangers associated with lack of sleep and work to find successful alternatives."

Natural Ways to Get a Good Night's Sleep

Now for the good news: there are a variety of natural substances that can help you get a good night's sleep.

CHAMOMILE TEA. This soothing drink has helped people sleep better for thousands of years, and recent scientific research has confirmed that it has a calming effect that prepares the body and mind for slumber. One Japanese study found that chamomile extract is as effective as a dose of benzodiazepine (a tranquilizing medication) as a sleep aid. Even the US Food and Drug Administration (FDA) has deemed it safe, with usually no side effects.

VALERIAN ROOT. The powdered extract from this medicinal plant is a powerful sedative and anxiety reducer that has been a used by traditional healers since the Roman Empire. A recent analysis of more than a dozen studies found that it helps people fall asleep faster and sleep more deeply than pills.

MAGNESIUM. Even small deficiencies in this essential compound can prevent the brain from calming down at night, research shows. Many Americans don't get enough magnesium, which might explain why so many have sleep problems. It is found in green leafy vegetables, wheat germ, pumpkin seeds, and almonds and is available in supplements.

CALCIUM. Warm milk not only is a comfort food, long recommended for a good night's sleep, but is also loaded with calcium, which plays a key role in sleep. In addition, milk and other dairy products contain tryptophan, an amino acid that drives the production of serotonin and melatonin—brain chemicals that help you relax and sleep.

ZINC. Numerous studies have found that zinc supplements are natural sleep aids. A recent study involving seniors living in a long-term care facility found that residents who received a nightly dose of zinc—along with melatonin and magnesium—had improvements in the quality of their sleep and were more alert during the day.

In addition to these natural compounds, the following strategies can help you get a good night's sleep by establishing good "sleep hygiene":

- **Change your diet.** Eat organic foods low in sugar and high in protein and vegetable fats to keep weight in check. Try having an earlier or lighter evening meal (salad, soup), which will help you sleep better.
- **Eliminate alcohol, caffeine, and sugar.** Skip desserts and refrain from consuming too much alcohol or caffeinated drinks at night.
- **Exercise early in the day.** Hormones released during exercise boost energy and might make it difficult to relax and fall asleep.
- **Settle down before bedtime.** Meditating and listening to calming music are good ways to prime the mind and body for bedtime.
- **Consider alternative medicine.** Acupressure, acupuncture, cognitive therapy, biofeedback, Reiki, and energy work have all been shown to improve the quality and quantity of sleep.
- **Make your bedroom a sanctuary.** Reserve your bed for sleep and sex only.
- **Keep a regular schedule.** Go to bed and wake up at the same time every day.
- **Take only short naps.** Avoid daytime naps longer than fifteen to twenty minutes, which can make it harder to get to sleep at night.
- **Beware of "blue light."** Unfortunately, the growing bedtime use of electronic devices such as TVs, computers, cell phones, and iPads has proven to be an efficient sleep robber. That's because such devices emit high amounts of "blue light"—equivalent to sunlight—which impedes the body's natural ability to produce melatonin. It's best to avoid such devices near bedtime.

"It is clear what a combination of healthy lifestyle choices—good diet, regular exercise, relaxation techniques, better sleep hygiene—can do to enhance sleep quality and quantity," Schwartz notes. "Give some of these suggestions a try and you'll soon be getting better shut-eye.

"Too many people rely on sleeping pills for all the wrong reasons. When you don't get sleep because you are up all night working or partying, a change in lifestyle is in order, not a drug prescription. If you are stressed, work night shifts, or suffer jet lag from frequent traveling, sleeping pills rarely will help."

Why Sleep Aids Do More Harm than Good
An astounding 60 percent of American adults report that they experience disrupted or unrefreshing sleep *every night* or *almost every night*, according to a recent survey. That's in addition to the millions who suffer from chronic insomnia or more serious

disorders such as sleep apnea, which causes potentially life-threatening respiratory pauses during slumber.

That short or disrupted sleep can lead to a host of problems:

- weight gain and metabolic syndrome
- diabetes and heart disease
- impaired immunity and infectious diseases
- cancer
- reduced motor skill function and an increased risk of accidents

Worst of all, getting less than the recommended seven to eight hours of shut-eye per night can lead to premature death. To cope, many people resort to nighttime sleep medications. But such drugs are a double-edged sword.

Many of the most common prescription and OTC sleep medications are best used occasionally to promote sleep. But when used routinely over long periods of time, they can lead to cognitive decline, brain shrinkage, and an increased risk of Alzheimer's disease, studies show.

These include prescription benzodiazepines such as Xanax (alprazolam) and traditional tricyclic antidepressants such as Elavil (amitriptyline). Alarming recent research suggests that antihistamines such as Benadryl (diphenhydramine), which are often found in OTC sleep medications, also are associated with such effects, particularly in middle-aged and older people.

Such drugs can deplete the brain's supply of the essential neurotransmitter acetylcholine. That's why they're collectively referred to as anticholinergic drugs. One of the hallmarks of Alzheimer's disease is a deficiency of acetylcholine. Anticholinergic drugs also can affect speech, gastrointestinal (GI) health, and sexual health.

In most studies, high doses of such drugs are associated with the worst side effects, which generally occur after about three years. The picture is more complicated with melatonin, a popular OTC dietary supplement that contains a hormone naturally released by the body in preparation for sleep. Although melatonin supplements have no anticholinergic effects, studies show mixed results on their ability to promote sleep. There is no data showing the optimal dose, time of administration, or long-term safety.

Nondrug remedies are best for promoting good sleep, such as establishing good sleep hygiene.

Vitamin D Might Be Your Key to Better Sleep

If you follow all the usual rules of sleep hygiene—such getting at least seven hours of slumber and keeping to the same schedule each night—and still have trouble getting enough shut-eye, your problem might be a suboptimal level of vitamin D. That's the upshot of the latest sleep research. But the solution might not be as simple as popping more vitamin D supplements.

What most people don't realize is that vitamin D is naturally produced from exposure to sunlight, and it acts on multiple systems in the body. If you get too little—which can happen during winter months—or too much, it can have many adverse effects.

It's a delicate balancing act, explains Dr. Stasha Gominak, a Texas-based neurologist who has extensively studied the effects of vitamin D on sleep. Even if you achieve what she considers an optimal level of sleep, you might experience deficiencies in other nutrients that need to be corrected.

During the past decade, Gominak has observed the effects of vitamin D supplementation in patients who have neurologic symptoms such as headaches, seizures, back pain, dizziness, and balance problems, as well as abnormal sleep. She wanted to see if vitamin D supplementation could help her patients avoid common and bothersome sleep remedies such as prescription medications.

In 2012, Gominak published the results of a study of 1,500 patients, showing that certain levels of vitamin D are associated with significant improvements in neurologic symptoms as well as sleep quality. This recommendation jives with levels recommended by the Vitamin D Council (40–80 ng/ml) and the Endocrine Society (30–100 ng/ml).

That said, few issues in modern medicine are as controversial as those surrounding vitamin D. Although no one disagrees that vitamin D is essential for good health, especially bone health, there is widespread disagreement about what constitutes an optimal level of vitamin D and the best ways to achieve it.

Like most vitamin D experts, Gominak recommends frequent measurement of vitamin D levels in order to determine a correct dose. "Medicare and all the insurance companies will pay for it four times a year," she says.

She states that most people can achieve an optimal level with daily vitamin D3 supplementation of 1,000–5,000 IU in summer and 5,000–7,000 IU in winter. Since vitamin D requirements can vary dramatically by factors such as age, skin type, geographical location, sun exposure, and general health, these are only general guidelines, she cautions.

"Vitamin D by itself can be very destructive to your sleep and to your health," she says. "You have to be extremely careful with the dose."

Gominak's latest research suggests that even optimal vitamin D supplementation and levels might have only a short-lived effect on sleep and health: "It works for about two years at most, and it doesn't work for everybody."

After normal sleep is reestablished, the body uses D vitamins to make repairs. Over time, this increased demand might result in a deficiency of B vitamins, which can adversely affect both sleep and health. Correcting a deficiency might require a complicated regimen of intermittent B-vitamin supplementation, Gominak explains.

Several other studies have suggested a link between vitamin D and sleep disorders. Among them is a 2014 analysis of data from more than 4,500 participants in the National Health and Nutrition Examination Survey (NHANES). This study showed that adequate vitamin D intake is associated with a significantly increased ability to maintain a full night's sleep.

Here's the bottom line on vitamin D and happy dreams:

- Get tested to determine your blood levels of vitamin D.
- Supplement as needed to maintain a level of 60–80 ng/ml.
- Be aware that a level of more than 150 ng/ml can have toxic effects.
- For more information, visit the Vitamin D Council website at http://www.vitamindcouncil.org/.

Six Tips for Making Your Bedroom More Sleep Friendly

You spend about a third of your life here, and it might be the one place that—more than any other—holds the key to your overall health. It's your bedroom and, sadly, health experts say it is the dirtiest room in the homes of many Americans.

"Most people are surprised to learn that the bedroom is one of the dirtiest rooms in the house because that's the furthest thing from their mind when they want to rest and relax," says Robin Wilson, a designer who specializes in creating healthy homes and the author of *Clean Design: Wellness for Your Lifestyle*.

Wilson, a spokesperson with the Asthma and Allergy Foundation of America (AAFA), says that keeping your bedroom clean, free of allergens, and sleep-friendly is a critical factor in your health. She offers these top tips:

Manage floor dust. Vacuum and mop it regularly to keep it clean.

Buy a quality mattress. The cheaper the mattress, the more chemicals it has inside, so spend a bit more to get the best quality mattress you can afford. A washable mattress cover is also a good idea to combat dust mites.

Choose hypoallergenic pillows. You should also use a zippered cover (wash it every three weeks), wash the pillow every three months, and replace it after three years.

Use eco-friendly products. Go with bedding and fabrics made from cotton, silk, and other natural fibers made without formaldehyde and toxic chemicals.

Avoid clutter. Pollen, mold, dust, and other allergens settle on knickknacks and other items, so it's best to keep belongings in boxes, bins, drawers, and cabinets.

Avoid bed bugs. When you return home from a trip, wash everything immediately and do not store your luggage in your bedroom closet.

Is Moisture in Your CPAP Device Putting You at Risk?

Millions of Americans use a continuous positive airway pressure (CPAP) device to treat sleep apnea, a common sleep disorder that causes brief but potentially dangerous interruptions of breathing. But if you don't use a humidifier with the unit—or distilled water—you could be asking for trouble.

CPAP devices help sleep apnea sufferers sleep through the night, says Dr. Brandon Peters. But it's important to be sure that you use one with a humidifier and distilled water to be safe.

Q: Why Use a CPAP humidifier?

A: CPAP devices are more comfortable and tolerable if you use the heated humidifier. Delivering more humidity ensures there is less dryness—especially in the nose and sinuses—which can reduce the risks of nasal congestion and nosebleeds.

Q: What about moisture control?

A: When using standard tubing with a humidifier, there also can be a problem with condensation within the tubes, particularly when the bedroom is cool. That can lead to moisture getting into the device. To control condensation, try what is called a "climate line" or "heated tubing," which will keep moisture levels low.

Q: Can you use tap water?

A: Most CPAP humidifier manufacturers recommend using distilled water to keep the risks low. Boiling water will kill microbes, but it will not remove minerals or chemical contaminants that can get into the system. Filtered water might remove some contaminants but not living organisms or other chemicals. Bottled water that has been distilled is the safest option.

Q: How about on the road?

A: If you're traveling to a part of the world with a water supply of questionable safety, take distilled water with you for the humidifier.

AMA Warns LED Streetlights Cause Sleeplessness

Here's a new reason New York is the city that never sleeps: high-intensity light-emitting diode (LED) streetlights in Gotham—as well as Seattle, Los Angeles, Houston, and elsewhere—emit unseen "blue light" that can seriously disturb natural wake-sleep cycles. And insomnia isn't the only concern; LED light exposure might also increase the risk of serious health conditions tied to sleep deprivation, including cancer and heart disease.

That's the upshot of a new warning from the American Medical Association (AMA), which also cautioned that LED lights can impair nighttime driving vision.

How serious is the risk? No one can say. Not yet, anyway. But the AMA report adds to rising concerns about the dangers of so-called blue light emitted by LED lighting—as well as TVs, computer screens, mobile phones, and tablets. Such fears are even prompting some cities to reevaluate the intensity of LED lights they install as a precaution.

"Much has been learned over the past decade about the potential adverse health effects of [LED] light exposure, particularly at night," noted Dr. Louis Kraus, chairman of the AMA Council on Science and Public Health, which produced the new report. "The core concern is disruption of circadian rhythmicity," he said, explaining that nighttime light interferes with the body's natural wake-sleep cycles.

About 10 percent of US roadway lighting is now LED, according to the US Department of Energy. But the number of cities embracing LED lights is rising because they use half as much energy as traditional sodium streetlights and last up to twenty years—ten times longer than the lights they replace. As a result, the AMA report suggests it's critical to spotlight growing potential public health risks linked to LED lighting.

"The [AMA] council is undertaking this report to assist in advising communities on selecting among LED lighting options in order to minimize potentially harmful human health and environmental effects," Kraus said in the new report.

Why Darkness Is Essential to Health

There's a reason we sleep at night and individuals who work night shifts have increased risks for cancer, heart, disease, obesity, and other mental and physical health disorders. Darkness triggers the release of the natural sleep-inducing hormone, melatonin, as well as drops in body temperature and hunger—all of which induce drowsiness. But artificial light—and blue light in particular—blocks this process, which is essential for health, by messing with the body's internal biological clock.

"A number of controlled laboratory studies have shown delays in the normal transition to nighttime physiology from evening exposure to tablet computer screens, backlit e-readers, and room light typical of residential settings," Kraus explained.

By contrast, natural light from the moon, candles, and wood fires don't cause such disruptions. Even low-wattage incandescent bulbs are safe, research shows.

"In human studies, a short-term detriment in sleep quality has been observed after exposure to [blue] light before bedtime. Although data are still emerging, some evidence supports a long-term increase in the risk for cancer, diabetes, cardiovascular disease, and obesity from chronic sleep disruption or shiftwork and associated with exposure to brighter light sources in the evening or night."

Are LED Risks Overstated?

Some officials, including those in Seattle and other cities, have dismissed the AMA's health concerns. They say there's little evidence LED streetlights are significantly harmful or that they emit more blue light than a typical TV, iPad, or computer screen.

In fact, brighter lights installed over the past decade to illuminate city streets and residential neighborhoods deter criminal activities that certainly pose a greater risk to city residents, they argue. They have also resulted in better witness descriptions of criminal suspects, some law enforcement authorities say.

Others, including officials in New York, have responded aggressively to the growing health concerns and resident complaints by replacing high-intensity white LED bulbs with lower-intensity lights the AMA considers safer.

At the same time, Phoenix and other municipalities have attempted to strike a middle ground—going with a mix of the intense lights for major intersections and park areas that need very bright light and softer lighting for residential areas. But even those efforts have been made with a healthy dose of skepticism.

Whether other cities will follow the AMA's guidance is anyone's guess. But as the debate rages, the take-home message is clear: there is no downside to drawing your blinds at night and making sure your bedroom is as dark as possible, health experts say.

For now, until more evidence confirms (or rejects) the notion that the risks of LED lighting are enough to keep you up at night—*literally*—that's the best advice to take to heart.

Nighty-night.

THYROID DISORDERS

The US obesity rate is at an all-time high, with the US Centers for Disease Control and Prevention (CDC) estimating that nearly a third of all Americans weigh too much. At the same time, the nation's top-selling prescription drug is the thyroid medication Synthroid (levothyroxine).

A coincidence? Probably not, health experts say.

In fact, thyroid problems are a common reason for unexplained weight gain—as well as low energy, hair loss, cognitive problems, cardiovascular issues, high blood pressure, and a host of other maladies.

Federal health statistics show that thyroid disorders and cancer rates have been soaring in recent decades. It is estimated that more than twenty-seven million Americans suffer from thyroid disease, and at least half of them are undiagnosed. The American Cancer Society (ACS) estimates that there are 56,460 new cases of thyroid cancer a year—twice as many as in 1990 and three times the rate in 1970.

Dr. Richard Shames, a leading expert and author of *Thyroid Mind Power*, believes that these health statistics only tell part of the story and might actually underestimate the number of people with thyroid problems. He says that if all Americans took the gold standard thyroid-stimulating hormone (TSH) blood test—with an upper limit at 3.0 as recommended by the American Association of Clinical Endocrinologists (AACE)—the number of people affected by thyroid disease could be as high as 20 percent of the population. "Both high and low thyroid disease, as well as thyroid cancer, are autoimmune diseases," he says. "The underlying cause of the increase in autoimmunity across the board is the incessantly increasing pollution of our air, food and water with thousands of hormone and immune disrupting synthetic chemicals."

Dr. Alan Christianson, author of *The Complete Idiot's Guide to Thyroid Disease*, agrees, adding that the thyroid is the only organ that concentrates all the chemicals found in the body. "There is genetic factor to thyroid disease, but the toxic levels of chemicals in the thyroid gland can be one hundred times higher than in the brain, for example," he explains. "Your thyroid is the only part of the body that needs iodine, so it has a built-in pump that pulls this mineral from the blood. But in doing so, it also pulls in toxic chemicals that lead to malfunction."

What's Driving the Thyroid Epidemic?

One reason that hypothyroidism, or underactive thyroid disease, is out of control is due to the drop in iodine intake along with increased fluoride intake, say many specialists. Stress also triggers thyroid disorders—the most common of which are Graves' disease (hyper- or overactive thyroid) and Hashimoto's thyroiditis (hypo- or underactive thyroid).

"When your immune system is strong, it can ward off attackers and keep dangerous bacteria, viruses, and fungi from getting into your body," Christianson says. "Stressors that are either physical or psychological can disrupt the immune response that protects the thyroid."

Iodine is an essential element necessary for the proper function of the thyroid gland as well as virtually every cell in the human body.

We cannot live without adequate production of thyroid hormone, and the thyroid gland cannot produce thyroid hormone without sufficient iodine stores. Thyroid problems that could be tied to iodine deficiency have been linked to several dozen symptoms and health problems. Among the most common are the following:

- fatigue
- coldness
- dry skin
- constipation
- hair loss
- unexplained weight gain
- brain fog
- headaches
- menstrual problems and PMS
- high cholesterol
- infertility
- arthritis

Drugs Only One Way to Treat Thyroid Disorders

Fortunately, drugs aren't the only way to correct thyroid disorders. In fact, most conditions can be easily treated with iodine supplementation or dietary supplements taken as part of a healthy diet and other lifestyle changes.

All thyroid hormones contain iodine, for instance. The most common thyroid hormone, thyroxine (T4), contains four iodine atoms per molecule. Iodine from kelp and as potassium iodide are among the most supportive for thyroid health. But to combat iodine deficiency, it is important to use other nutrients along with iodine, including unrefined salt, which differs from refined salt. Refined salt is 99 percent sodium and chloride, along with additives such as ferrocyanide and aluminum. But unrefined salt contains as much as 2 percent trace minerals, which makes it healthier than refined salt.

Iodine: Casualty of America's Modern Diet

The American diet today has less than half the iodine levels of diets of thirty to forty years ago. That's because iodine-rich baked goods that were once American staples have been replaced by processed foods that no longer contain it.

Until the 1970s, bread and baked goods were a significant source of iodine because it was an ingredient in dough conditioner used by bakeries. But since then, bromine, which blocks our bodies from absorbing it, has replaced iodine as an additive in many commercially available flours and oils.

Chemically, bromine is somewhat similar to iodine. As a result, bromine attaches to the thyroid gland, stops it from absorbing iodine, and triggers iodine excretion. Bromine also blocks other cells from absorbing iodine and thyroid hormone. To avoid it, buy foods and beverages made with organic or unbrominated ingredients (without the words *bromine*, *bromide*, or *bromate*).

Iodized table salt contains iodine, but most Americans get most of the salt in their diets from processed foods, which don't contain beneficial iodine. Adding iodized table salt to our diets might help, but it won't solve the problem because only about 10 percent of the iodine in salt is absorbed.

Other Vital Nutrients

In addition to iodine, these nutrients can boost thyroid function.

HERBS. Ashwagandha balances thyroid and adrenal function. Forskohlii and guggul gum extract optimize thyroid performance. (Amounts vary by formulation.)

L-TYROSINE (300 MG DAILY). The amino acid is a key building block of thyroid hormone.

METHYLSULFONYLMETHANE (MSM; 50 MG DAILY). MSM is a form of sulfur that helps regulate the hormone.

ESSENTIAL VITAMINS AND MINERALS. Vitamins A (2,500 IU), D (300 IU), and E (100 IU); riboflavin (5 mg); niacinamide (30 mg); magnesium (15 mg); zinc (5 mg); selenium (30 mcg); copper (0.1 mg); and manganese (2 mg) work in various ways to stimulate hormone production or convert it to the active form, or to protect the thyroid gland.

Testing Your Thyroid Function

Several at-home and doctor-administered tests are available to diagnose thyroid problems.

AT HOME. Take your temperature first thing in the morning. When measured under the arm, normal levels range between 97.8 and 98.2 degrees Fahrenheit and one degree higher with a rectal thermometer. Below-normal morning temperature can indicate that your thyroid is likely underactive.

AT THE DOCTOR. Thyroid hormone levels can be measured with blood tests, but conventional tests that measure only TSH miss thyroid problems in some patients. TSH is secreted by the pituitary gland and triggers hormone production and release in the thyroid gland. When TSH is elevated, thyroid function is low, but it might be considered "normal" even when there is a problem. As a result, Brownstein recommends measuring TSH as well the following:

- **T4.** This is an inactive form of thyroid hormone that is released by the thyroid gland.
- **T3.** This is T4 converted to the active form of the hormone, which is used by all the cells in the body.
- **Reverse T3.** If high, this might indicate that T4 is not being converted to T3 and thyroid function is low.
- **Thyroid antibodies (TPO) and antithyroglobulin antibodies.** These can indicate inflammation in the thyroid.

Best Ways to Treat Thyroid Disorders

Treatment includes replacing hormones with medication such as Synthroid for hypoactive thyroid disease or using radioactive ablation for hyperactive conditions. Sometimes a hyperactive thyroid will reset itself. In cancerous cases, the gland is removed followed by radioactive ablation. Symptoms of thyroid disorders include unexplained fatigue, weight gain, and hair loss. But commonsense prevention strategies and natural remedies can sidestep the need for medication.

A MONTHLY CHECKUP. Your thyroid is located between your Adam's apple and your sternum. Put your right hand against your neck and move downward. Aside from muscle tissue, if you feel anything unusual, check with your doctor. Next, swallow a glass of water. This moves the trachea and the esophagus in such a way that the thyroid is pushed out, which would expose any lumps or bumps.

WATCH FOR ABNORMALITIES. If you see or feel anything unusual, ask your doctor for an ultrasound. If you have had thyroid disease, your risk of getting cancer is higher, so schedule regular ultrasounds.

SUPPLEMENTS. Take a multivitamin that includes 100 mcg of iodine. Eat seafood but avoid processed food that contains too much sodium but no iodine. And don't take in too much iodine either, says Christianson. "It's like Goldilocks—too little or too much iodine can damage the thyroid gland."

CONSUME SELENIUM. This mineral helps your body utilize thyroid hormones. Eat a handful of Brazil nuts each week.

MINIMIZE MERCURY. Beware of high-mercury seafood. The biggest no-no is eating tuna daily. Avoid mercury amalgams. Getting new fillings? Go for porcelain or ceramic.

AVOID PERCHLORATE. This is a toxic by-product from rocket and jet fuels. It usually ends up in our water supply and is absorbed through our skin and intestines. Once in our bodies, it prevents our thyroid gland from absorbing iodine. Drink purified water only, not tap water. Ideally, use a filter for your shower too. We can also get this toxic product from dry cleaning, so when you bring your clothes home, take them out of the bag ASAP and ideally let them off-gas in the sunshine before wearing.

EXERCISE. The more aerobic activity you do, the lower your odds of developing thyroid disease.

GET TESTED. If you or someone you love has possible thyroid symptoms, have a complete panel of tests done, including TSH, thyroid antibodies, free T3, and free T4. Look for your TSH to be in the *optimal* range of 0.3–1.5. In the case of suspected thyroid disease or any other symptoms, never assume that you need to suffer. Educate yourself and see your doctor so that you can feel your best.

Metabolic Disorder Tied to Underactive Thyroid

Diabetes has long been linked to lack of exercise, poor diet, and genetic factors. But a landmark new study suggests another factor might be at work: a growing epidemic of underactive thyroid.

The condition, called hypothyroidism, affects millions of Americans, according to Dr. Raphael Kellman, a leading expert on thyroid disease who runs the Kellman Center for Integrative and Functional Medicine in New York City. He says the findings confirm a link he's suspected for many years.

About 12 percent of the nation's population have diseased thyroids, with many people unaware that their thyroid glands might be responsible for other health problems, according to the ATA. This butterfly shaped endocrine gland, found in the lower front of the neck, plays a critical role in keeping vital organs—including the brain and heart—working normally.

Restoring thyroid glands to normal function can help stall development of other diseases. According to another expert on hypothyroidism, endocrinologist Dr. Minisha Sood, director of inpatient diabetes care at New York City's Lenox Hill Hospital, evidence now confirms suspicions of a link between deficient thyroids and diabetes. "Most endocrinologists now screen for thyroid disease in patients with prediabetes and diabetes," she says, "because it's known that thyroid disease is more prevalent in these populations."

New Call for Diabetes Screening

The latest study was conducted by Dutch researchers at Rotterdam's Erasmus University Medical Center, who tracked about 8,500 people over eight years. A team led by Dr. Layal Chaker found that 1,100 study participants developed prediabetes—modestly raised blood sugar levels but not high enough to be considered diabetes—before the study ended and 798 developed the chronic disease more seriously.

Overall, Chaker's researchers found underperforming thyroid glands increased chances of developing diabetes by a worrying 13 percent. "This finding suggests we should consider screening people with prediabetes for low thyroid function," she comments.

The work was presented at a recent meeting in Boston of the Endocrine Society—which boasts 18,000 members in 122 countries. While the study pinpointed the close relationship between underactive thyroid glands and diabetes, it didn't shed any new light on why this link exists.

Symptoms of possible thyroid disease include depression, difficulty losing weight, fatigue, hair loss, inability to concentrate, and heightened sensitivity to cold, among others. According Kellman, the first step for people who suspect that they might have thyroid disease is to have levels of hormones known as T3, T4, and TSH checked through simple blood tests. It's essential to seek professional advice, he emphasizes.

While some doctors favor drugs to treat high blood sugar, Kellman leans heavily toward health supplements, which have been successful in reinstating thyroid heath. His center's treatments encompass evaluating patients' physiology, environment, nutrition, and other factors that might impact the thyroid's ability to function normally. "Vitamins and nutrients can help fight the underlying cause of thyroid disorders, such as autoimmune processes and inflammation, and help improve dysfunctional thyroids," he says.

Among treatments he has used successfully are selenium (a mineral found in the soil), ashwagandha (a powerful herb long used by practitioners India's traditional Ayurvedic medicine), compounded T3 and T4 hormone supplements, and Armour thyroid (a natural medication made from pigs' thyroids). Some patients are treated with more than one of these, depending on identified causes of hypothyroidism. Kellman also stresses the importance of gut health, noting that the body's bacteria are crucial in "creating by-products that can help insulin sensitivity and protect against inflammation."

Other nutrients some doctors find effective include iodine, vitamins B and D (a strong association has been found between vitamin D deficiency and hypothyroidism), zinc, tyrosine, and probiotics. "The microbiome [microorganisms found in the body] in the gut play critical roles in many physiological processes, including thyroid function," observes Kellman. "I don't necessarily recommend the [probiotic] supplement with the highest number of bacteria—although that's important—but supplements with the most diversity."

Beating hypothyroidism is an important step in preventing the onset of diabetes, he argues.

CONTRIBUTORS

David Alliot, Lynn Allison, Rick Ansorge, Sylvia Booth Hubbard, Eric Caplan, Stacey Colino, Frances Chamberlain, Michele Bender, Shellie Faulkner, Gary Greenberg, Charlotte Libov, Marti Lotman, Emily Netburn, David A. Schwartz, Vera Tweed.

INDEX

ABOUT THE AUTHOR

Nick J. Tate is an award-winning journalist, best-selling author, and sought-after public speaker specializing in medicine, healthcare, business, technology, finance, and consumer affairs. He is the Health Editor with Newsmax Media Inc. in South Florida. His work has appeared in Newsmax magazine, The Miami Herald, South Florida Sun Sentinel, Atlanta Journal-Constitution, Boston Herald, and other print and online publications. He is also a regular on Newsmax TV.

Tate's *ObamaCare Survival Guide* ranked among the nation's top sellers. It was on the *Publishers Weekly* and *The New York Times Best Sellers* lists for 22 weeks—reaching No. 1 on *The Times* list for paperback advice books. He's also the author of *DaVinci's Baby Boomer Survival Guide: Live, Prosper, and Thrive in your Retirement.* His first book, *The Sick Building Syndrome* was the result of a year-long journalism fellowship at the Harvard School of Public Health.

In addition to his work as a multimedia journalist, Tate is an experienced educator whose background includes teaching health/science journalism as an adjunct professor at Emory University in Atlanta. He has also led a variety of training seminars on healthcare reform, consumer-health issues, and media relations for college students, scientists, doctors, business executives, and public relations specialists.

Find him at: www.linkedin.com/in/nicktate1.